Quality of Life in Asia

Volume 7

Series Editors
Alex C. Michalos
University of Northern British Columbia, British Columbia, Canada
Daniel T.L. Shek
The Hong Kong Polytechnic University, Hunghom, Hong Kong, China
Doh Chull Shin
University of California, Irvine, California, U.S.A.
Ming-Chang Tsai
National Taipei University, Taipei, Taiwan

This series, the first of its kind, examine both the objective and subjective dimensions of life quality in Asia, especially East Asia. It unravels and compares the contours, dynamics and patterns of building nations, offering innovative works that discuss basic and applied research, emphasizing inter- and multi-disciplinary approaches to the various domains of life quality. Thus, the series appeals to a variety of fields in humanities, social sciences and other professional disciplines. Asia is the largest, most populous continent on Earth, and it is home to the world's most dynamic region, East Asia. In the past three decades, East Asia has been the most successful region in the world in expanding its economies and integrating them into the global economy, offering lessons on how poor countries, even with limited natural resources, can achieve rapid economic development. Yet while scholars and policymakers have focused on why East Asia has prospered, little has been written on how its economic expansion has affected the quality of life of its citizens. The series publish several volumes a year, either single or multiple-authored monographs or collections of essays.

More information about this series at http://www.springer.com/series/8416

Tak Yan Lee • Daniel T.L. Shek
Rachel C.F. Sun

Editors

Student Well-Being
in Chinese Adolescents
in Hong Kong

Theory, Intervention and Research

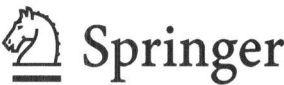 Springer

Editors
Tak Yan Lee
City University of Hong Kong
Kowloon, Hong Kong, China

Daniel T.L. Shek
The Hong Kong Polytechnic University
Hung Hom, Hong Kong, China

Rachel C.F. Sun
The University of Hong Kong
Pok Fu Lam, Hong Kong, China

ISSN 2211-0550 ISSN 2211-0569 (electronic)
Quality of Life in Asia
ISBN 978-981-10-1269-3 ISBN 978-981-287-582-2 (eBook)
DOI 10.1007/978-981-287-582-2

Springer Singapore Heidelberg New York Dordrecht London
© Springer Science+Business Media Singapore 2015
Softcover re-print of the Hardcover 1st edition 2016

Printed on acid-free paper

Springer Science+Business Media Singapore Pte Ltd. is part of Springer Science+Business Media (www.springer.com)

Preface

A survey of the scientific literature shows that there is a paucity of research studies on the development of junior secondary school students in Hong Kong. Besides, there are several limitations of the existing studies. First, most studies focus on psychological symptoms and problems in which a narrow conception of student well-being was used. In particular, there are few studies adopting the positive youth development approach to examine the protective factors in different adolescent developmental issues. Second, the major trends of developmental issues among early adolescents in Hong Kong over time are seldom examined. With reference to these limitations in the field, this book focuses on several developmental issues faced by early adolescents in Hong Kong, including relationships with peers and family, resilience in the face of adversity, face-to-face and cyberbullying, drug use, Internet addiction, sex behaviors, and sex education, as well as money literacy and concept of success. Besides, the links between positive youth development and such developmental issues are addressed.

Third, there are few studies that combine theory and practice. This is the first work that offers a comprehensive theory-driven program for the implementation of a positive youth development program targeting common developmental issues for early adolescents in a Chinese context. After reviewing the nature of common adolescent developmental issues in Hong Kong, we then present the theoretical background, conceptual framework, and implementation of a comprehensive positive youth development project (named "P.A.T.H.S. to Adulthood: A Jockey Club Youth Enhancement Scheme," with P.A.T.H.S. denoting Positive Adolescent Training through Holistic Social programs) in the form of in-class teaching and learning activities. Previous studies suggest that the project is able to promote the holistic development of early adolescents in Hong Kong.

Fourth, most of the existing studies are cross-sectional studies, and there are few longitudinal studies. Besides, large and representative samples are not common in Chinese research studies. As such, this book reviews the published longitudinal evaluation findings on the effectiveness of the prevention program on five common developmental issues. Furthermore, papers on the developmental trends based on longitudinal data collected within the context of the Project P.A.T.H.S. are included.

In short, being one of the titles in the series *Quality of Life in Asia*, this book offers theory, practice, and research of a large-scale preventive program with reference to the positive youth development framework to promote the quality of life of early adolescents in the Chinese context in Hong Kong.

The positive youth development program was initiated by the Hong Kong Jockey Club Charities Trust to promote the holistic development of adolescents in Hong Kong. In collaboration with the Government's Social Welfare Department, Education Bureau, and five universities in Hong Kong, the initial phase of this pioneer project was conducted between 2005 and 2012 with more than 210,000 adolescent participants. Its goal was to help students meet various challenges in their path to adulthood, with a focus on their psychosocial competencies, developmental assets, healthy relationships, and their well-being. We would like to acknowledge the initiation and generous financial support by the Hong Kong Jockey Club Charities Trust.

Edited by the researchers of the project, this book reviews the theories regarding the common developmental issues among Chinese adolescents in Hong Kong (Chaps. 1, 2, 3, 4, 5, 6, 7, 8, and 9), the application of positive youth development constructs to a large-scale positive youth development program in Hong Kong (Chaps. 10, 11, 12, 13, 14, 15, 16, and 17), and longitudinal research findings on five common developmental issues (Chaps. 18, 19, 20, 21, and 22). Using multiple perspectives, materials, and research findings, this book presents the overall constructs and framework underlying the Project P.A.T.H.S. in response to the various psychosocial needs of adolescents in Hong Kong. This book provides a clear picture on theory, practice, and evidence of success of the school-based prevention program in promoting students' well-being.

In the first part of this book, each chapter starts with an in-depth analysis of a common developmental issue among early adolescents. Specifically, each chapter of part 1 includes (a) literature review of the definitions, significance, and relevance of the issue today in different cultures and societies, (b) a critical analysis of its impact on adolescents and society, (c) a re-contextualization of the developmental issue in Hong Kong and Chinese societies, and (d) an analysis of the risk and protective factors at different levels (individual, group, society, etc.) and for the different stakeholders involved (families, teachers, peers, etc.). In the second part, each chapter presents (a) an analysis of the theoretical framework structuring the units of the P.A.T.H.S. program on each topic; (b) an analysis on how the relevant positive youth development constructs have been implemented and operationalized in the in-class activities; and (c) an analysis of major criticalities and resistance from students, teachers, families, and institutions. Detailed description and analysis of the program content are necessary for replication in other contexts. Finally, in the last part, results from the 4-year longitudinal study based on the extension phase of the program covered in this book addressed the question of how positive youth development attributes are related to measures of adolescent well-being across the junior high school years.

To conclude, the P.A.T.H.S. program is designed by professionals (psychologists, educators, and social workers) for the professionals (school teachers and school social workers); it provides a comprehensive theoretical framework for students to develop their quality of life. This program is designed to help young adolescents in developing and managing positive knowledge, values, and skills for social, emotional, cognitive, and spiritual wellness through the acquisition of knowledge and experiences, clarifying conflicting values and sharing in a safe and enjoyable manner. These knowledge, values, and skills are especially geared for finding direction and purpose in life. It is a program that allows students to make positive choices in creating and maintaining a healthy lifestyle and well-being. It advocates a positive approach to life and health that helps maximize the students' potential and their quality of life. As our work is pioneer with evidence of success, it can contribute to the Chinese and global database, and it can be used for research and teaching purposes.

We believe this book will be of keen interest to a wide range of professionals who need to design preventive or positive youth development programs to reduce risk factors for adolescents. Professionals such as social workers, psychologists, policy makers, education administrators, teachers, as well as mental health practitioners will find this book valuable in their work. The positive youth development program, in particular the curriculum units based on the positive youth development constructs, can be adopted and used in the formal school curriculum, after school programs, mental health services, and youth programs. We hope that this book will also serve as a resource for researchers and practitioners who are involved in the development and evaluation of preventive programs using positive youth development concepts for adolescents in an attempt to promote student well-being.

Hong Kong, China   Tak Yan Lee
Hong Kong, China   Daniel T.L. Shek

Contents

Contributors

Diego Busiol, Ph.D. is Italian and currently working in the Department of Applied Social Sciences, City University of Hong Kong. After graduating in clinical psychology (Italy and Germany), he specialized in psychotherapy (Italy). He worked for several years in different psychiatric community residences as a social worker and a psychologist. Later, he came to Hong Kong to do research on the relations between psychoanalysis and Chinese culture. His research and publications cover psychoanalytic theory and practice, cross-cultural studies, psychoanalysis in Chinese contexts, counseling, and mental health.

Chau Kiu Cheung, Ph.D. is an associate professor in the Department of Applied Social Sciences, the City University of Hong Kong, China. He has recently published articles concerning civility, social inclusion, resilience, character education, moral development, peer influence, and class mobility. His current research addresses issues of grand-parenting, drug abuse, risk society, and Internet use.

Xinli Chi, Ph.D. is a postdoctoral research fellow in the Department of Applied Social Sciences, the Hong Kong Polytechnic University. She obtained her Ph.D. degree from the Department of Education, the University of Hong Kong. Research in educational psychology generates strong interest in adolescent and young people development for her. Specifically, her research interests involve youth mental health and positive development, behavior prevention and intervention, and youth development program evaluation.

Eadaoin K. Hui, Ph.D. is an Honorary Associate Professor at the Faculty of Education, the University of Hong Kong, mainly engaging in doctoral supervision. She is the former Division Head of the Faculty. She is internationally known for her research in forgiveness education, school guidance and counseling, affective education, student school and life satisfaction, positive youth development and teacher stress. As an Educational Psychologist, she serves the Catholic Diocese of Hong Kong as the Consultant to its Educational Psychology Service. She also contributes to effective school leadership and management as School Supervisor of Marymount Secondary School and Marymount Primary School.

Wai Man Kwong, Ph.D. is an associate professor of the Department of Applied Social Sciences, City University of Hong Kong. He graduated from the University of Hong Kong with a B.Sc. degree in 1973 and an M.S.W. degree in 1975. He received counselor education at the University of Toronto and graduated with M.Ed. degree in applied psychology in 1982. He obtained his Ph.D. at the University of Bristol in 2002. He is currently the leader of the Master in Social Sciences in Counselling Programme. He teaches courses on counseling theories and practice, laboratory training of counseling skills, research methods in counseling, and providing supervision to student research projects and research degree students.

Ben M.F. Law, Ph.D. is an assistant professor of the Department of Social Work and Social Administration at the University of Hong Kong. His teaching is in positive youth development, human behavior and social environment, social work with young people, and group work. His research covers youth volunteerism, coping of adolescents with reading disability, and psychological well-being of adolescents. Before joining the university, he had been a social worker for more than 15 years in school social work service, family service, and project management with children with reading disability. He is editorial board member of *Research on Social Work Practice* and *Child and Adolescent Social Work Journal*.

Tak Yan Lee, M.S.W., Ph.D. is an associate professor of the Department of Applied Social Sciences at the City University of Hong Kong. His teaching and research interests are in group work, positive youth development, and practice teaching and learning. His research covers adolescent prostitution, positive youth development, parent–child communication, parental control, and resilience of children and the elderly. He had provided consultancy to statutory bodies and social service agencies on civic awareness, youth development indices, moral values and behavior, socio-cultural beliefs, gambling behavior, and compensated dating. He had also conducted research on fieldwork learning strategy and field instruction.

Mary T.W. Leung, R.S.W., M.S.W., Ed.D. is currently teaching in the Department of Applied Sciences, City University of Hong Kong. She participated in founding Baptist Oi Kwan Social Service and served as its chief executive, from 1984 to 2003. From 2006 she served as the general secretary for Hong Kong Bible Society and consultant (part time) for family and community service of the Haven of Hope Christian Service. Dr. Leung has put much effort in developing innovative services, including life education for schools, family resource, and service center for relatives of the ex-mentally ill.

Hildie Leung, Ph.D. is a research assistant professor in the Department of Applied Social Sciences at The Hong Kong Polytechnic University. She obtained her Ph.D. degree in psychology at the Chinese University of Hong Kong. Her research centers on positive youth development and its application to the promotion of healthy adolescent development and the prevention of problem behaviors among children and adolescents. Her work appears in journals such as *Social Indicators Research*, *International Journal on Disability and Human Development*, and *Journal of Behavioral and Decision Making*. She has also co-authored book chapters in the area of positive youth development and positive psychology.

Jianqiang Liang, Ph.D. is a postdoctoral fellow of the Department of Applied Social Sciences at The Hong Kong Polytechnic University. He earned his Ph.D. degree at PolyU and MSW at Washington University. He has actively engaged in the research and teaching on young people. His research areas include positive youth development, youth unemployment, social work practice, education, and staff development in China. His work appears in *Journal of Social Work*, *International Journal on Disability and Human Development*, and *China Journal of Social Work*. He teaches in the areas of leadership and intrapersonal development and the service learning of university students.

Li Lin, Ph.D. is an instructor in the Department of Social Sciences of the Hong Kong Polytechnic University, Hong Kong. She received her Ph.D. degree in psychology from the Chinese University of Hong Kong. Her main research interests involve adolescent development, parent–child relationship, positive youth development and related intervention program, and sociocultural influence.

Cecilia M.S. Ma, Ph.D. is an assistant professor in the Department of Applied Social Sciences at the Hong Kong Polytechnic University. She received her Ph.D. from the University of South Carolina. Her research interests include psychometrics, structural equation modeling, and program evaluation. She has published peer-reviewed papers in journals such as *Research on Social Work Practice*, *Social Indicators Research*, *Child Indicators Research*, and *International Journal on Disability and Human Development*. She has also coauthored book chapters and articles in the area of Chinese adolescents' psychological development. Her current research projects focus on positive youth development programs and the development of a university leadership program.

Daniel T.L. Shek, Ph.D., B.B.S., S.B.S., J.P. is associate vice president (undergraduate program) and chair professor of Applied Social Sciences at the Hong Kong Polytechnic University, advisory professor of East China Normal University, and honorary professor of Kiang Wu Nursing College of Macau. He is chief editor of *Journal of Youth Studies* and editorial board member of several international refereed journals, including *Journal of Adolescent Health*, *Social Indicator Research*, *International Journal of Behavioral Development*, and *International Journal of Adolescent Medicine and Health*. He is chairman of the Action Committee Against Narcotics and Family Council of the Government of Hong Kong Special Administrative Region, P.R.C.

Rachel C.F. Sun, Ph.D. got her B.Soc.Sc. and Ph.D. at the University of Hong Kong, Hong Kong. She is assistant professor of the Faculty of Education at the University of Hong Kong. She is a principal investigator of school misbehavior research studies and coprincipal investigator of positive youth development programs and a service leadership program in Hong Kong. Her research areas include academic achievement motivation, school satisfaction, life satisfaction, positive youth development, problem behavior, school misbehavior, adolescent suicidal ideation, and psychological health. She is a member of the editorial boards of *Research on Social Work Practice* and *Frontiers in Child Health and Human Development*.

Sandra K.M. Tsang, Ph.D., J.P. is an associate professor of the Department of Social Work and Social Administration of the University of Hong Kong. She is a registered clinical psychologist, a fellow of the Hong Kong Psychological Society, a registered social worker, and an accredited family mediator. Her research, publications, and media profile focus on parent education, children with special educational needs, children and youth development, and drug prevention. She was awarded the HKU Teaching Fellowship for outstanding teaching, the Chief Executive's Commendation for Community Services, and the 2011 Medal of the Hong Kong Paediatrics Society for contributions in child health.

Qiuzhi Xie, Ph.D. completed her Ph.D. study in psychology at the University of Hong Kong. Her Ph.D. focuses on cognitive and learning styles that address individual differences in learning and information processing. Her postdoctoral research mainly focuses on positive youth development and adolescent risk behavior. She had a broad range of research interests in psychology, in particular in the area of learning and cognition, and would like to bridge different research areas.

Lu Yu, Ph.D. is an assistant professor of the Department of Applied Social Studies, the Hong Kong Polytechnic University. She was trained in clinical medicine, psychiatry, education, and positive psychology. Her research interests include positive youth development, mental health and addiction, leadership, cross-cultural studies, gender development, and instrument development and validation. Her work appeared in *Personality and Individual Differences*, *Archives of Sexual Behaviors*, *Journal of Autism and Developmental Disorders*, *BMC Public Health*, *International Journal of Disability and Human Development*, *Journal of Pediatric and Adolescent Gynecology*, *Journal of Sex Research*, *Sex Roles*, *The Scientific World Journal*, *Asian Journal of Counseling*, and *International Journal of Child Health and Human Development*.

Introduction

Tak Yan Lee and Daniel T.L. Shek

Abstract The organization of various chapters covered in this book is outlined. In the first part of the book, several adolescent developmental issues (including substance abuse, sexual behavior, exposure to pornographic materials, self-harm, and Internet addiction) are discussed with respect to different theoretical explanations, related phenomena in Hong Kong and other countries, and protective factors as well as related effective prevention programs. In the second part of the book, the teaching units developed in the Project P.A.T.H.S. with reference to these developmental issues are presented and the evaluation findings in the previous studies are discussed. In the third part of the book, several chapters based on four waves of longitudinal data collected for the Project P.A.T.H.S. are presented. Throughout the book, it is argued that positive youth development attributes can promote student well-being, and it is important to nurture positive youth development attributes in young people to protect them from engaging in risk behavior.

This book offers the theory, intervention program materials, and related research findings within the context of a positive youth development program to tackle common adolescent developmental issues in Hong Kong. Specifically, five key issues – substance abuse, sexual behavior, exposure to pornographic materials, self-harm, and Internet addiction – were selected for discussion. To give the readers a roadmap for the chapters included in this book, this chapter offers a brief description of the organization of the content in this book.

Author contributed equally with all other contributors.

The preparation for this chapter and the Project P.A.T.H.S. were financially supported by The Hong Kong Jockey Club Charities Trust.

T.Y. Lee (✉)
Department of Applied Social Sciences, City University of Hong Kong,
Kowloon, Hong Kong, China
e-mail: ty.lee@cityu.edu.hk

D.T.L. Shek
Department of Applied Social Sciences, The Hong Kong Polytechnic University,
11 Yuk Choi Road, Hung Hom, Kowloon, Hong Kong, China

In Part I of the book, the selected adolescent developmental issues are examined in terms of different theoretical perspectives with reference to the most up-to-date scientific literature. Basically, the first five chapters follow a somewhat similar structure: (a) presentation of the theoretical conceptions of the issue and why it matters, (b) presentation of findings from Hong Kong as well as the recent trends and differences with reference to other geographic areas, and (c) discussion of protective factors and guidelines for effective prevention programs. In Chap. 1, we discuss why the youth drug problem in Hong Kong is escalating, what drugs are most used in Hong Kong, and what theories may explain the drug use and abuse. Chapter 2 addresses the question of why young people today have an earlier onset of puberty than the previous generations. Following this, a review of the main sex education approaches in the United States, the United Kingdom, and the Netherlands is conducted and how this can be relevant for Hong Kong is discussed. Chapters 3 and 4 examine the problem of bullying and cyberbullying in different parts of the world and in Hong Kong, with a particular focus on the role of bystanders; some of the major anti-bullying intervention approaches are also presented. Chapter 5 presents the different types of Internet addiction, how Internet addiction is increasing among youths in recent years, and what consequences on socialization it can have. Chapter 6 presents the issue of money literacy, which is particularly relevant in the context of the pragmatic and materialistic culture of Hong Kong, and what conflicting values are involved. Chapters 7 and 8 examine the concept of bonding among youths, particularly when they are with their peers or with their family members. Besides psychological theories, related cultural issues and values that may affect interpersonal bonding are discussed. Finally, Chap. 9 presents the key concept of resilience, what it is, why it is essential to a positive youth development, and what its relationships with other positive youth development constructs are.

The Project P.A.T.H.S. covers a total of 15 constructs (including cognitive, social, moral, emotional, and behavioral competencies, bonding, resilience, self-efficacy, self-determination, clear and positive identity, belief in the future, spirituality, prosocial norms, prosocial involvement, and recognition of positive behavior) that have been identified as crucial and effective elements of successful positive youth development programs (Catalano et al. 1998). While the first six chapters focus on developmental issues, the next three chapters provide a discussion on two major sources of protective factors, i.e., coping and adaptation, resilience, and human social capital (Gullotta 2015) which have been found as crucial to promoting health and psychosocial wellness among adolescents. According to Gullotta (2015), prevention means "taking actions that encourage resiliency, coping, adaption, and developing human social capital" (p. 4). We therefore review the literature on resilience and bonding with peers and family in the context of positive youth development.

In Part II of the book, each of the previous chapter is expanded (except the chapter on prevention of bullying and cyberbullying) so as to present the development and implementation of the P.A.T.H.S. program in Hong Kong. For each construct, the related conceptual framework is presented. The operationalization of the constructs, the linkage between related curriculum units, the overall structure of the curriculum in Grade 7 to Grade 9, and the implementation of the protective factors in the curriculum are also presented. Concept maps and tables are used to illuminate the positive youth development program.

In Part III of the book, the focus is put on five common developmental issues, namely, substance abuse, sexual behavior, self-harm, Internet addiction, and consumption of pornographic materials. Findings based on the first four waves of a 6-year longitudinal study among adolescents in Hong Kong in the extension phase of the project are presented. Basically, a total of 3,328 Secondary 1 (Grade 7) students were recruited from 28 schools in Hong Kong in the 2009/2010 academic year. Students were then assessed at intervals of 1 year. Finally, 2,682 students completed the questionnaires in all 4 years and were then included in the longitudinal data analysis.

Chapter 18 investigates some of the risk and protective factors related to the increasing substance abuse among youths. Results showed that gender, age, and family intactness were significantly related to initial status of substance abuse, while economic disadvantage and family intactness were significantly related to the growth trajectory of substance abuse, with adolescents from poor and non-intact families at higher risk of substance abuse. Chapter 19 examines sexual behavior and intention to engage in sexual behavior among adolescents. Results showed that adolescents from economically disadvantaged and non-intact families engaged in sexual behavior at a faster rate than their counterparts. Furthermore, family functioning and positive youth development influenced adolescent sexual behavior and intention. Chapter 20 examines the prevalence and psychosocial correlates of consumption of pornographic materials. Results showed that older male adolescents from non-intact families consumed more pornography than others. Results also indicated that positive youth development and family functioning are protective factors against consumption of pornographic material. Chapter 21 examines Internet addiction and its related psychosocial correlates. Results showed that economic disadvantage and family non-intactness are risk factors, whereas family functioning and positive youth development are protective factors. Finally, Chap. 22 examines the influence of family attributes, family functioning, and positive youth development on self-harm and suicidal behaviors. Analyses revealed that family intactness but not economic disadvantage was related to initial deliberate self-harm and suicidal behavior. By contrast, positive youth development and adaptive family functioning are protective antecedents of decreased adolescent deliberate self-harm and suicidal signs, respectively.

Why Do Positive Youth Development Programs Work?

We would like to approach this question from two levels. First, adoption of evidenced-based principles can promote success in program implementation. As a positive youth development program, the design, implementation, and evaluation of the Project P.A.T.H.S. followed closely the 15 principles identified by Borkowski et al. (2006). Second, we also used appropriate technologies in the design and implementation of the program to maximize the program effectiveness.

In their summary of the major principles associated with effective preventive research, Borkowski et al. (2006) identified three groups of principles: treatment, procedural, and design and evaluation. Treatment principles relate to the specific curriculum and related components of an intervention. They include theory-driven, comprehensive, varied teaching methods, positive relationships, and sociocultural relevance principles. Procedural principles correspond to how that intervention program is implemented. They cover sufficient dosage, appropriate timing, well-trained staff, programmed generalization, and treatment fidelity. Design and evaluation principles refer to an appropriate and convincing evaluation of program effectiveness. They cover interpretative standards, outcome evaluation, internal validation, adequate effect size, and clinical and social significance. Based on the works of Ramey and Ramey (1992) and Nation and colleagues (2003), Borkowski et al. (2006) identified these 15 principles and demonstrated that they have been shown to lead to important scientific and clinical outcomes.

Adoption of Principles of Effective Preventive Research

Since 2005, a huge number of publications on the Project P.A.T.H.S. have been published. These include more than 600 titles in English and Chinese, including books, book chapters, manuals, journal papers, conference papers, and special issues.

About half of the publications cover curriculum development and implementation. First, some adolescent developmental issues in Hong Kong are presented and discussed (Shek 2006a), with an extensive literature review and analysis dedicated to the understanding of the possible causes, consequences, and potential risk and protective factors for such issues among youths. Consequently, a number of articles focus on each single positive youth development (PYD) construct, such as prosocial involvement (Cheng et al. 2006a), recognition for positive behavior (Cheng et al. 2006b), self-determination (Hui and Tsang 2006), emotional competence (Lau 2006a), spirituality (Lau 2006b), bonding (Lee 2006a), resilience (Lee 2006b), behavioral competence (Ma 2006a), moral competence (Ma 2006b), social competence (Ma 2006c), prosocial norms (Siu et al. 2006), beliefs in the future (Sun and Lau 2006), cognitive competence (Sun and Hui 2006), self-efficacy (Tsang and Hui 2006), and positive identity (Tsang and Yip 2006). Finally, papers on the conceptual framework and program design were also published (Shek 2006b, c; Shek and Ma 2006; Shek et al. 2006).

More than 50 publications are specifically dedicated to the training of the program, which include mainly manuals and journal papers. Among these, the most substantial one is the series edited by Shek and Ma (2013a, b, c, d, e, f, g, h, i, j, k, l, m, n) titled *P.A.T.H.S. to Adulthood: A Jockey Club Youth Enhancement Scheme*, which includes 12 activity handbooks and one project learning handbook. These handbooks are practical and detailed manuals designed for teachers and/or instructors with clearly defined activities for each teaching unit during the 3 years of junior secondary school. These tools are particularly flexible because they can operationalize complex theoretical concepts into easy activities using simple and straightforward language. Furthermore, the structure of the handbooks enables teachers to adapt the program to their needs and schedules, as they can decide the number of modules to deliver (as well as the in-class activities, discussions, games, etc.). These training manuals have some undeniable advantages. For example, they allow teachers and instructors in the 237 secondary schools to have a reference manual for all. This not only implies the delivery of a more effective training to teachers, but as a consequence this also means that the same program will be delivered to all participating students.

The remaining 40 % of the publications are composed of evaluative studies about the efficacy of the program, which in most cases are in the form of journal papers and book chapters. Among these, the most important evaluation studies are longitudinal research that normally analyzes students' progress over three or more waves of data on issues such as drug abuse (Shek and Ma 2011), gambling (Shek and Sun 2011), consumption of pornographic materials (Ma and Shek 2013; Shek and Ma 2012), delinquency and problem behavior (Shek et al. 2012), Internet addiction (Shek and Yu 2012a), self-harm and suicide attempts (Law and Shek 2013; Shek and Yu 2012b), compensated dating (Lee and Shek 2013), sexual behavior, and intention to engage in sexual behavior (Shek 2013). The reliability of measurements is high, because they are based on data from more than 3,000 Hong Kong adolescents from 28 secondary schools, and the same questionnaire was used every year in the study.

Making Use of Effective Technology

To answer the question from a technology perspective, the Project P.A.T.H.S. made use of three out of the four essential technologies identified by Gullotta (2015). They are (a) education, (b) promotion of social competency, and (c) natural caregiving. Effective technologies for education include the provision of information and knowledge, anticipatory guidance (so as to educate a particular group prior to some expected events), and personal self-management of behavior (with methods that can vary from skills training to psychotherapeutic strategies). Social competency means a sense of belonging and a willingness to contribute to the group through a positive self-esteem, an internal locus of control, a sense of self-efficacy, and an attitude of caring for others (Catalano et al. 1998; Gullotta 2015). Finally, natural caregiving could be in the form of a mutual self-help group in which individuals serve as both caregivers and care receivers. Indigenous trained caregivers such as teachers and mentors provide advice, comfort, and support. Peers who are capable can also share knowledge, experiences, compassionate understanding, companionship, and, if needed, confrontation (Bloom 1996).

Education is the core of the Project P.A.T.H.S., although education alone is not sufficient for producing a significant change. As commented by Gullotta (2015), "the most often used of all prevention's technologies, alone it rarely, if ever, is effective.

Table 1 Teaching and learning activities designed for use in the Project P.A.T.H.S.

Instructors	Individuals (students)
Experience sharing (one-way)	Individual activities
Short tutorial (one-way)	Individual creative activities
Raising questions (two-way)	Individual reflections
Groups	**The whole class**
Group sharing	Class discussion
Group discussion (including presentation)	Class sharing
Group games	Class games
Group creative activities	
Role-plays	

The reason for this is that while education increases knowledge, only occasionally does it affect attitudes, and it almost never changes behavior" (p. 6). The Project P.A.T.H.S. provides basic education through (1) teaching and learning activities (increased knowledge), (2) learning activities using real-life examples (anticipatory guidance), and (3) skills development (personal self-management of behavior). Basic knowledge is provided partly by instructors in a one-way mode of teaching; these are universal information about different issues (e.g., effects of drug abuse), which are available to everyone. However, this information is always provided within a specific context (i.e., drug prevention) and serves as a basis for students to elaborate *their own* opinion about that specific issue through role-play, debate, or discussion, so that they can be prepared to face it in the future. This is anticipatory guidance. Finally, the Project P.A.T.H.S. teaches adolescents a set of practical skills that can be used in multiple settings for multiple purposes (Gullotta 2015). Youths can learn and train these skills in role-playing activities, where they can practice different roles simulating real-life cases, for example, how to say no to socially undesirable requests. Table 1 summarizes the teaching and learning activities designed for use in the preventive program. Adolescents learn new behaviors effectively in small groups where they can practice and test what they learn in small groups and natural caregiving can be developed (Gullotta 2015).

Another form of instruction of the Project P.A.T.H.S. is "Project Learning." "Project Learning" is an exploratory learning method for a specific topic which is related to students' daily lives. It aims to develop students' independent learning capacities and self-learning attitudes. There are five "Project Learning" in P.A.T.H.S., including romantic relationships, bullying prevention, religion and life values, success and materialistic orientation, and national/ethnic identity and acceptance. Each Project Learning can be divided into three stages: preparatory (instructors arrange activities so as to arouse students' interest), implementation (students collect data, make conclusions, and write reports), and concluding (students use different formats to present their results). Here, students are required to have some information and skills (knowledge as a base for education) for participating. However, they are then required to experience and share with others and develop their critical thinking. Experiential learning begins with a concrete experience, is followed by a reflective observation, an abstract conceptualization, and ends with an active experimentation, which can also be the starting point for a new experience of learning. The Project P.A.T.H.S. adopts an experiential learning perspective, which means (a) knowledge is constructed and acquired through experience; (b) knowledge is constructed in an individual mind, and it can be expressed and transferred to new situations; (c) learners can choose their own goals and can learn by asking questions and doing experiments; and (d) instructors can help students reflect on their experience and reexamine their personal assumptions. New behaviors are then learned by lived experiences. Experiential learning provides chances for adolescents to control the learning experience, to change its content, and to modify its intensity and duration (Gullotta 2015).

Promotion of psychosocial skills of the youth is an essential component of the P.A.T.H.S. program. Indeed, literature review (Catalano et al. 2012) on previous prevention programs has revealed that among 25 successful programs, 24 were based on the training of social or cognitive-behavioral skills. The curriculum for junior secondary school students was designed considering that development of adolescents at this stage in life goes through different domains, including physical development, cognitive development, personality and psychological development, social development, and relationships with the family and peers. The Project P.A.T.H.S. pursues the principles of "whole person education" and "whole person development" (Shek and Ma 2006). The project adopts both an ecological and a developmental perspective. Based on ecological models, adolescent developmental outcomes are determined by personal factors and environmental factors (family, peer, school, community, and cultural context). Based on life-span developmental theories, there are different developmental assets that need to be developed by an adolescent. Hence, adolescents need to learn different skills. The Project P.A.T.H.S. aims at helping adolescents develop their own abilities and enhance their ability to bond with others. After participating in this project, students will (a) enhance connections with healthy adults and peers (connection); (b) enhance social, emotional, cognitive, behavioral, and moral competence (competence); (c) enhance self-determination, self-efficacy, resilience, and beliefs in the future (confidence); (d) develop a clear identity and enhance their spirituality (character); (e) care for others (caring); (f) be more compassionate toward others (compassion); and (g) contribute to society (contribution). Indeed, longitudinal studies on the effectiveness of P.A.T.H.S. showed an increase in all major psychosocial indicators (Shek and Ma 2011, 2012; Shek et al. 2012; Shek and Sun 2013, 2014; Shek and Yu 2012a, b).

One of the constructs used in the curriculum is behavioral competence. Students are assisted to develop the ability to use verbal and nonverbal strategies to perform socially acceptable and normative behavior in social interactions (Ma 2006a). Based on a positive or prosocial motivation, students are taught to be courteous, graceful, and fair. The behavioral curriculum units cover three types of behaviors: applause, criticism, and apology. By providing opportunities to discuss and role-play, students were able to say no to socially undesirable requests.

Finally, the curriculum of P.A.T.H.S. is designed in such a way that students can gradually become more active indigenous caregivers within their groups. Teaching methods are an important factor for achieving this goal. In the Secondary 1 curriculum, there are mainly group and class discussions, which aim to enhance students' communication skills. The Secondary 2 curriculum adds role-playing, class games, and class sharing as teaching methods to increase students' learning interest and enhance their learning experience. Finally, as Secondary 3 students are becoming more mature, individual activities are increased so that students can learn more about themselves, observe their achievement, and prepare for future positive development (Shek and Sun 2013). However, it also means that Secondary 3 students are more likely to be ready to give their contribution to their groups, as they have developed a personal opinion or knowledge that they can share with others. At this stage, they are more likely to be in the position to become not only group members but also caregivers toward others.

What role can a massive preventive program using the positive youth development approach play in addressing developmental issues of early adolescents? That is the central question addressed in this book. Previous research findings have showed that positive youth development attributes are positively related to student well-being (Sun and Shek 2010, 2012, 2013). It is hoped that the theoretical discussion, practical intervention program manuals, and research findings provided in these chapters will serve as a stepping stone on the journey to promoting the well-being of early adolescents.

References

Bloom, M. (1996). *Primary prevention practices*. Thousand Oaks: Sage.

Borkowski, J. G., Akai, C. E., & Smith, L. E. (2006). The art and science of prevention research: Principles of effective programs. In J. G. Borkowski & C. M. Weaver (Eds.), *Prevention: The science and art of promoting healthy child and adolescent development* (pp. 1–16). Baltimore: Paul H. Brookes.

Catalano, R. F., Berglund, M. L., Ryan, J. A. M., Lonczak, H. S., & Hawkins, J. D. (1998). *Positive youth development in the United States: Research findings on evaluation of positive youth development programs*. Retrieved from http://aspe.hhs.gov/hsp/PositiveYouthDev99

Catalano, R. F., Fagan, A. A., Gavin, L. E., Greenberg, M. T., Irwin, C. E., Jr., Ross, D. A., & Shek, D. T. L. (2012). Worldwide application of prevention science in adolescent health. *The Lancet, 379*(9826), 1653–1664.

Cheng, H. C. H., Siu, A. M. H., & Leung, M. C. M. (2006a). Prosocial involvement as a positive youth development construct: Conceptual bases and implications for curriculum development. *International Journal of Adolescent Medicine and Health, 18*(3), 393–400.

Cheng, H. C. H., Siu, A. M. H., & Leung, M. C. M. (2006b). Recognition for positive behavior as a positive youth development construct: Conceptual bases and implications for curriculum development. *International Journal of Adolescent Medicine and Health, 18*(3), 467–473.

Gullotta, T. P. (2015). Understanding primary prevention. In T. P. Gullotta & G. R. Adams (Eds.), *Handbook of adolescent behavioral problems: Evidence-based approaches to prevention and treatment* (pp. 17–26). New York: Springer.

Hui, E. K. P., & Tsang, S. K. M. (2006). Self-determination as a positive youth development construct: Conceptual bases and implications for curriculum development. *International Journal of Adolescent Medicine and Health, 18*(3), 433–440.

Lau, P. S. Y. (2006a). Emotional competence as a positive youth development construct: Conceptual bases and implications for curriculum development. *International Journal of Adolescent Medicine and Health, 18*(3), 355–362.

Lau, P. S. Y. (2006b). Spirituality as a positive youth development construct: Conceptual bases and implications for curriculum development. *International Journal of Adolescent Medicine and Health, 18*(3), 363–370.

Law, B. M. F., & Shek, D. T. L. (2013). Self-harm and suicide attempts among young Chinese adolescents in Hong Kong: Prevalence, correlates, and changes. *Journal of Pediatric and Adolescent Gynecology, 26*(3S), S26–32.

Lee, T. Y. (2006a). Bonding as a positive youth development construct: Conceptual bases and implications for curriculum development. *International Journal of Adolescent Medicine and Health, 18*(3), 483–492.

Lee, T. Y. (2006b). Resilience as a positive youth development construct: Conceptual bases and implications for curriculum development. *International Journal of Adolescent Medicine and Health, 18*(3), 475–482.

Lee, T. Y., & Shek, D. T. L. (2013). Compensated dating in Hong Kong: Prevalence, psychosocial correlates, and relationships with other risky behaviors. *Journal of Pediatric and Adolescent Gynecology, 26*(3S), S42–48.

Ma, H. K. (2006a). Behavioral competence as a positive youth development construct: Conceptual bases and implications for curriculum development. *International Journal of Adolescent Medicine and Health, 18*(3), 387–392.

Ma, H. K. (2006b). Moral competence as a positive youth development construct: Conceptual bases and implications for curriculum development. *International Journal of Adolescent Medicine and Health, 18*(3), 371–378.

Ma, H. K. (2006c). Social competence as a positive youth development construct: Conceptual bases and implications for curriculum development. *International Journal of Adolescent Medicine and Health, 18*(3), 379–385.

Ma, C. M. S., & Shek, D. T. L. (2013). Consumption of pornographic materials in early adolescents in Hong Kong. *Journal of Pediatric and Adolescent Gynecology, 26*(3S), S18–S25.

Nation, M., Crusto, C., Wandersman, A., Kumpfer, K. L., Seybolt, D., Morrisey-Kane, E., & Davino, K. (2003). What works in prevention: Principles of effective prevention programs. *American Psychologist, 58*(6–7), 449–456.

Ramey, S. L., & Ramey, C. T. (1992). Early educational interventions with disadvantaged children – To what effect? *Applied and Preventive Psychology, 1*(3), 131–140.

Shek, D. T. L. (2006a). Adolescent developmental issues in Hong Kong: Relevance to positive youth development programs in Hong Kong. *International Journal of Adolescent Medicine and Health, 18*(3), 341–354.

Shek, D. T. L. (2006b). Conceptual framework underlying the development of a positive youth development program in Hong Kong. *International Journal of Adolescent Medicine and Health, 18*(3), 303–314.

Shek, D. T. L. (2006c). Construction of a positive youth development program in Hong Kong. *International Journal of Adolescent Medicine and Health, 18*(3), 299–302.

Shek, D. T. L. (2013). Sexual behavior and intention to engage in sexual behavior in junior secondary school students in Hong Kong. *Journal of Pediatric and Adolescent Gynecology, 26*(3S), S33–41.

Shek, D. T. L., & Ma, H. K. (2006). Design of a positive youth development program in Hong Kong. *International Journal of Adolescent Medicine and Health, 18*(3), 315–327.

Shek, D. T. L., & Ma, C. M. S. (2011). Substance abuse in junior secondary school students in Hong Kong: Prevalence and psychosocial correlates. *International Journal of Child Health and Human Development, 4*(4), 433–442.

Shek, D. T. L., & Ma, C. M. S. (2012). Consumption of pornographic materials among early adolescents in Hong Kong: A replication. *The Scientific World Journal*. Available from http://www.hindawi.com/journals/tswj/2012/406063/ref/

Shek, D. T. L., & Sun, R. C. F. (2011). Prevention of gambling problems in adolescents: The role of problem gambling assessment instruments and positive youth development programs. In J. L. Derevensky, D. T. L. Shek, & J. Merrick (Eds.), *Youth gambling: The hidden addiction* (pp. 231–243). Berlin: De Gruyter.

Shek, D. T. L., & Sun, R. C. F. (2013). Helping adolescents with greater psychosocial needs: The extension phase of the project P.A.T.H.S. in Hong Kong. *International Journal of Adolescent Medicine and Health, 25*(4), 425–432.

Shek, D. T. L., & Sun, R. C. F. (2014). Positive youth development programs for adolescents with greater psychosocial needs: Subjective outcome evaluation over three years. *Journal of Pediatric and Adolescent Gynecology, 27*, S17–25.

Shek, D. T. L., & Yu, L. (2012a). Internet addiction phenomenon in early adolescents in Hong Kong. *The Scientific World Journal, 2012,* Article ID 104304, 9 pages. Available from http://www.hindawi.com/journals/tswj/2012/104304/

Shek, D. T. L., & Yu, L. (2012b). Self-harm and suicidal behaviors in Hong Kong adolescents: Prevalence and psychosocial correlates. *The Scientific World Journal, 2012,* Article ID 932540, 14 pages. Available from http://www.hindawi.com/journals/tswj/2012/932540/

Shek, D. T. L., Siu, A. M. H., Lee, T. Y., Cheng, H., Tsang, S., Lui, J., & Lung, D. (2006). Development and validation of a positive youth development scale in Hong Kong. *International Journal of Adolescent Medicine and Health, 18*(3), 547–558.

Shek, D. T. L., Ma, C. M. S., & Tang, C. Y. P. (2012). Delinquency and problem behavior intention among early adolescents in Hong Kong: Profiles and psychosocial correlates. *International Journal of Disability and Human Development, 11*(2), 151–158.

Shek, D. T. L., & Ma, H. K. (Series Eds.), Ma, H. K., Shek, D. T. L., Law, B. M. F., Lam, C. M., & Lau, P. S. Y. (Eds.). (2013a). *P.A.T.H.S. to adulthood: A Jockey Club youth enhancement scheme. Activity handbook 9: Secondary three curriculum special teaching units.* Hong Kong: Centre for Innovative Programmes for Adolescents and Families, The Hong Kong Polytechnic University.

Shek, D. T. L., & Ma, H. K. (Series Eds.), Ma, H. K., Shek, D. T. L., Lee, T. Y., Lam, C. M., & Lau, P. S. Y. (Eds.). (2013b). *P.A.T.H.S. to adulthood: A Jockey Club youth enhancement scheme. Activity handbook 11: Secondary two curriculum updated teaching units.* Hong Kong: Centre for Innovative Programmes for Adolescents and Families, The Hong Kong Polytechnic University.

Shek, D. T. L., & Ma, H. K. (Series Eds.), Ma, H. K., Shek, D. T. L., Sun, R. C. F., Lam, C. M., Hui, E. K. P., & Lau, P. S. Y. (Eds.). (2013c). *P.A.T.H.S. to adulthood: A Jockey Club youth enhancement scheme. Activity handbook 2: Secondary one curriculum original teaching units.* Hong Kong: Centre for Innovative Programmes for Adolescents and Families, The Hong Kong Polytechnic University.

Shek, D. T. L., & Ma, H. K. (Series Eds.), Ma, H. K., Shek, D. T. L., Sun, R. C. F., Lam, C. M., Hui, E. K. P., & Lau, P. S. Y. (Eds.). (2013d). *P.A.T.H.S. to adulthood: A Jockey Club youth enhancement scheme. Activity handbook 4: Secondary two curriculum original teaching units.* Hong Kong: Centre for Innovative Programmes for Adolescents and Families, The Hong Kong Polytechnic University.

Shek, D. T. L., & Ma, H. K. (Series Eds.), Ma, H. K., Shek, D. T. L., Sun, R. C. F., Lam, C. M., Hui, E. K. P., & Lau, P. S. Y. (Eds.). (2013e). *P.A.T.H.S. to adulthood: A Jockey Club youth enhancement scheme. Activity handbook 6: Secondary three curriculum original teaching units.* Hong Kong: Centre for Innovative Programmes for Adolescents and Families, The Hong Kong Polytechnic University.

Shek, D. T. L., & Ma, H. K. (Series Eds.). Shek, D. T. L., & Sun, R. C. F. (Eds.). (2013f). *P.A.T.H.S. to adulthood: A Jockey Club youth enhancement scheme. Users' manual.* Hong Kong: Centre for Innovative Programmes for Adolescents and Families, The Hong Kong Polytechnic University.

Shek, D. T. L., & Ma, H. K. (Series Eds.), Shek, D. T. L., Ma, H. K., Lee, T. Y., Law, B. M. F., & Siu, A. M. H. (Eds.). (2013g). *P.A.T.H.S. to adulthood: A Jockey Club youth enhancement scheme. Activity handbook 12: Secondary three curriculum updated teaching units*. Hong Kong: Centre for Innovative Programmes for Adolescents and Families, The Hong Kong Polytechnic University.

Shek, D. T. L., & Ma, H. K. (Series Eds.), Shek, D. T. L., Ma, H. K., Lee, T. Y., & Siu, A. M. H. (Eds.). (2013h). *P.A.T.H.S. to adulthood: A Jockey Club youth enhancement scheme. Activity handbook 8: Secondary two curriculum special teaching units*. Hong Kong: Centre for Innovative Programmes for Adolescents and Families, The Hong Kong Polytechnic University.

Shek, D. T. L., & Ma, H. K. (Series Eds.), Shek, D. T. L., Ma, H. K., Sun, R. C. F., Lee, T. Y., Siu, A. M. H., & Tsang, S. K. M. (Eds.). (2013i). *P.A.T.H.S. to adulthood: A Jockey Club youth enhancement scheme. Activity handbook 5: Secondary three curriculum original teaching units*. Hong Kong: Centre for Innovative Programmes for Adolescents and Families, The Hong Kong Polytechnic University.

Shek, D. T. L., & Ma, H. K. (Series Eds.), Shek, D. T. L., Ma, H. K., Sun, R. C. F., Lee, T. Y., Siu, A. M. H., & Tsang, S. K. M. (Eds.). (2013j). *P.A.T.H.S. to adulthood: A Jockey Club youth enhancement scheme. Activity handbook 1: Secondary one curriculum original teaching units*. Hong Kong: Centre for Innovative Programmes for Adolescents and Families, The Hong Kong Polytechnic University.

Shek, D. T. L., & Ma, H. K. (Series Eds.), Shek, D. T. L., Ma, H. K., Sun, R. C. F., Lee, T. Y., Siu, A. M. H., & Tsang, S. K. M. (Eds.). (2013k). *P.A.T.H.S. to adulthood: A Jockey Club youth enhancement scheme. Activity handbook 3: Secondary two curriculum original teaching units*. Hong Kong: Centre for Innovative Programmes for Adolescents and Families, The Hong Kong Polytechnic University.

Shek, D. T. L., & Ma, H. K. (Series Eds.), Shek, D. T. L., Ma, H. K., Tsang, S. K. M., Hui, E. K. P., & Sun, R. C. F. (Eds.). (2013l). *P.A.T.H.S. to adulthood: A Jockey Club youth enhancement scheme. Activity handbook 10: Secondary one curriculum updated teaching units*. Hong Kong: Centre for Innovative Programmes for Adolescents and Families, The Hong Kong Polytechnic University.

Shek, D. T. L., & Ma, H. K. (Series Eds.), Shek, D. T. L., Ma, H. K., Tsang, S. K. M., & Hui, E. K. P. (Eds.). (2013m). *P.A.T.H.S. to adulthood: A Jockey Club youth enhancement scheme. Activity handbook 7: Secondary one curriculum special teaching units*. Hong Kong: Centre for Innovative Programmes for Adolescents and Families, The Hong Kong Polytechnic University.

Shek, D. T. L., & Ma, H. K. (Series Eds.), Shek, D. T. L., Ma, H. K., & Sun, R. C. F. (Eds.). (2013n). *P.A.T.H.S. to adulthood: A Jockey Club youth enhancement scheme. Activity handbook 13: Project learning*. Hong Kong: Centre for Innovative Programmes for Adolescents and Families, The Hong Kong Polytechnic University.

Siu, A. M. H., Cheng, H. C. H., & Leung, M. C. M. (2006). Prosocial norms as a positive youth development construct: Conceptual bases and implications for curriculum development. *International Journal of Adolescent Medicine and Health, 18*(3), 451–457.

Sun, R. C. F., & Hui, E. K. P. (2006). Cognitive competence as a positive youth development construct: Conceptual bases and implications for curriculum development. *International Journal of Adolescent Medicine and Health, 18*(3), 401–408.

Sun, R. C. F., & Lau, P. S. Y. (2006). Beliefs in the future as a positive youth development construct: Conceptual bases and implications for curriculum development. *International Journal of Adolescent Medicine and Health, 18*(3), 409–416.

Sun, R. C. F., & Shek, D. T. L. (2010). Life satisfaction, positive youth development, and problem behaviour among Chinese adolescents in Hong Kong. *Social Indicators Research, 95*(3), 455–474.

Sun, R. C. F., & Shek, D. T. L. (2012). Positive youth development, life satisfaction and problem behaviour among Chinese adolescents in Hong Kong: A replication. *Social Indicators Research, 105*(3), 541–559.

Sun, R. C. F., & Shek, D. T. L. (2013). Longitudinal influences of positive youth development and life satisfaction on problem behaviour among adolescents in Hong Kong. *Social Indicators Research, 114*(3), 1171–1197.

Tsang, S. K. M., & Hui, E. K. P. (2006). Self-efficacy as a positive youth development construct: Conceptual bases and implications for curriculum development. *International Journal of Adolescent Medicine and Health, 18*(3), 441–449.

Tsang, S. K. M., & Yip, F. Y. Y. (2006). Positive identity as a positive youth development construct: Conceptual bases and implications for curriculum development. *International Journal of Adolescent Medicine and Health, 18*(3), 459–466.

Part I
Student Well-Being and Developmental Issues: Theory

Prevention of Drug Abuse Among Young People: A Conceptual Framework

Tak Yan Lee and Diego Busiol

Abstract Recent research shows that the youth drug problem in Hong Kong is escalating. Ketamine is the most abused drug, followed by ecstasy, ice, cocaine, and cannabis. There are biological and psychological as well as sociological theories of drug use. Each theory provides a partial explanation for drug use and has important prevention, treatment, and policy implications. With the explanations provided by biologists, psychologists, and sociologists, an integrated model of factors contributing to adolescents' use and abuse of psychotropic drugs is presented. Adopting an ecological and positive youth development perspective, the protective and risk factors against drug use will be discussed, with a specific focus on youth in Hong Kong. Finally, a set of guidelines for conducting anti-drug prevention with students will be presented.

Introduction

Recent research shows that the youth drug problem in Hong Kong is escalating (Tsang 2011). The total number of reported drug abusers increased from 3.3 % in 2004/05 to 4.3 % in 2008/2009, and the number of drug abusers aged 21 and younger increased 51 % (Lam et al. 2011). This increase was particularly remarkable because it ran counter to the overall declining trend of reported drug abusers for the previous decade (Narcotics Division 2008).

The preparation for this work and the Project P.A.T.H.S. were financially supported by The Hong Kong Jockey Club Charities Trust.

This paper is partially based on an article originally published by *The Scientific World Journal*: Lee, T. Y. (2011). Construction of an integrated positive youth development conceptual framework for the prevention of the use of psychotropic drugs among adolescents. *The Scientific World Journal, 11*, 2403–2417.

T.Y. Lee (✉) • D. Busiol
Department of Applied Social Sciences, City University of Hong Kong,
Kowloon, Hong Kong, China
e-mail: ty.lee@cityu.edu.hk

© Springer Science+Business Media Singapore 2015
T.Y. Lee et al. (eds.), *Student Well-Being in Chinese Adolescents in Hong Kong*,
Quality of Life in Asia 7, DOI 10.1007/978-981-287-582-2_2

In a study population of 26,111 Hong Kong students, aged 10–19 years, recruited from 48 primary (primary grades 4–6) and secondary schools (secondary grades 1–7), 2.1 % of students had inhaled glue and 1.2 % had inhaled glue on one or more occasion (i.e., current use). Moreover, 1.1 % of students had used cough syrup for nonmedical (recreational) use, and 0.5 % had used cough syrup on one or more occasions (current use) (Lee and Tsang 2004). In the USA, one study of a nationally representative sample of 10,123 adolescents showed that 9.6 % of those aged 13–14 years reported lifetime illicit drug use (Swendsen et al. 2012). In Hong Kong, 28.3 % of youths used psychoactive substances for the first time when they were between 13 and 14 years old (Hong Kong Legislative Council Secretariat 2009).

General Theories of Drug Use and Abuse

There are biological and psychological as well as sociological theories of drug use. Although theories from these disciplines might seem competitive or even conflicting, an examination emphasizing their complementary nature is crucial. Each theory provides a partial explanation for drug use and has important prevention, treatment, and policy implications. Indeed, a comprehensive explanation could involve a combination of factors. For example, although we know that certain types of adolescent drug abuse are concentrated in areas of relative social and economic deprivation, most adolescents in similar situations do not abuse drugs.

The Neurological Perspective

From the neurological perspective, the immature brain of adolescents can explain why they show risky behavior. The part of the brain (prefrontal cortex) which deals with the ability to make sound judgments and calm unruly emotions develops slowly. As a result, when determining risk versus reward, the immature adolescent brain tends to emphasize benefits while discounting dangers (Goldstein and Volkow 2002). Different labels are given to this and related cognitive constraints, including damaged decision-making ability or weak analytical ability, psychological barriers, or weak emotional control and expression. Neuroscientists found that the orbitofrontal cortex and anterior cingulated cortex activate in addicts while they are craving, intoxicated, and bingeing. When an addict goes through treatment to withdraw his or her addiction, these areas deactivate. This system accounts for the addict's overvaluing his or her favored drug and the total failure of any inhibition in seeking it out because prefrontal areas provide the overly positive appraisal of the drug and disable the neuronal arrays for inhibition of impulse (Ellis 1990). Research also reveals that the adolescent brain is more responsive to drugs and thus more vulnerable to drug abuse than the adult brain, and it drives an interest in novelty that vastly exceeds that of children and adults (Whitten 2007). In short, the immaturity of the adolescent brain can explain their risky behavior, weak will power, and relapse of drug addiction.

The Pharmacological Perspective

As a major theory from the biological perspective, arousal theory describes the adolescent drug user as a person whose body is malfunctioning with regard to the production of crucial neurotransmitters, making drug use self-medicating or as a way of coping (Logan et al. 2006). As a result of the interaction between the pharmacological properties and the feeling experienced, the adolescent drug user's central nervous system habituates to the drug due to a neurotransmitter malfunction and is then reinforced for engaging in the drug. Biological vulnerabilities may manifest in any of a number of physical and mental health problems. The typical cyclical processes may go like this: a stress-producing mental health problem diminishes appropriate responses to stress, which increases stress levels, resulting in a more severe mental health problem; increased stress contributes to biological vulnerabilities and drug abuse, which then can affect physical and mental health (Volkow 2006).

Genetic Predisposition

According to the National Institute on Drug Abuse (NIDA), research evidence reveals that an individual's genetic makeup is one of the major factors related to vulnerability to drug abuse (Comings 1996). While drug abuse is the result of a complex interplay of biochemical, psychological, social, and environmental factors, genetic variance plays an important role in the susceptibility of adolescents' drug use and abuse. It is also claimed that the more severe the abuse, the greater the role of genetic factors (Crabbe 2002; Logan et al. 2002). While social and environmental factors may determine whether an adolescent is exposed to drugs, genetics may help to explain why only some of those adolescents who are exposed use and abuse drugs.

To summarize, biological theories of drug use and abuse, including genetics, neurological, and pharmacological perspectives, provide explanations in terms of trauma and coping factors. These factors are almost identical to the model of factors contributing to victimization and substance abuse among women presented by Logan et al. (Volkow 2006; Abadinsky 2011) after an extensive review of the literature. Specifically, these factors include genetic and biological vulnerabilities, drug use as a coping mechanism as well as physical and mental health problems. In the original model (Abadinsky 2011), the last factor is named "child and adolescent victimization." These factors are shown in a revised model which is adopted with some revisions (like the name of the drug-dependent factor) and presented in Fig. 1.

Psychological Theories

Behaviorism builds its foundations in the laboratory of experimental psychology and is based on learning theory (Bandura 1977). All forms of behavior are conditioned, the results of learned responses to certain stimuli. Behavior is strengthened

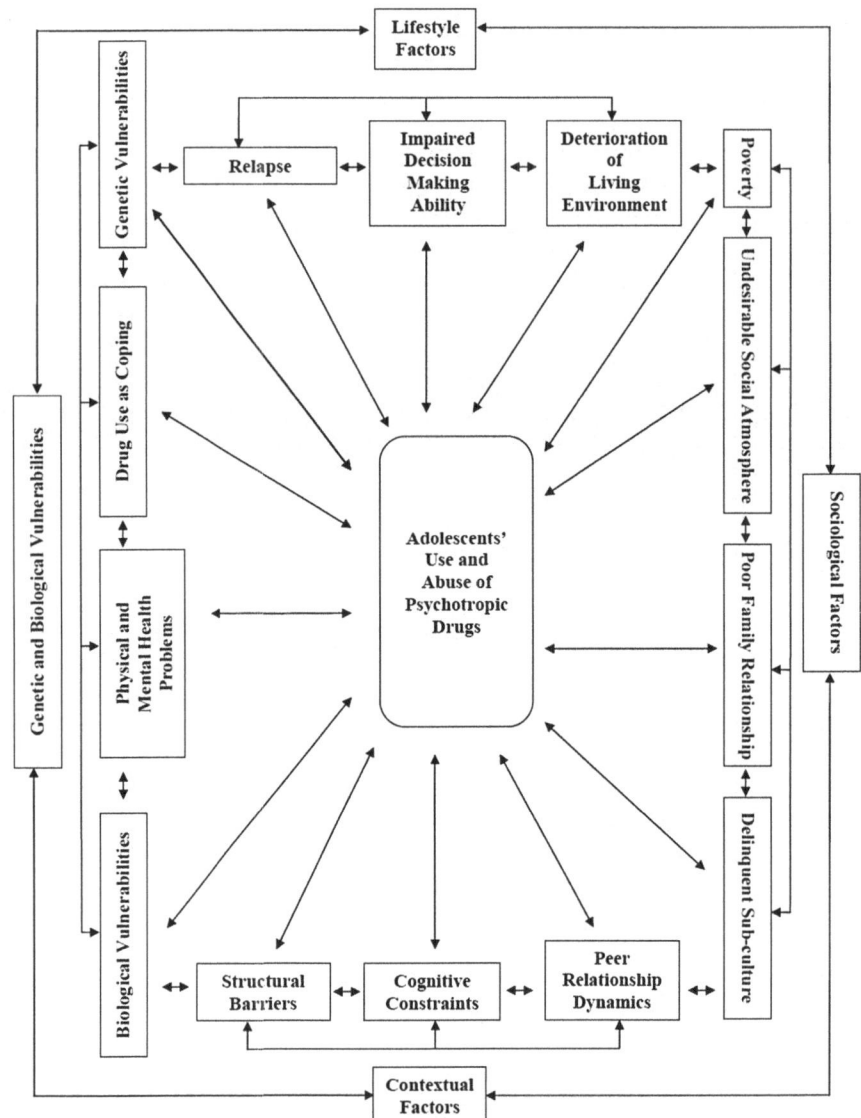

Fig. 1 A revised model of factors contributing to adolescents' use and abuse of psychotropic drugs

by its consequences and can be modified by operant conditioning: positive and negative reinforcement. Drugs can be used as powerful reinforcers, while withdrawal symptoms provide negative reinforcement. However, some adolescents manage to quit using drugs even after a pleasurable experience. Those who keep on using are more likely to be from an impoverished environment (Glassner and Loughlin 1987). This leads to a sociological perspective.

The model presented by Logan et al. (Volkow 2006; Abadinsky 2011) covers two categories of factors, that is, contextual and lifestyle factors. Although there are minor differences in terms of the specific content of the two versions, these two factors are in general closely related to psychological theories of drug use and abuse, which offer explanations including cognitive constraints, impaired decision-making abilities, peer relationship dynamics, and relapse. These specific factors are shown in the revised model of factors contributing to adolescents' use and abuse of psychotropic drugs presented in Fig. 1.

Sociological Theories

Sociological theory is concerned with social structures and social behavior. It examines adolescents' drug use and abuse in its social context. A sociological perspective often views drug use and abuse as the product of social conditions and relationships that cause despair, frustration, hopelessness, and general feelings of alienation in the most socially disadvantaged. Sociological theories, including anomie (a strong sense of strain among the socially disadvantaged causing the individual to abandon all attempts to reach conventional social goals), differential association (the existence of excessive deviant associations with drug abusers over nondeviant or prosocial associations), social control theory (the individual's weak bond to society), subcultures and cultural deviance (subcultures not conducive to conventional types of achievement), and symbolic interactionism (societal reaction stigmatizing drug users thus causing a damaged self-image, deviant identity, and a host of negative social expectations), all provide plausible explanations. Many sociological studies have found that drug use among adolescents is motivated by intermittent feelings of boredom and depression and that, like other aspects of adolescence, drug use may be abandoned when the person reaches adulthood. Furthermore, contrary to conventional wisdom, research has found that drug use is typically a group activity of socially well-integrated youngsters (The National Institute on Drug Abuse 1987). That is, different from some psychological views, some adolescent drug users are socially competent.

To summarize, sociological theories of adolescents' drug use and abuse provide explanations as sociological factors (including poverty, undesirable social atmosphere, poor family relationship, and delinquent subculture), lifestyle factors (deterioration of living environment), and contextual factors (including peer relationship dynamics and structural barriers such as the availability of drugs, unavailability, and/or unwillingness to seek help as well as poor social support network). These specific factors under the three domains are shown in the revised model presented in Fig. 1.

The National Institute on Drug Abuse (Peele 1981) outlines the lifestyle, contextual, sociological, as well as trauma and coping factors that are associated positively with adolescent substance abuse. The factors that are frequently found in deprived socioeconomic environments include:

1. Families whose members have a history of alcohol abuse and/or histories of antisocial behavior or criminality
2. Inconsistent parental supervision, with reactions that swing from permissiveness to severity
3. Parental approval or use of dangerous substances
4. Friends who abuse drugs
5. Children who fail in school during their late elementary years and show a lack of interest in school during early adolescence
6. Children who are alienated and rebellious
7. Children who exhibit antisocial behavior, particularly aggressive behavior, during early adolescence

The above examination shows the complementary nature of different theories and demonstrates the need for a biopsychosocial perspective, although the effect of the interaction of neurological and psychosocial factors is not yet clear. For example, the availability of choice of "novelty" for adolescents often depends on the social and economic situation as well as child-rearing practice of the family. This supports both psychological and sociological theories of drug use and abuse. From the psychosociological perspective, drug use depends on the actor who must learn that ingesting certain chemicals is desirable. Studies on subjective experience of drug abuse support the notion that intoxication is not inherently pleasurable (Coombs and Ziedonis 1995). Expectations based on learning influence the direction of drug use. This shows the interrelatedness of both biological and psychological theories.

Hypothesis

The amount of ethically based testing that can be done by social and behavioral scientists is limited since we cannot subject human beings to high levels of stress, expose them to drugs, and then find out whether they become drug addicts. The social or behavioral sciences have to study the etiology of drug addiction in a more indirect manner. Therefore, Abadinsky's (Bukstein et al. 1989) hypothesis is commonly accepted: what promotes adolescents' drug use and abuse is a biologically and psychologically vulnerable adolescent – that is, having a tendency of neurotransmitter deficiency and an additive personality resulting from problematic family relationships, inappropriate reinforcement, the lack of healthy role models, contradictory parental expectations, and/or an absence of love and respect living in deprived social circumstances with exposure to certain psychoactive chemicals.

Reasons for Psychotropic Drug Abuse in Hong Kong

According to the Narcotics Division of the Security Bureau of the Government of Hong Kong (Narcotics 2010), the main reasons for drug use of the reported drug abusers aged under 21 in Hong Kong in 2009 were peer influence/to identify with peers

(66.7 %), relief of boredom/depression/anxiety (51.1 %), curiosity (43.0 %), seeking euphoria or sensory satisfaction (33.6 %), and avoiding the discomfort due to its absence (15.2 %). Other reasons reported by the literature include: personal problems, unhappy experiences, failures, desire to escape from reality, low self-image, and lack of life (Lam et al. 2011). The percentages among different causes are not much different from that of similar surveys conducted in the last 10 years. However, these self-reported reasons are only overt reasons that youths themselves can realize. The underlying reasons for drug abuse are much more complex. For example, although some young people mentioned that they abused drugs because they wanted to relieve their depression, the data do not show what made them depressed. With these overt reasons in mind, a critical examination of the theoretical underpinnings of adolescents' use and abuse of psychotropic drugs is presented in the next section.

What Drugs Are Most Used in Hong Kong?

Different drugs, at different times, can become more or less popular in different societies and among different populations. The use of a specific drug may be characteristic of a (sub)culture more than others, and variations in drug use can be revealing of a shift in the social discourse. Then, it is important to understand what drugs are mostly used for by the population in question, and how their consumption changes over time. In Hong Kong, drugs abused by young people under the age of 21 are mainly psychotropic substances, particularly ketamine, followed by ecstasy, ice, cocaine, and cannabis (Lam et al. 2011). According to Joe-Laidler and Hunt (2008), the total number of reported drug users under the age of 21 using ketamine grew from less than 1 % in 1999 to 60 % in 2001 (overtaking the proportion of ecstasy use – 53 %) and reached 73 % by 2006. Reported ice and cocaine use has been comparatively lower. The percentage of polydrug use among all reported young persons grew from 16 % in 1997 to 51 % in 2006. Other research confirms that ketamine gained popularity and overtook ecstasy to be the commonest abused psychotropic drug in Hong Kong (HK) since 2001 (Cheung et al. 2010).

In a study commissioned by the action committee against narcotics (Lam et al. 2004), two samples of drug abusers ($N=201$) and students from one secondary school ($N=223$) were compared. Most of the drug abusers (88.6 %) were polydrug users and abused more than three kinds of drugs on average. The three most popular drugs were ketamine (89 %), ecstasy (84 %), and cannabis (79 %). Another study investigated the habits of 202 Hong Kong adolescents (aged 9 to 18) who were psychotropic substance abusers (Lau and Yung 2011). The study considered the following psychotropic substances: ketamine (K-Jai), methyl amphetamine (ice), cocaine (coke), cannabis (grass), ecstasy (E Jai), nimetazepam (5 jai), flunitrazepam (cross), triazolam (blue gremlin), midazolam (blue), zopiclone (white seed), LSD (black sesame), and codeine (robo). Of them 75.7 % reported to take ketamine, 8.2 % were aged between 9 and 12 years old, 40.6 % were aged 13–15 years old, and 51.1 % were aged 16–18 years old; 63.1 % were students; 70.4 % and 41.8 % were current smokers and drinkers, respectively.

Following Shek et al. (2011), ketamine abuse in Hong Kong could be regarded as quite unique because this drug is not commonly abused in other parts of the world. Joe-Laidler and Hunt argue that ketamine's popularity "may also be due to its ability to transcend the boredom and stress experienced by working class young persons, albeit temporarily, and float and be free in a variety of social spaces including leisure, school, and work. In a society in which freedom may be increasingly elusive, ketamine's liberating qualities may be particularly attractive. Ecstasy, as users themselves report, is intimately tied to the dance scene and has not been deemed as appropriate outside of that context" (2008, pp. 8–9).

A Revised Model of Factors Explaining Adolescents' Use and Abuse of Psychotropic Drugs

Over the years, scholars have summarized a set of risk and protective factors for drug use (Volkow 2006; Abadinsky 2011; Levinthal 2010; Pagliaro and Pagliaro 1996; Catalano et al. 1998). It is difficult to categorize the factors because drug abuse results from the interplay between biological, psychological, and sociological factors. According to system theory, to understand individuals' behavior, we have to understand the individuals, the environment around them, and the interactions between the individuals and the environment (Bukstein et al. 1989).

With the explanations provided by biologists, psychologists, and sociologists, the model of factors contributing to adolescents' use and abuse of psychotropic drugs developed by Logan et al. (Abadinsky 2011; Volkow 2006) is adopted after minor revisions and presented in the next section.

In the revised model, there are three levels, that is, macro-, mezzo-, and microlevels:

(1) The macro-level (dimensions)

Four dimensions are included: genetic and biological vulnerabilities, contextual factors, sociological factors, and lifestyle factors. These four dimensions interplay and cover all risk factors of adolescent drug abuse.

(2) The mezzo-level (factors)

Under the broad coverage of biological (factor (A), Fig. 1) and genetic (factor (D), Fig. 1) vulnerabilities, there are also two psychosocial factors, that is, factor (B), physical and mental health problems, and factor (C) – drug use as a coping mechanism. Under contextual factors, there are three factors: peer relationship dynamics (factor (L)), cognitive constraints (factor (M)), and structural barriers (factor (N)). Poverty (factor (H)), undesirable social atmosphere (factor (I)), poor family relationship (factor (J)), and delinquent subculture (factor (K)) are grouped under sociological factors. Finally, impaired decision-making ability (factor (F)), deterioration of living environment (factor (G)), and relapse (factor (E)) are treated as lifestyle factors.

(3) **The microlevel (causes)**

At this level, perceived reasons provided by adolescent drug abusers and causes used in laymen terms are presented. These perceived reasons or alleged causes are easily understandable and are manifestations of the real causes. Under the dimension of genetic and biological vulnerabilities, there are two visible factors, that is, physical and mental health problems and drug use as coping. Within these two factors, there are five self-reported reasons, including curiosity and ostentation, boredom, low self-esteem, peer pressure, and weak problem-solving ability. Contextual factors, the second dimension, include three causes, that is, (1) complex situations associated with structural barriers (factor (N), which means complicated situations confronted by the adolescent including the availability of drugs, unavailability and/or unwillingness to seek help, present and/or past abusive relationships, and the lack of social support); (2) weak emotional control and expression associated with cognitive constraints (factor (M)); and (3) difficult interpersonal relationships generated from peer relationship dynamics (factor (L)). Sociological factors, the third dimension, covers four causes, that is, (1) obtaining quick money (e.g., through engaging in drug trafficking to relieve poverty, factor (H)), (2) social exclusion (e.g., being isolated, bullied, or rejected) as a manifestation of undesirable social atmosphere (factor (I)), (3) alienated family relationships due to poor family relationships (factor (J)), and (4) the influence of delinquent peers as a result of differential association with delinquent subculture. The last dimension, lifestyle factors, covers three causes, that is, (1) weak will power associated with relapse (factor (E)), (2) weak analytical ability as a result of impaired decision-making ability (factor (F)), and (3) weak resilience associated with deterioration of one's living environment (factor (G)). The linkage between factors at the mezzo-level and causes at the micro-level is shown in Fig. 2.

Protective and Risk Factors for Youth in Hong Kong

As reported by the literature, youth at risk of drug use normally have limited social and relational skills. Vulnerable groups are generally unattached or unengaged youth, underachievers, and those excluded from schools and nondrug-using peer groups. The Hong Kong Youth Health Behaviors Survey (Tam 2014) was targeted at two cohorts of students, 14 years old (secondary 2) and 16 years old (secondary 4), within the Hong Kong public school system. A total of 31 secondary schools participated in the study and 2,084 secondary 2 and 1,466 secondary 4 students completed the survey. Findings showed that: (1) both values and self-efficacy contribute negatively to drug abuse; (2) protective factors against drug abuse are parental, school, and peer support (with school support as the most prominent factor); (3) risk factors are psychosomatic symptoms, study stress, and peer influence (with peer influence particularly influential); and (4) resilience strengthens protective factors and weakens risk factors. A survey on cough medicine abuse among young people in Hong Kong,

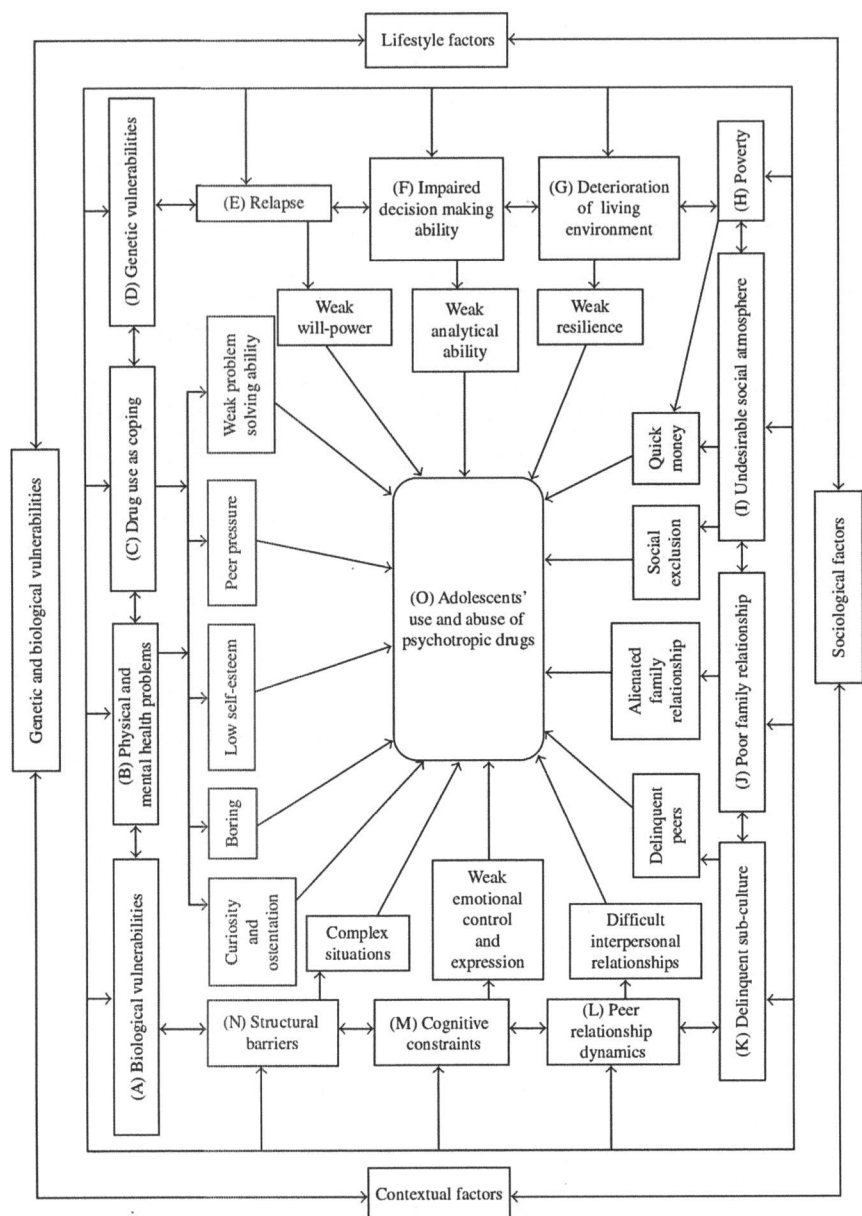

Fig. 2 A revised model of causes of adolescents' use and abuse of psychotropic drugs at the microlevel

conducted on 225 individuals (Tung Wah Group of Hospitals 2004), found that: "curiosity" (76.3 %), "peer influence" (67.5 %), and "seeking stimulation, pleasure, or euphoria" (50.6 %) are the first three reasons for abusing cough medicine for the first time. In addition, "peer influence" (56.3 %); "seeking stimulation, pleasure, or euphoria" (53.1 %); and "reducing stress, unhappiness, or boredom" (46.9 %) are the first three reasons for continued abuse of cough medicine. Furthermore, 93.1 % of respondents continued to abuse cough medicine after the first use. The first three common venues for abusing cough medicine are electronic game centers (73.1 %), one's home (43.8 %), and friends' homes (39.4 %). Adolescents having friends who endorse cough medicine abuse are more likely to abuse cough medicine. Respondents who reported a better perceived relationship with their mother had lower levels of endorsement of cough medicine abuse. Against this, researchers suggested to: (1) raise awareness of the harmful effects of cough medicine, (2) help professionals train them to identify the high-risk cases, and (3) educate parents about the signs of cough medicine abuse, help them to understand the peers of their children, and alert them to pay attention to how their children use money. Other research on 969 adolescents in Hong Kong (Tang et al. 1996) found a high correlation between drug use and psycho-social variables like: sensation seeking, peer drug use, family drug use, susceptibility to peer pressure, perceived control to gain access to drugs, intention to try other substances, and perceived adverse consequences of drug use. It was clearly shown that the use of substances is largely dependent on social influence. Indeed, it can be said that substance use in adolescents is a social behavior that is developed and maintained in deviant peer reference groups.

It is not always clear whether drug abuse is the cause or consequence of youth disengagement; some have interpreted drug abuse in youths as a symptom of disengagement from social life and emotional involvement (Tam 2011). According to Lam et al. (2011), the school is a domain of particular significance for Hong Kong adolescents, because Chinese parents expect them to work hard and do well in school and have a strong aspiration for academic achievement. As a consequence, school performance and school results can have significant effects on young people's drug use. Also a poor teacher-student relation and negative labeling by teachers, suspension from school, and frequent school changes are factors associated with later drug use (Cheung 1997). Finally, other risk factors for drug abuse in Hong Kong are sociodemographic factors (such as being in a single-parent family); mental health problems (such as social isolation, depression, anxiety, and stress); childhood experience of school suspension, physical maltreatment, corporal punishments, and peer influence (for a review, see Lau 2013); and low self-control (correlated with delinquency in Chinese settings, Lam et al. (2011)).

Results from a study on 40 female ex-ketamine abusers aged from 13 to 29 (Cheung et al. 2010) showed that female ketamine users had more frequent high-risk sexual relations, more liberal sexual attitudes (30.6 % of participants had their first sexual intercourse at the age of 13 or below), more termination of pregnancy, and more STDs than a control group. Results also showed that female ketamine users had severe lower urinary tract symptoms, which affected their quality of life. Commonly reported adverse effects were reduced functional bladder capacity, detrusor over activity, ulcerative cystitis, decreased bladder compliance, and vesico-ureteric reflux. According to the researchers, ketamine users may falsely believe that adverse physical consequences will resolve after termination of drug consumption.

Furthermore, they reported psychiatric morbidity. Altogether, 32 subjects completed the psychiatric assessment: 21 (66 %) of them had lifetime psychiatric diagnoses, the most common being substance-induced mood disorder (47 %), followed by substance-induced psychotic disorder (16 %) and specific phobias (13 %); 14 out of 15 of those suffering from substance-induced mood disorders were depressive types and one was of mixed type; finally, major depressive disorder, obsessive-compulsive disorder, and posttraumatic stress disorder all stood at 3 %. In a previous study from 2005 (Chen et al. 2005), of 95 ketamine abusers recruited from nightclubs and drug counseling centers, 26.3 % had lifetime psychiatric diagnoses and substance use disorders. The two most common diagnoses were depressive disorder (12.6 %) and drug-induced psychotic disorder (6.3 %).

A study of 222 at-risk youth served by the Hong Kong Christian Service and the Hong Kong Children and Youth Services (CityU Professional Services 2011) aimed at investigating the (mis)understanding of drugs by adolescents. It was found that youth express interest for drugs in terms of: playfulness ("like to play everything, try everything, do whatever that is playful," "a mentality for seeking excitement"), perceived benefits of drug abuse to the body ("slimming quickly," "increasing strength," "killing pain, reducing pain"), spirit ("feeling full of spirit, not easy to get tired"), interpersonal relationships ("able to open windows in our minds," "having more topics to talk with friends who use drugs"), and mood ("making people have more courage to court persons of the opposite sex," "relieving boredom"). They primarily reflected three types of misunderstanding, pertaining to: (1) need for drug abuse, (2) benefits of drug abuse, and (3) controllability over drug abuse.

Comparing a drug user group with a control group (Lam et al. 2004), it was found that the drug user group had a higher single-parent rate (23.4 %) than the school comparison group (7.3 %). Furthermore, it was found that drug abusers had less purpose in life than nondrug users. Further findings from this research highlighted the strong peer-related and in-group nature of this kind of drug consumption. Respondents might abuse drugs in different locations: in organized, structural, and commercialized settings (small-scale discos/dance clubs); in spontaneous and self-initiated ways (at home, at karaoke bars, at video game centers, in public parks or country parks); and in various places (beaches, cinemas, and podiums of public housing). Lastly, an association between unemployment and substance abuse has been reported.

An Effective Approach to Drug Prevention

Providing correct information regarding the potentially harmful effects of substance use should be the basis of a well-designed and acceptable prevention program (Abdullah et al. 2002). However, recent research on anti-drug programs reported that comprehensive approaches have higher efficacy than approaches which focus solely on one aspect of drug consumption (for a review, see Tobler 2000). Substance abuse has multiple causes (Greenberg et al. 1999), so an effective program needs to address both individual and contextual risk and protective factors (Catalano et al. 1998). Particularly, literature shows that multicomponent programs are more effective when they are informed by theory and research (Nation et al. 2003) and when they extend across a number of years (Greenberg et al. 2003). Anti-drug education should not be imposed but rather be cultivated together with youth. The goal of a drug-prevention course should be creating an anti-drug culture in an atmosphere of openness and acceptance and not just the normalization of some "deviant behavior" or the cure of some "pathology." Undue attachment of responsibility and blaming of the individual should be avoided (Hage et al. 2007). Also, an exclusive focus on risks has been criticized, for pathologizing, whereas instead it has been demonstrated that protective factors may reduce the probability of negative outcomes (Kaplan 2000). Finally, an effective approach should: (1) be comprehensive and not just focused on the substance or the individual, (2) strengthen the protective factors, (3) reduce the risk factors, and (4) enhance one's own resilience.

Information provided should not be exaggerated with the intention to scare youth; likewise, privacy and confidentiality must be protected. In 2009, a school drug-testing survey on youth was conducted among 700 students (Salvation Army and Community Services 2009). Results showed that: (a) 76.4 % of respondents to the questionnaire agreed that "schools are required to consult the views of students before deciding to participate in school drug-testing programs"; (b) 84.9 % of respondents agreed that "schools are required to explain clearly the details to students before participating in school drug testing"; (c) 64.2 % of respondents agreed that "the implementation of school drug-testing programs must obtain the consent of both parents and students"; (d) 83.7 % of the respondents expressed concern regarding "level of confidentiality of test results," and 48.8 % showed great concern; (e) 80.9 % of the respondents expressed concern over "level of confidence in the test results," and 41.0 % showed great concern; (f) 77.8 % of the respondents expressed concern over "the consequences of students who have been confirmed to have taken drugs," and 37.7 % showed great concern; (g) 81.4 % of respondents expressed concern about "police prosecution," and 45.9 % showed great concern; (h) 80.3 % of respondents expressed concern about "the confidentiality of the results," and 48.3 % showed great concern; and (i) 77.9 % of respondents expressed concern about "the school requires students to drop out," while 39.7 % showed great concern. Finally, the researchers suggested a set of guidelines for conducting anti-drug prevention with students: (1) the government should formulate clear privacy protection measures; (2) before recommending drug testing to students, they should be invited to fill out a letter of intent with respect to their intentions; (3) the school should set up an independent professional team to collaborate with the school drug-testing team to provide further evaluation to those students in need; (4) the school should explain clearly to all students their corresponding actions to students who test positive and should also emphasize that drug-test results should not be inconsistent with their basic rights to education and to be a student; and (5) the school is proposed to provide counseling to parents who feel frustrated with the students' results.

References

Abadinsky, H. (2011). *Drug use and abuse: A comprehensive introduction* (7th ed.). Belmont: Wadsworth.

Abdullah, A. S. M., Fielding, R., & Hedley, A. J. (2002). Patterns of cigarette smoking, alcohol use and other substance use among Chinese university students in Hong Kong. *The American Journal on Addictions, 11*(3), 235–246.

Bandura, A. (1977). *Social learning theory*. Englewood Cliffs: Prentice Hall.

Bukstein, O. G., Brent, D. A., & Kaminer, Y. (1989). Comorbidity of substance abuse and other psychiatric disorders in adolescents. *American Journal of Psychiatry, 146*(9), 1131–1141.

Catalano, R. F., Berglund, M. L., Ryan, J. A. M., Lonczak, H. S., & Hawkins, J. D. (1998). Positive youth development in the United States: Research findings on evaluation of positive youth development programs. Retrieved from http://aspe.hhs.gov/hsp/PositiveYouthDev99

Chen, R. Y. L., Lee, A. M., Chen, R. C. K., Chen, E. Y. H., & Tang, S. W. (2005). *A study on the cognitive impairment and other harmful effects caused by ketamine abuse*. Hong Kong: Security Bureau of Hong Kong, Narcotics Division.

Cheung, Y. W. (1997). Family, school, peer, and media predictors of adolescent deviant behavior in Hong Kong. *Journal of Youth and Adolescence, 26*(5), 569–596.

Cheung, R. Y. K., Chan, S. S. C., Lee, J. H. S., Pang, A. W. L., & Choy, R. K. W. (2010). *Research report on prospective observational study of urinary symptoms, sexual behaviors and psychiatric symptoms in ketamine misusers*. Hong Kong: The Chinese University of Hong Kong, Faculty of Medicine, Department of Obstetrics & Gynaecology, submitted to Beat Drug Fund Association.

CityU Professional Services Limited. (2011). *Research report on effective ways to dispel misunderstandings about psychotropic substances in youth at risk for drug abuse problems*. Hong Kong: CityU Professional Services Ltd, submitted to Beat Drug Fund Association.

Comings, D. E. (1996). Genetic factors in drug abuse and dependence. In H. W. Gordon & M. D. Glantz (Eds.), *Individual differences in the biochemical etiology of drug abuse* (pp. 16–38). Rockville: National Institute on Drug Abuse.

Coombs, R. H., & Ziedonis, D. (1995). *Handbook on drug abuse prevention: A comprehensive strategy to prevent the abuse of alcohol and other drugs*. Boston: Allyn and Bacon.

Crabbe, J. C. (2002). Genetic contributions to addiction. *Annual Review of Psychology, 53*, 435–462.

Ellis, L. (1990). Universal behavioral and demographic correlates of criminal behavior: Toward common ground in the assessment of criminological theories. In L. Ellis & H. Hoffman (Eds.), *Crime in biological, social, and moral contexts* (pp. 36–49). Westport: Praeger.

Glassner, B., & Loughlin, J. (1987). *Drug use in adolescent worlds: Burnouts to straights*. Houndmills: Macmillan.

Goldstein, R. Z., & Volkow, N. D. (2002). Drug addiction and its underlying neurobiological basis: Neuroimaging evidence for the involvement of the frontal cortex. *American Journal of Psychiatry, 159*(10), 1642–1652.

Greenberg, M. T., Domitrovich, C., & Bumbarger, B. (1999). *Preventing mental disorders in school-age children: A review of the effectiveness of prevention programs*. Washington, DC: U.S. Department of Health and Human Services.

Greenberg, M. T., Weissberg, R. P., O'Brien, M. U., Zins, J. E., Fredericks, L., Resnik, H., Elias, M. J., et al. (2003). Enhancing school-based prevention and youth development through coordinated social, emotional, and academic learning. *American Psychologist, 58*(6–7), 466.

Hage, S. M., Romano, J. L., Conyne, R. K., Kenny, M., Matthews, C., Schwartz, J. P., et al. (2007). Best practice guidelines on prevention practice, research, training, and social advocacy for psychologists. *The Counseling Psychologist, 35*(4), 493–566.

Hong Kong Legislative Council Secretariat. (2009). *The youth drug abuse problem in Hong Kong*. Hong Kong: Hong Kong Legislative Council.

Joe-Laidler, K., & Hunt, G. (2008). Sit down to float: The cultural meaning of ketamine use in Hong Kong. *Addiction Research & Theory, 16*(3), 259–271.

Kaplan, R. M. (2000). Two pathways to prevention. *American Psychologist, 55*, 382–396.

Lam, C. W., Boey, K. W., Wong, O. O. A., & Tse, S. K. J. (2004). *A study of substance abuse in underground rave culture and other related settings.* Hong Kong: The Action Committee Against Narcotics (ACAN), Research Sub-committee.

Lam, C. M., Lau, P. S., Law, B. M., & Poon, Y. H. (2011). Using positive youth development constructs to design a drug education curriculum for junior secondary students in Hong Kong. *The Scientific World Journal, 11*, 2339–2347.

Lau, J. T. (2013). *Study on drug abuse situation and service needs of non-engaged youths in Hong Kong.* Hong Kong: The Chinese University of Hong Kong, Faculty of Medicine, School of Public Health and Primary Care, submitted to Narcotics Division, Security Bureau.

Lau, J. T. F., & Yung, T. K. C. (2011). *Research report on the dietary intake and body weight status of adolescent psychotropic substance abusers in Hong Kong: An explorative study for improving drugs rehabilitation programme.* Hong Kong: The Chinese University of Hong Kong, Faculty of Medicine, Division of Health Improvement School of Public Health and Primary Care, submitted to Research Advisory Group.

Lee, A., & Tsang, C. K. K. (2004). Youth risk behaviour in a Chinese population: A territory-wide youth risk behavioural surveillance in Hong Kong. *Public Health, 118*(2), 88–95.

Levinthal, C. F. (2010). *Drugs, behavior, and modern society* (6th ed.). Boston: Allyn and Bacon.

Logan, T. K., Walker, R., Cole, J., & Leukefeld, C. G. (2002). Victimization and substance abuse among women: Contributing factors, interventions, and implications. *Review of General Psychology, 6*(4), 325–397.

Logan, T. K., Walker, R., Jordan, C. E., & Leukefeld, C. G. (2006). *Women and victimization: Contributing factors, interventions, and implications.* Washington, DC: American Psychological Association.

Narcotics Division. (2008). *Report of the task force on youth drug abuse.* Hong Kong: Security Bureau.

Narcotics Division (2010). *Drug statistics.* Retrieved from http://www.nd.gov.hk/en/crdaess.htm

Nation, M., Crusto, C., Wandersman, A., Kumpfer, K. L., Seybolt, D., Morrissey-Kane, E., Davino, K., et al. (2003). What works in prevention: Principles of effective prevention programs. *American Psychologist, 58*(6–7), 449.

Pagliaro, A. M., & Pagliaro, L. A. (1996). *Substance use among children and adolescents.* New York: John Wiley & Sons.

Peele, S. (1981). Addiction to an experience: A social-psychological theory of addiction. In D. J. Lettieri, M. Sayers, & H. W. Pearson (Eds.), *Theories of drug abuse: Selected contemporary perspectives* (pp. 142–144). Rockville: National Institute on Drug Abuse.

Salvation Army Youth, Family and Community Services (2009). *School drug testing survey report in youth.* Retrieved from http://www.breakthrough.org.hk/ir/youthdatabank/de/de_01.htm#C1-472

Shek, D. T. L., Ma, H. K., & Sun, R. C. F. (2011). A brief overview of adolescent developmental problems in Hong Kong. *The Scientific World Journal, 11*, 2243–2256.

Swendsen, J., Burstein, M., Case, B., Conway, K. P., Dierker, L., He, J., Merikangas, K. R., et al. (2012). Use and abuse of alcohol and illicit drugs in US adolescents. *Archives of General Psychiatry, 69*, 390–398.

Tam, W. M. (2011). Hidden school disengagement and its relationship to youth risk behaviors in Hong Kong. *Educational Research Journal, 26*(2), 175–198.

Tam, F. W. M. (2014). A structural equation model of drug abuse among secondary students in Hong Kong. *International Journal of Mental Health and Addiction, 13*, 1–15.

Tang, C. S., Wong, C. S., & Schwarzer, R. (1996). Psychosocial differences between occasional and regular adolescent users of marijuana and heroin. *Journal of Youth and Adolescence, 25*(2), 219–239.

The National Institute on Drug Abuse. (1987). *Drug abuse and drug abuse research.* Rockville: NIDA.

Tobler, S. N. (2000). Lesson learned. *Journal of Primary Prevention, 20*(4), 261–274.

Tsang, S. K. (2011). Parent engagement in youth drug prevention in Chinese families: Advancement in program development and evaluation. *The Scientific World Journal, 11*, 2299–2309.

Tung Wah Group of Hospitals (2004). *Cough medicine abuse among young people in Hong Kong.* Retrieved from http://www.breakthrough.org.hk/ir/youthdatabank/de/de_01.htm#C1-311

Volkow, N. D. (2006). NIDA Director's report to CPDD meeting: Progress, priorities, and plans for the future. In W. L. Dewey (Ed.), *Problems of drug dependence. Proceedings of the 67th annual scientific meeting, the College on problems of drug dependence* (pp. 70–79). Bethesda: U.S. Department of Health and Human Services, National Institutes of Health, National Institute on Drug Abuse.

Whitten, J. L. (2007). Behavioral response to novelty foreshadows neurological response to cocaine. *NIDA Notes, 21*(3), 1–6.

Principles for the Construction of a School-Based Sex Education Program

Diego Busiol, Mary T.W. Leung, and Tak Yan Lee

Abstract Recent research showed that today an increasing number of adolescents have an active sex life in Hong Kong. However, the emerging needs of adolescents are not met, as today's standard of sex education is both variable and inconsistent in Hong Kong. Other countries such as the USA, Britain, Germany, France, and the Netherlands have put much effort into introducing or expanding sex education in schools; these experiences will be critically presented and analyzed. Protective and risk factors are defined as factors that can both directly influence behavior and moderate the relationship between risk and behavior. Protective and risk factors will be presented in detail, highlighting those which can be addressed in the context of a school-based program. Finally, in light of the previous literature, a conceptual framework for a prevention program will be proposed.

Introduction

Recent research showed that today many young people in China have active sex lives. Increasing premarital sexual activities (Gao et al. 2001; Wang et al. 2005; Zhang et al. 1999) characterized by nonuse of contraception and condoms, multiple partners, and casual sex experiences have been reported (Lou et al. 2002; Tu et al. 1998; Wang et al. 2002; Zheng et al. 2001). As a consequence, sexually transmitted infections (STIs) and HIV/AIDS, unwanted pregnancy, and induced abortion are also observed (Hu 1996; Li 2000; Cao et al. 2000; Tu et al. 1998).

Research findings showed a similar situation in Hong Kong (Hong Kong Family Planning Association 1991; Hong Kong Federation of Youth Groups 1995; Lam 1997a, b), leading some to say that young people today have an earlier onset of puberty than their predecessors (Fok 2005). However, although increasing, the number of Hong Kong

---

The preparation for this work and the Project P.A.T.H.S. were financially supported by The Hong Kong Jockey Club Charities Trust.

D. Busiol • M.T.W. Leung • T.Y. Lee (✉)
Department of Applied Social Sciences, City University of Hong Kong,
Kowloon, Hong Kong, China
e-mail: ty.lee@cityu.edu.hk

© Springer Science+Business Media Singapore 2015   31
T.Y. Lee et al. (eds.), *Student Well-Being in Chinese Adolescents in Hong Kong*,
Quality of Life in Asia 7, DOI 10.1007/978-981-287-582-2_3

youth having sexual intercourse remains limited; particularly, percentages are low if compared to other societies. For example, according to a study conducted in 1995 by the Boys' & Girls' Clubs Association of Hong Kong, only 3 % of interviewees (among more than 4,000 secondary school students) reported that they had had sexual intercourse (BGCA 1996). Other studies showed similar results. In 1999–2000, a large survey on youth risky behavior was carried out among 15–18-year-old students from 21 schools in Hong Kong; a total of 8,382 students completed the questionnaire (with a 99.7 % response rate), showing that only 377 students (4.7 %) (198 males and 179 females) claimed to have had sexual intercourse (Wong et al. 2006). Lee and Tsang (2004) examined a sample of 26,111 Hong Kong students aged 10–19 years old and found that only 3.4 % of them reported experience of sexual intercourse; however, only less than half of them reported the use of a contraceptive device. Finally, in 2011 the Family Planning Association of Hong Kong (2012) examined over 3,700 S1 to S7 students and found that 4.7 % had sexual intercourse experience. Data from Hong Kong show a different picture from what happens; for example, in the USA, according to the Youth Risk Behavior Surveillance 2011 (Eaton et al. 2012), 47 % of Grade 9 to Grade 12 students (equivalent to S3 to S6 in Hong Kong) indicated that they had sexual intercourse experience.

Similarly, when considering the teen pregnancy rates, Hong Kong scores among the lowest in the world (3.2/1,000 in 2008), together with China and other culturally close societies such as Korea and Japan. Hong Kong's teenage pregnancy rate is much lower than that of other Asian countries like Nepal, Bangladesh, India, and Sri Lanka, where socioeconomic factors, low educational attainment, and cultural and family structure are all consistently identified as risk factors for teenage pregnancy (Acharya et al. 2010). Switzerland and the Netherlands, which are the European countries with the lowest teenage pregnancy rates (5.5/1,000), come immediately after Hong Kong. Instead, quite surprisingly, technologically advanced countries like the UK and USA have much higher rates. So, generally speaking the overall data from Hong Kong are not alarming. However, the low teen pregnancy rate here is not necessarily the effect of good sex education and high consciousness among youth; young people in Hong Kong are not necessarily better prepared in their knowledge about sex than youth of the same age from other countries. Instead, it is more likely that social, cultural, and familial factors prevent youth from having sexual intercourse and thus from experiencing sex-related problems.

According to Wong et al. (2006) the sexual knowledge of young Chinese people remains rather limited and the incidence of unsafe sex practices has increased. Many youth lack sexual knowledge, and many of them have a sense of inferiority about themselves (Fok 2005). On the other hand, they would like to: (a) receive more information about sex; (b) have proactive teaching about courtship, marriage, and parenthood; (c) develop self-esteem, unbiased gender roles, and the ability to play a constructive role in the family; and (d) clarify values and make responsible decisions on issues relating to sex (Fok 2005). However, the emerging needs of adolescents are not met, as sex remains a taboo in many Chinese families and open discussions are discouraged. The majority of the adult population have received little sex education themselves and do not know how to approach sex-related issues. On the other hand, today's standard of sex education is both variable and inconsistent in Hong Kong (Wong et al. 2006).

Development of Sex Education in the USA, the UK, and the Netherlands

What is sex education and how has it been approached in different countries? During the second half of the last century, many industrialized countries such as the USA, Britain, Germany, France, and the Netherlands have put much effort into introducing or expanding sex education in schools (Kawahara 2000).

In the USA, most states adopt an abstinence-only policy, as defined by Section 510 of Title V of the Social Security Act. Abstinence is generally intended as abstinence from sexual intercourse and is proposed as a public health issue; however, most supporters of this option have moral or religious grounds (Santelli et al. 2006; Constantine et al. 2007). The federally funded abstinence-only-until-marriage grant program prohibits instruction in or promotion of the use of contraceptive methods (Constantine et al. 2007). Funding for abstinence-only education is increasing (Lindberg et al. 2006). California is the only state that opted out of this program from the beginning (eight other states followed), advocating instead "comprehensive sex education," which aims at providing "complete, accurate, positive and developmentally appropriate information on human sexuality, including the risk reduction strategies of abstinence, contraception and STD protection; it promotes the development of relevant personal and interpersonal skills; and it includes parents or caretakers as partners with teachers" (Constantine et al. 2007).

Religious values have also largely affected the debate on sex education in the UK, where "the old determination to instill traditional Christian morality in respect of the family using the vehicle of sex education in schools re-surfaced during the prolonged period of Conservative rule [...] during the 1980s and 1990s" (Lewis and Knijn 2002). Different concerns have contributed to the unclear definition of what sex education is and what it is for. In the words of Simon Blake, the director of the Sex Education Forum: "In sex education it still hasn't been worked out if it's meant to prevent teen pregnancies, make teenagers understand their bodies, or contribute to personal and social development." Lewis and Knijn (2002) take the UK and the Netherlands as two paradigmatic examples of the two opposite approaches to sex education, the former being mainly the expression of moral or religious values and the latter mainly based on scientific evidence. According to the authors, the confusion and conflicts of different levels and needs are what resulted in some countries (like the UK) having unclear definitions of sex education and, as a consequence, less effective policies. Indeed, looking at the statistics, the more conservative countries like the USA and UK have the highest rate of STDs and teen pregnancy. For example, in the UK the policymakers struggled over whether family change should be addressed or not, while instead in Holland they took a more pragmatic approach and by the end of the 1970s marriage and family were no longer the central planks in Dutch sex education (Lewis and Knijn 2002). This means that in some countries sex education involves different interested parties, like professional groups, but also churches; in contrast, countries like Holland opted to base sex education on scientific evidence alone, firmly rejecting any moral or judgmental approach about individual choices. Findings from previous research suggest that those countries with pragmatic sex education policies (the Netherlands) have better sexual health-related statistics than those countries where sex education is largely affected by religion (the UK) and the USA with its sexual abstinence-based policy (Weaver et al. 2005). Furthermore, Schaalma et al. (2004) observe that "teaching social skills relevant to sexual behavior in classroom settings requires specialist expertise both in program design and in delivery by teachers or facilitators" (p. 265). This is, for example, the case of the Netherlands, where the Dutch government has tended to pass the issue of sex education out to the professionals in the field or voluntary organizations.

Development of Sex Education in Mainland China and in Hong Kong

Mainland China

For a long time in Chinese societies, attitudes toward sex and sexuality have been largely influenced by Confucianism, Taoism, and Buddhism. For Confucius, sex should not interfere with social stability and harmony in human relations; for Taoism sex contributes to health and longevity (Ruan 1991). However, during the Qin and Han dynasties (207 BC–220 AD), interpretation of the classics became more moralistic and attitudes toward sexuality more negative and repressive (Brotto et al. 2005). Only sex within marriage for the purpose of procreation was approved, and it was viewed as having a merely procreative role. This trend continued during the succeeding dynasties and sex education was banned during the Cultural Revolution, as love and open discussion of sexual matters were considered part of the "bourgeois culture" (Zhang et al. 2007). In the late 1970s, the introduction of the one-child policy led to the emergence of more comprehensive sex education. In 1988, the Ministry of Education and the State Family Planning Commission required that sex education be incorporated into middle school curricula nationwide. In 1993, the Ministry of Education issued the Guideline to Health Education for University Students, but only in 2002 did the government officially become committed to providing sex education to middle school students (Li et al. 2004). First comprehensive courses have been made available in middle schools of major Chinese cities like Chongqing, Guangzhou, Harbin, Shanghai, Wuhan, and Xi'an. These cities produced their own textbooks on sexual behavior, ethics, procreation and contraception, anti-drug warnings, and AIDS prevention (Ho 2006). Adopting popular culture to promote sex education was the strategy initially adopted by the Ministry of Education. In 2004, more than 50 Shanghai secondary schools adopted new textbooks on love that were based on stories and poems by both ancient and contemporary Chinese and foreign writers. China also published its first cartoon book series on puberty and sex education in April 2002, based on South Korea's series of books for young students entitled, *I Want to Know Myself* (Ho 2006). In addition, more traditional sex education programs, including information on abstinence, contraception, and healthy sexual behavior were implemented (Wang et al. 2005), demonstrating that community-based interventions may be effective in reaching large numbers of Chinese youth and in promoting sexual negotiation, contraceptive use, and pregnancy and STI/HIV prevention.

Hong Kong

Hong Kong presents a more complex picture, where sexual practices have come under both traditional Chinese and Judeo-Christian influence (Tsang 1987; Ng and Ma 2001).

Public sex education in Hong Kong started around the 1950s, predominantly with the work by the government-subvented Family Planning Association of Hong Kong (Ying Ho and Tsang 2002). A first attempt by the Education Department to introduce sex education in schools is dated 1971; however, the first Guidelines on Sex Education in Secondary Schools were published only in 1986. The guidelines comprehended more detailed recommendations on sex education topics, resources, and references than the memorandum of 1971. In 1987, 1990, and 1994, the Advisory Inspectorate of the Education Department assessed the implementation of the guidelines in schools but found no improvement in sex education. Indeed, coverage of sex education was not broad enough and many schools avoided the most sensitive areas (Fok 2005). Thus, the guidelines were revised again in 1997, which is a significant year as Hong Kong was also making a transition to a new political status. To some (Fok 2005) the new guidelines reflected changes in social values leading to more open sex education, covering different aspects of human sexuality and suggesting teaching strategies. Apparently, greater attention was given to sex equity, gender roles, and human rights (Fok and Tung 2000). However, others (Ying Ho and Tsang 2002) have pointed out that "the 1997 Guidelines showed a strong bias towards teaching young people socially accepted morality while aspects of human sexuality were largely confined by discourses on emotional well-being and human relationships." Ng (1998) found the guidelines to be "heavily skewed toward moral indoctrination, emotion, self-images, interpersonal and family relationships. Sexual anatomy and physiology, sexual behavior and psychology and sexual medicine were limited to very basic and there was nothing on controversial issues like sexual variation, prostitution and pornography" (p. 32). Some scholars suggested that sex education would best be taught as an independent subject to ensure that students are able to receive adequate coverage of related knowledge. In 1998, the government set up topics on the stages of learning and stage-based learning objectives for sex education. The policy papers suggested teachers to use a creative and realistic "life events" approach to share the following topics with their students:

• Personal hygiene and disease
• Understanding of human growth and development, gender-specific characteristics of puberty, sexual intercourse, and pregnancy

- Respect for others' bodies, their rights to decision-making, and privacy
- Differentiation between love, friendship, and other relationships
- Handling sexual impulses and ways to deal with sexual harassment (Curriculum Development Council 1998)

The above content placed sex education within the umbrella of interpersonal relationships. The topics included skills, attitudes, and ethical explorations with emphases placed on students' ability to both understand and apply the knowledge and concepts. From 1997 to 2000, the government spearheaded and implemented many major reforms in education. From 2003 onward the government began the implementation of the 12-session "life education" classes in primary schools in order to enhance students' self-knowledge, self-care, and interpersonal skills. The 12-session course covered topics on self-understanding, managing self, relating to others and planning for the future. Schools have the option to incorporate sex education content into life education, from teachers' classes, religious education lessons, or biology lessons. Nongovernment organizations like the Family Planning Association and the Society for Truth and Light offered support to primary and secondary teachers. However, results from research found that the level of sex education in Hong Kong was not satisfactory. Ying Ho and Tsang (2002) found discourses on sexuality to be under vigilant surveillance in high schools, even within the context of sex education courses. Others (Ng 1998; Wong 2000) observed that sex education in Hong Kong's high schools was just an attempt to control sexual expression. Although the Hong Kong Education Department has advised for many years that primary and secondary schools were to include sex education in their curricula, programs were seldom implemented by schools or at best as extracurricular activities (Ip et al. 2001). Indeed, each school has the freedom to choose if and how to implement sex education and who will deliver the courses. Most of the schools claim that some form of sex education is given, but not all actually do so (Fok 2005). In 1993, research found that half of school principals were not aware of the AIDS prevention programs offered in their schools (Lau and Lee 1993). The same research also found that only 60 % of schools made use of the teaching kits they received. Interestingly, most resistance to sex education is from adults, not pupils. For example, some teachers were found to be too embarrassed to teach sex education; in contrast, students reported that the current level of sex education is inadequate and that they would require more information and opportunities to learn (Lau and Lee 1993; Fok 2005). In most cases teachers complained that they first did not receive adequate training in sex education (which is also one of the main reasons why sex education units were included in PATHS). However, there is consensus among different observers that young students demand more sex education in schools, as they have little chance to receive information within the family, which leads them in most cases to refer to the Internet only, with all the consequences that this may bring. A survey commissioned by the Education Department (Lam 1997a) showed that among the 4,087 pupils who responded to the questionnaire, 61.2 % of them thought that sex education was necessary and a further 28.1 % thought that it was absolutely necessary. Regarding the appropriate persons or institutes to conduct sex education, 61.1 % of the secondary school pupils favored guidance from teachers and social workers.

The Education Bureau has recently issued some guidelines on the production of learning and teaching resources on sex education. Great emphasis is given to the transmission of moral and civic values. Precisely, it is stated that "Topics and objectives of the learning and teaching material should be designed to help students cultivate the priority values recommended by the Education Bureau, in addition to other relevant positive values and attitudes, and to achieve the expected learning outcomes relating to sex education under the Revised Moral and Civic Education Curriculum Framework (2008)." Furthermore, it is specified that areas to be covered by learning and teaching material are (compulsory areas) "(i) Media literacy and sex education, (ii) Life-skills-based education on prevention of sexual transmitted disease and AIDS, (iii) Gender equality, (iv) Sexual minority and (v) Family and love." In addition, other areas of sex education and new topics can be introduced to help students cope with the rapid changes of society.

Peculiarities of Hong Kong

Compared to the opposite cases of Holland and the USA, it can be said that Hong Kong lies in the middle. It can be said that for Hong Kong, there seems to be endless debate about whether the priority should be moral education (enhancing individual awareness of moral issues) or civic/democratic education (one's rights and responsibilities as citizens of the community) at this moment in time. Likely, this is related to the particular structure of Hong Kong society. Generally speaking, in the Chinese context, the development of self is seen by scholars (Tu 1985) to start with the development of the virtues of a person, extending to the family and then taking up responsibilities for the country. Emphasis has been placed on young people achieving prescribed roles to fulfill conventional expectations from elders.

Part of the struggle for the developing young person is how to balance the rights and responsibilities for self and others. Then, at a later stage, one must also struggle to balance the concern for the needs of oneself as compared to the needs and priorities of one's family and neighbors and the needs of the community or nation as a whole (Fig. 1).

The figure represents an overall view of defining how citizenship is seen to be reflective of the approach adopted by the Curriculum Development Council of the Hong Kong Government:

> Some societies place stronger emphasis on individualism, while others collectivism. However, the two are not necessarily dichotomized and mutually exclusive...In societies where individualism is more obviously valued, the significance of common interests, common will and common good is also valued. Likewise, in societies where collectivism seems to be dominant, there are various extents of respect for individuality, and self-realization. In the Chinese tradition, even though collectivism has been a dominant social value, self has been seen as the starting point of civic values. (Curriculum Development Council 1996, p. 15)

The government has tried to demonstrate its efforts to address the importance of citizenship education as one of the major goals of the education reforms beginning

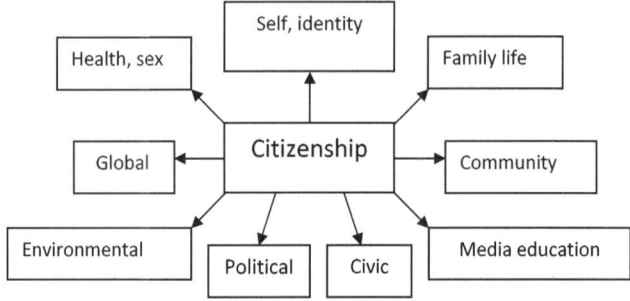

Fig. 1 Citizenship: balancing rights and responsibilities for self and others

even before the change of sovereignty of 1997 in the area of "moral and civic education." The name "personal, social, humanity education" is used to provide direction for this broad area which is also used as a cross curricula theme in both secondary schools and primary schools.

Case Study

A very popular course for all students, named "Sex, Love, and Relationships," of a local university may shed further light on this important topic. The curriculum is based on psychology, science, and evolution, and the teachers are either psychologists or social workers. The course emphasizes research using the scientific methods (using observation, asking questions, collecting data, carrying out experiments, analyzing the results, and drawing conclusions). Besides lectures, students are asked to study in small groups and make presentations on a topic of their choice to the class and complete a written report. Below is the schedule of content:

- Love, friendship, affection defined
- What factors bring about attraction (socialization processes and gender roles)
- Finding a mate (long-term, short-term) for males and females
- How culture, traditions, trends affect our views on sex and love
- Sex and sexuality, including homosexuality
- Infidelity and jealousy
- Ending relationships

Since there is adequate classroom time, the teacher can introduce concepts on Piaget's cognitive development stages as well as Kohlberg's moral development stages for the students' reference, in addition to evolution theory and the scientific point of view. The added material challenges the students to think about their own growth in reasoning, emotion, and moral development. The class can also be presented with how cultures and various religions look at sex and intimate relationships, in addition to the Asian or Chinese view on the subject. Use of role-play and video clips is useful to bring the concepts "closer to home."

Besides covering the concepts, teachers can select some controversial topics or practical topics to help students as they face important matters related to sex and intimacy. For example, socialization processes can be described as lively portrayal – how to dress themselves to attract the attention of the opposite sex, how boys try to protect their companions, or how to practice skills to deal with rivals, the process of socialization in gender roles in society, and the common labels. Other more challenging content includes how to recognize and deal with "sexual impulses," how to respect and consider the needs of partners in intimate moments, and how girls can politely "say no" to sexual advances or requests. In these sessions, the discussion could be brought to touch on the skills aspect as well as attitudes toward sex.

Teachers could use various methods to cover the curriculum in a lively and realistic manner, and group discussions could be offered two to three times in class, so that students have the opportunity to freely reflect on the concepts, carry out discussions, and share the group's conclusion. Use of short films, music and lyrics, role-playing, and other methods is helpful to bring out some themes. The use of small groups allows students to carry out such experiences as trust walk and trust fall, as they explore the importance of intimacy and friendship. Willingness to share the findings of a group allows students to maintain their privacy, avoiding embarrassment yet allowing them to hear the views of their classmates.

Use of actual life events allows students to explore emotions, intellect, and values related to sex and relationships. Attitudes of teachers to deal with these issues, the level of comfort, and proficiency demonstrated will have an effect on students. Familiarity and comfort with the subject matters require practice and hard work in preparation.

Students' requests bring about a sharing of decision-making skills toward the end of the course. Practical steps on making decisions are outlined to students to support their struggles in making decisions. Steps include: pondering short-term and long-term consequences before taking the step, balancing the need for emotional and rational aspects, and finally thinking about others and the community before finalizing their choice.

Guiding Principles for the Construction of the Curriculum of a School-Based Prevention Program

Youth should not be considered mainly as being at a problematic age of turmoil. Instead, adolescence is a very valuable resource, a critical period of life, and a phase full of potential (Anthony 2011). Adolescence is a positive age of life characterized by rapid physical growth and development, and adolescents should be given the opportunity to experiment with different methods of coping and explore their needs. Indeed, a course on sexual education in secondary schools should be inspired by the principles of positive psychology, grounded on recognizing strengths rather than focusing on concepts like normality/pathology (Shek and Ma 2006; Shek et al. 2007).

After this literature review, it can be said that in Hong Kong there is no specific concern related to youth sex behavior, such as HIV/AIDS or early childbearing as in other parts of the world. Furthermore, research has shown that it is not productive to focus on one isolated type of behavior without addressing a broader set of adolescent sexual and health concerns. Lastly, an effective program should aim at enhancing protective factors of young people and not simply try to reduce the risk factors.

Protective and Risk Factors for Youth Sexual Behavior

Protective and risk factors are defined as factors that can both directly influence behavior and moderate the relationship between risk and behavior (Jessor et al. 1995). A school-based program that aims to be effective should be able to tackle some risk factors. Factors that may increase an adolescent's odds of early sexual debut and risky sexual behavior are easily available pornography, money attraction, low self-esteem, sexually active peers, adolescents' serious delinquency, drug and alcohol use, school truancy or problems, low monthly family income, low levels of maternal education, being born to a teenage mother, and poor neighborhood quality (for a systematic review, see Buhi and Goodson 2007). In a study on a large sample of 26,023 American students in grades 7–12 (13–18 years old), lower levels of sexual activity were associated with: dual-parent families, higher socioeconomic status (SES), better school performance, greater religiosity, absence of suicidal thoughts, feeling that adults or parents cared, and high parental expectations. Furthermore, variables significantly associated with delayed onset of sexual activity for both males and females included: dual-parent families, higher socioeconomic status, residing in rural areas, higher school performance, concerns about the community, and higher religiosity. On the contrary, high levels of body pride were associated with higher levels of sexual activity for all age and gender groups. Other risk factors included: emotional status (males), higher suicide risk, smoking, moderate/high drug use (marijuana), and moderate/high alcohol use (Lammers et al. 2000).

However, only a few risk factors might be addressed in the context of a school-based program (factors such as socioeconomic status, parenting style, or demographics are variables that cannot be influenced); in addition, existing problems of drug or alcohol abuse should be addressed in different contexts than in in-class activities, as they might require therapeutic settings and different kinds of interventions. Ideally, the elective goal of a school-based program should be prevention. Thus, an effective and comprehensive program should focus on developing and reinforcing protective factors, rather than assessing disorders and treating problematic youth.

Knowledge can be a protective factor, whereas a lack of adequate sex-related knowledge can be a risk factor for sexual behavior. In Hong Kong, many youths lack appropriate sexual knowledge (Fok 2005). Providing sex-related knowledge to youth may be the cornerstone of a sex education course.

Connectedness, defined as adolescents' belief that adults care about them as individuals, has been found to be a very salient protective factor for adolescent health and well-being (Resnick et al. 1993). Other studies also confirmed that emotional health and connectedness with friends and adults in the community, including school, church, and police personnel, were protective factors for male adolescents against sexually aggressive behavior, and academic achievement was a protective factor for female adolescents (Borowsky et al. 1997). Resnick and colleagues (1997) found that connectedness to family and parental disapproval of intercourse and contraception, greater religiosity, better grades, having taken a virginal pledge, and a slower than average pubertal tempo were all associated with delay of sexual intercourse.

Self-efficacy, which refers to one's confidence in being able to carry out specific behavior (e.g., resist sexual advances and negotiate condom use with a partner; see, e.g., To et al. 2013), was found to be associated with a range of health behavior, including actions to prevent HIV transmission in a survey among 1,720 Texas ninth graders (Basen-Engquist and Parcel 1992).

Results from analyses conducted on data from 491 predominantly African-American adolescents (61 % of whom were boys) show that educational goals, self-concept, future time perspective, orientation to health, self-efficacy, outcome expectations, parental involvement/support, communication, values, prosocial activities, and peer values are protective factors for sexual behavior among adolescents (DiLorio et al. 2004).

Several studies reported that sexually inactive adolescent boys are more interested in school, have higher academic success, and have greater educational expectations than sexually active adolescent boys and girls (for a review see Lohman and Billings 2008).

Conceptual Framework for a Prevention Program

According to the ecological perspective the course should:

- Affirm a positive self and a positive approach to sexuality
- Be participatory and interactive in nature
- Not be fear based or prescriptive
- Make use of life-skills-based education
- Be comprehensive regarding sexuality in broad terms
- Be culturally sensitive and tailor-made for the reality of Hong Kong
- Be oriented to promote strengths and personal thinking rather than being normative
- Support students to articulate their issues, express their curiosity, and learn about their rights and responsibilities

As can be seen in Fig. 2, on one hand a prevention program is expected to: (a) lower the risk factors that affect adolescents (easily available pornography, money

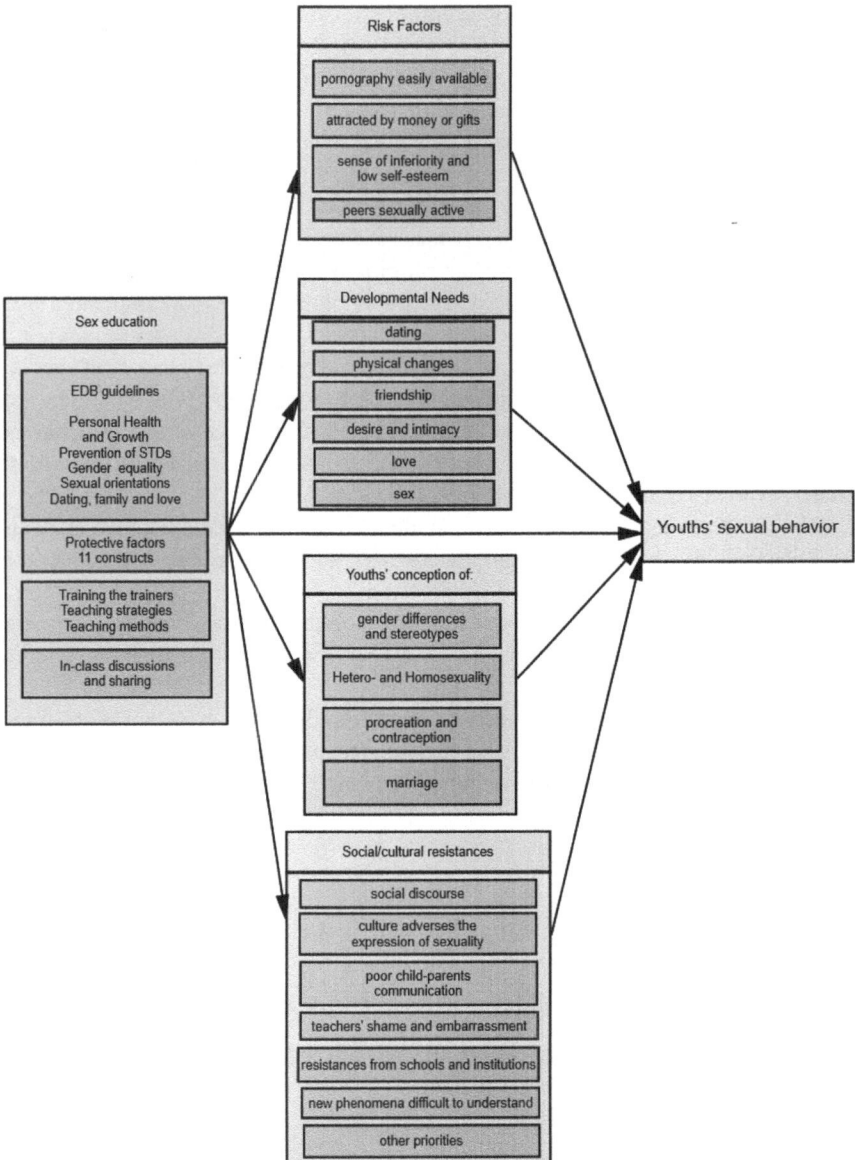

Fig. 2 Conceptual framework

attraction, low self-esteem, sexually active peers); (b) help students to better under-stand their developmental needs from proper perspectives (dating, physical changes, friendship, desire and intimacy, love, sex); (c) help students to reflect on their implicit conception of gender differences and stereotypes, heterosexuality and homosexuality, procreation and contraception, and marriage; (d) enhance students' social/relational/cognitive/emotional skills and help them to develop a positive attitude toward sex-related issues; (e) understand the sociocultural/cultural resistances that affect the various actors and institutions around the youth (social discourse, cultural resistance, poor child–parent communication, teachers' shame and embarrassment, resistance from schools and institutions, new phenomena difficult to understand like compensated dating, different priorities than sex education); and (f) possibly weaken such resistance by giving teachers and schools new training opportunities and tools.

On the other hand, the course should aim at strengthening the protective factors highlighted by the literature thanks to the PYD constructs. Then, the course is expected to have direct influence on the sexual (and nonsexual) development of youth. A prevention program implicitly assumes that youth have resources that can be strengthened; from this perspective, enhancing protective factors is even more important than weakening risk factors. Enhancing protective factors is more from a perspective of growth, whereas risk factors are likely more related to the contingent and the past; as such, simply tackling the risk factors cannot guarantee proper development. Then, the Positive Youth Development embraces a more comprehensive perspective of growth, in which pupils not only learn how to face current changes but also acquire skills for facing future challenges.

References

Acharya, D. R., Bhattaria, R., Poobalan, A. S., van Teijlingen, E., & Chapman, G. N. (2010). Factors associated with teenage pregnancy in South Asia: A systematic review. *Health Science Journal, 4*(1), 3–14.

Anthony, D. (2011). *The state of the world's children 2011 – adolescence: An age of opportunity.* New York: United Nations Publications.

Basen-Engquist, K., & Parcel, G. S. (1992). Attitudes, norms, and self-efficacy: A model of adolescents' HIV-related sexual risk behavior. *Health Education Quarterly, 19*(2), 263–277.

Borowsky, I. W., Hogan, M., & Ireland, M. (1997). Adolescent sexual aggression: Risk and protective factors. *Pediatrics, 100*, 1–8.

Boys' & Girls' Clubs Association of Hong Kong [BGCA]. (1996). *A research report on family roles — youth sex attitudes and behaviour.* Hong Kong: Boys' & Girls' Clubs Association of Hong Kong [BGCA].

Brotto, L. A., Chik, H. M., Ryder, A. G., Gorzalka, B. B., & Seal, B. N. (2005). Acculturation and sexual function in Asian women. *Archives of Sexual Behavior, 34*(6), 613–626.

Buhi, E. R., & Goodson, P. (2007). Predictors of adolescent sexual behavior and intention: A theory-guided systematic review. *Journal of Adolescent Health, 40*(1), 4–21.

Cao, C. S., Wang, Y. G., & Weng, R. J. (2000). Reproductive health investigation on 788 unmarried women. *Chinese Journal of Maternal and Child Health, 15*, 628–629.

Constantine, N. A., Jerman, P., & Huang, A. X. (2007). California parents' preferences and beliefs regarding school-based sex education policy. *Perspectives on Sexual and Reproductive Health, 39*(3), 167–175.

Curriculum Development Council. (1996). *Guidelines on civic education in schools.* Hong Kong: Curriculum Development Council, Education Department.

Curriculum Development Council. (1998). *Sex education key learning areas guide and stages of learning expectations.* Hong Kong: Curriculum Development Council, Education Bureau.

DiLorio, C., Dudley, W. N., Soet, J. E., & McCarty, F. (2004). Sexual possibility situations and sexual behaviors among young adolescents: The moderating role of protective factors. *Journal of Adolescent Health, 35*(6), 11–20.

Eaton, D. K., Kann, L., Kinchen, S., Shanklin, S., Flint, K. H., Hawkins, J., Harris, W. A., Lowry, R., McManus, T., Chyen, D., Whittle, L., Lim, C., & Wechsler, H. (2012). Youth risk behavior surveillance-United States, 2011. *Morbidity and Mortality Weekly Report. Surveillance Summaries, 61*(4), 1–162.

Family Planning Association of Hong Kong. (2012). *Youth sexuality study 2011: Secondary school survey*. (In Chinese) [Electronic version]. Retrieved from http://www.famplan.org.hk/fpahk/zh/press/press/20120619-press-chi.ppt

Fok, C. S. (2005). A study of the implementation of sex education in Hong Kong secondary schools. *Sex Education, 5*(3), 281–294.

Fok, S. C., & Tung, E. L. (2000). Reflection over the guidelines on sex education. In Y. C. Cheng, K. W. Chow, & K. T. Tsui (Eds.), *School curriculum change and development in Hong Kong*. Hong Kong: The Hong Kong Institute of Education.

Gao, Y., Lu, Z. Z., Shi, R., Sun, X. Y., & Cai, Y. (2001). AIDS and sex education for young people in China. *Reproductive Fertility Development, 13*, 729–737.

Ho, W. C. (2006). Popular culture in mainland Chinese education. *International Education Journal, 7*(3), 348–363.

Hong Kong Family Planning Association. (1991). *Youth sexuality study, in-school youth*. Hong Kong: Hong Kong Family Planning Association.

Hong Kong Federation of Youth Groups. (1995). *Teenage pregnancy*. Hong Kong: Hong Kong Federation of Youth Groups.

Hu, X. G. (1996). The study of STDs among 429 unmarried adolescents. *Chinese Journal of Prevention and Therapy of STDs/AIDS, 2*, 206–207.

Ip, W. Y., Chau, J. P., Chang, A. M., & Lui, M. H. (2001). Knowledge of and attitudes toward sex among Chinese adolescents. *Western Journal of Nursing Research, 23*(2), 211–222.

Jessor, R., Van Den Bos, J., Vanderryn, J., Costa, F. M., & Turbin, M. S. (1995). Protective factors in adolescent problem behavior: Moderator effects and developmental change. *Developmental Psychopathology, 31*, 923–933.

Kawahara, Y. (2000). Diverse strategies in classroom instruction: Sex education in secondary Japanese school. *Japanese Studies, 20*, 295–311.

Lam, M. P. (1997a). *A study on the knowledge, attitude and behaviours of secondary pupils relating to sex*. Hong Kong: The Education Department.

Lam, T. H. (1997b). *A research report on youth, proceeding of seminar on youth sex*. Hong Kong: The Hong Kong Family Association.

Lammers, C., Ireland, J., Resnick, M., & Blum, R. (2000). Influences on adolescents' decision to postpone onset of sexual intercourse: A survival analysis of virginity among youths aged 13 to 18 years. *Journal of Adolescent Health, 26*(1), 42–48.

Lau, J., & Lee, S. S. (1993). *Evaluation of AIDS educational programs for secondary schools in Hong Kong*. Paper presented at Yokohama conference on AIDS. Yokohama, Japan

Lee, A., & Tsang, C. K. K. (2004). Youth risk behaviour in a Chinese population: A territory-wide youth risk behavioural surveillance in Hong Kong. *Public Health, 118*(2), 88–95.

Lewis, J., & Knijn, T. (2002). The politics of sex education policy in England and Wales and the Netherlands since the 1980s. *Journal of Social Policy, 31*, 669–694.

Li, Z. P. (2000). Investigation on adolescent sex-related issues in Guangzhou. *Chinese Journal of School Health, 21*, 105.

Li, Y., Cottrell, R. R., Wagner, D. I., & Ban, M. (2004). Needs and preferences regarding sex education among Chinese college students: A preliminary study. *International Family Planning Perspectives, 30*(3), 128–133.

Lindberg, L. D., Santelli, J. S., & Singh, S. (2006). Changes in formal sex education: 1995–2002. *Perspectives on Sexual and Reproductive Health, 38*(4), 182–189.

Lohman, B. J., & Billings, A. (2008). Protective and risk factors associated with adolescent boys' early sexual debut and risky sexual behaviors. *Journal of Youth and Adolescence, 37*, 723–735.

Lou, C. H., Peng, M. G., & Tu, X. W. (2002). Premarital contraceptive use and its influencing factors. *Journal of Reproduction and Contraception, 22*, 226–230.

Ng, M. L. (1998). School and public sexuality education in Hong Kong. *Journal of Asian Sexology, 1*, 32–35.

Ng, M. L., & Ma, J. L. C. (2001). Hong Kong. In R. T. Francoeur (Ed.), *The international encyclopedia of sexuality* (Vol. 4). New York: Continuum.

Resnick, M. D., Harris, L. J., & Blum, R. W. (1993). The impact of caring and connectedness on adolescent health and well-being. *Journal of Paediatrics and Child Health, 29*(1), S3–S9.

Resnick, M. D., Bearman, P. S., Blum, R. W., Bauman, K. E., Harris, K. M., Jones, J., Tabor, J., Beuhring, T., Sieving, R. E., Shew, M., Ireland, M., Bearinger, L. H., & Udry, J. R. (1997). Protecting adolescents from harm. Findings from the National Longitudinal Study on Adolescent Health. *Journal of the American Medical Association, 278*, 823–832.

Ruan, F. F. (1991). *Sex in China: Studies in sexology in Chinese culture*. New York: Plenum.

Santelli, J., Ott, M. A., Lyon, M., Rogers, J., Summers, D., & Schleifer, R. (2006). Abstinence and abstinence-only education: A review of US policies and programs. *Journal of Adolescent Health, 38*(1), 72–81.

Schaalma, H. P., Abraham, C., Gillmore, M. R., & Kok, G. (2004). Sex education as health promotion: What does it take? *Archives of Sexual Behavior, 33*(3), 259–269.

Shek, D. T. L., & Ma, H. K. (2006). Design of a positive youth development program in Hong Kong. *International Journal of Adolescent Medicine and Health, 18*(3), 315–327.

Shek, D. T. L., Ma, H. K., & Merrick, J. (Eds.). (2007). *Positive youth development: Development of a pioneering program in a Chinese context*. London: Freund Publishing House.

To, S. M., Tam, H. L., & Chu, F. (2013). A qualitative study of the lived experiences of young Chinese females in condom use negotiations. *International Journal of Adolescence and Youth, 18*(4), 248–262.

Tsang, A. K. T. (1987). Sexuality: The Chinese and the Judeo-Christian traditions in Hong Kong. *Bulletin of the Hong Kong Psychological Society, 19*(20), 19–28.

Tu, W. M. (1985). *Confucian thought: Selfhood as creative transformation*. Albany: State University of New York Press.

Tu, X. W., Yuan, W., & Lou, C. H. (1998a). Women's first premarital sexual behavior in Shanghai. *China Public Health, 14*, 637–639.

Tu, X., Lou, C., Tao, J., & Gao, E. (1998b). The status of premarital pregnancy and its influencing factors among the tested women in Shanghai. *Medicine and Society, 11*, 8–11.

Wang, B., Lou, C. H., & Shen, Y. (2002). Sexual behavior and contraceptive use among unmarried youths in suburban Shanghai. *Journal of Reproduction and Contraception, 22*, 99–106.

Wang, B., Hertog, S., Meier, A., Lou, C., & Gao, E. (2005). The potential of comprehensive sex education in China: Findings from suburban Shanghai. *International Family Planning Perspectives, 31*, 63–72.

Weaver, H., Smith, G., & Kippax, S. (2005). School-based sex education policies and indicators of sexual health among young people: A comparison of the Netherlands, France, Australia and the United States. *Sex Education, 5*(2), 171–188.

Wong, V. (2000). A never-ending obsession with breasts. In V. Wong, W. Shiu, & H. Har (Eds.), *From lives to critique*. Hong Kong: Hong Kong Policy Viewers (In Chinese).

Wong, W., Lee, A., Tsang, K., & Lynn, H. (2006). The impact of AIDS/sex education by schools or family doctors on Hong Kong Chinese adolescents. *Psychology, Health & Medicine, 11*(1), 108–116.

Ying Ho, P. S., & Tsang, A. K. T. (2002). The things girls shouldn't see: Relocating the penis in sex education in Hong Kong. *Sex Education: Sexuality, Society and Learning, 2*(1), 61–73.

Zhang, K., Li, D., Li, H., & Beck, E. J. (1999). Changing sexual attitudes and behaviors in China: Implications for the spread of HIV and other sexually transmitted diseases. *AIDS Care, 11*(5), 581–589.

Zhang, L., Li, X., Shah, I. H., Baldwin, W., & Stanton, B. (2007). Parent-adolescent sex communication in China. *European Journal of Contraception and Reproductive Healthcare, 12*(2), 138–147.

Zheng, Z., Zhou, Y., Zheng, L., Yang, Y., Zhao, D., Lou, C., & Zhao, S. (2001). Sexual behaviour and contraceptive use among unmarried young women migrant workers in five cities in China. *Reproductive Health Matters, 9*(17), 118–127.

Preventing and Combating School Bullying: A Conceptual Review

Sandra K.M. Tsang and Eadaoin K. Hui

Abstract School bullying has become a spreading and explicit problem in Hong Kong schools and is an issue of growing concern for parents, teachers, and educators. It is one of the top three types of misbehavior in students, with increasing frequency and severity. Bullying refers to intentional, oppressive behavior against another person that causes physical and/or psychological harm. Research studies have shown that school bullying has detrimental effects on victims, bullies, and even bystanders, affecting their academic, social, emotional, mental, and psychological functioning as well as physical health. A number of variables have been found to correlate with victim and bullying behavior and will be presented. Finally, different bullying intervention approaches will be critically examined. Specifically, focus will be on (1) remedial, preventive, and developmental guidance; (2) interventions at individual student level, classroom level, and whole-school level; and (3) peer-led intervention.

Introduction

School bullying has become a spreading and explicit problem in Hong Kong schools and is an issue of growing concern for parents, teachers, and educators. It is one of the top three types of misbehavior in students, with increasing frequency and severity (Lam and Liu 2007; Ng and Tsang 2008; Wong 2004). However, most of the

The preparation for this work and the Project P.A.T.H.S. were financially supported by The Hong Kong Jockey Club Charities Trust. This paper is based on two articles originally published by The Scientific World Journal Hui et al. (2011): Combating school bullying through developmental guidance for positive youth development and promoting harmonious school culture. *The Scientific World Journal*, *11*, 2266–2277. Tsang et al. (2011). Bystander position taking in school bullying: the role of positive identity, self-efficacy, and self-determination. *The Scientific World Journal*, *11*, 2278–2286.

S.K.M. Tsang (✉)
Department of Social Work and Social Administration, The University of Hong Kong, Pok Fu Lam, Hong Kong, China
e-mail: sandratsang@hku.hk

E.K. Hui
Faculty of Education, The University of Hong Kong, Pok Fu Lam, Hong Kong, China

© Springer Science+Business Media Singapore 2015   47
T.Y. Lee et al. (eds.), *Student Well-Being in Chinese Adolescents in Hong Kong*,
Quality of Life in Asia 7, DOI 10.1007/978-981-287-582-2_4

programs and guidelines dealing with the problem have been highly remedial and reactive in nature (Olweus 1993). The present chapter discusses a more proactive approach to bullying prevention and intervention. Project P.A.T.H.S. is an example of a classroom guidance initiative that uses the positive youth development (PYD) paradigm as a way of combating school bullying. Delivered as a developmental guidance curriculum to all students, the program aims to strengthen young people's skills and competencies in interpersonal relationships and to cultivate a harmonious, nonviolent school culture.

What Is Bullying and Why It Matters

Following the definition of Olweus (1993), bullying refers to intentional, oppressive behavior against another person that causes physical and/or psychological harm. It is abusive behavior which is typically repeated over time; that is, such behavior is not a one-time occurrence. Bullying behavior is usually classified into one of four categories: (1) physical bullying refers to overt physical aggression such as hitting, pushing, kicking, spitting, and punching; (2) verbal bullying refers to overt verbal aggression such as name calling, teasing, insulting, and threatening speech; (3) social exclusion behavior aims to hurt victims by damaging their peer relationships or social standing. Such behavior includes ignoring the presence of the victims, spreading hurtful rumors, excluding the victims from a friendship group, or warning others not to play with the victims; and (4) extortion includes asking for money or others' property (Egan and Todorov 2009; Wong et al. 2008). Often, a real or perceived imbalance of power persists between the bullies and their victims (Olweus 1993; Rigby 2007). For example, the child bullies who are older have greater physical strength and are more socially or verbally adept than their victims. Also, bullies are more psychologically manipulative or have a higher social standing than their victims (Bauman and Hurley 2005; Egan and Todorov 2009).

Bullying in Hong Kong

In Hong Kong, recent studies and surveys have indicated the rising trend of bullying among youth (Hong Kong Family Welfare Society 2012; Hong Kong Playground and União Geral das Associações dos Moradores de Macau 2008; Ma 2005a, b; Wong 2004; Wurf 2010). The study on bullying behavior conducted by the Hong Kong Playground Association in 2008 showed that over 90 % of the respondents aged between 6 and 24 years had witnessed bullying events within the last 3 months. Over 50 % of the respondents reported having been spectators to three or more different counts of bullying. Furthermore, the report showed that the most common feeling of bullies after bullying is regret (32.2 %), followed by happiness (24.3 %), while findings have also suggested that their aggressive behavior may be reinforced by peer pressure.

It was found that conflicts and bullying behavior is more likely to occur among Primary 4 to Secondary 3 students (Hong Kong Family Welfare Society 2012). Among primary schoolchildren, 87 % reported witnessing verbal bullying in the past 6 months, with 30 % of them having seen it more than 10 times. Also, 68 % of the respondents had experienced physical bullying in the past half year, with 14 % experiencing it more than 10 times (Wong et al. 2008). Bullying continues to be commonplace as students enter secondary schools: according to a study on secondary school teachers' and students' perceptions of bullying, more than 50 % of the respondents had been involved in bullying, as bullies, victims, or bystanders (Wong 2004). In light of the proliferation of social media, many have also begun taking their aggressive behavior online. In a study on cyberbullying, 22 % of the respondents admitted to bullying others in cyberspace, 30 % of the respondents had been bullied, and nearly 60 % had witnessed cyberbullying in the past year (The Hong Kong Federation of Youth Groups 2010). This worrying trend demands immediate work on effective strategies for the amelioration and prevention of school bullying.

Consequences of Bullying and Characteristics of Those Involved

Research studies have shown that school bullying has detrimental effects on victims, bullies, and even bystanders, affecting their academic, social, emotional, mental, and psychological functioning as well as physical health. Problems arising from bullying may persist into adulthood (Cheng et al. 2010; Davis and Davis 2007; Ng and Tsang 2008; Rigby 2003, 2007).

Victims

Victims can be identified as passive (who seldom resist the bullies and will not react aggressively to the bullies) and reactive (who will normally react and attempt to get revenge). While the former type tends to be more anxious, less dominating, and less assertive, the latter tends to be emotional and have bad temperaments (Shek et al. 2011). Regardless of type, bullying produces significant and persistent effects on victims' emotional, mental, psychological, physical, social, and academic functioning (Kohut 2007; Ng and Tsang 2008; Olweus 1993; Rigby 1999). Oftentimes, students lack the skills and strategies to deal with incidents of bullying. Those who are bullied during childhood are more likely than non-victims to report depression, trait anxiety, social anxiety (Roth et al. 2002), social phobia (McCabe et al. 2003), as well as low self-esteem, loneliness, and relationship dysfunction (Schäfer et al. 2004). They show more sleeping problems, headaches, stomach aches, bed-wetting, and depression (Salmon et al. 1998; Williams et al. 1996) and have more frequent suicidal thoughts (Cleary 2000). In addition, these victims often develop intense anger and anxiety and suffer low self-esteem or depression (Fung and Wong 2007; Ng and Tsang 2008).

Bullies

According to Shek and his colleagues (2011), the main characteristics of typical bullies are (1) being less able to empathize with their victims; (2) tend to be impulsive, hyperactive, and often overreact to other's behavior and they have a need to dominate others; (3) believe in the effectiveness of aggression; (4) usually experience negative peer relations and negative teacher relations; (5) tend to have low academic achievement in school; and (6) usually come from a negative family social environment – a family that is less cohesive and less warm and often has a lot of conflicts among family members. Perpetrators of bullying are at risk of becoming increasingly short of compassion and concern for others. They are eventually desensitized to bullying, which then becomes part of their normal life (Wong 2002). They may indulge in the satisfaction from behaving aggressively instead of academic pursuits and thus are more likely to drop out of school and be involved in gangs, delinquent activities, and antisocial behavior (Davis and Davis 2007; Rigby 2007). They may have increased difficulty in maintaining healthy intimate interpersonal relationships and become abusive spouses and parents (Wong et al. 2008). Over the long term, they are at increased risk of depression and suicide (Kaltiala-Heino et al. 1999).

It is unclear whether anxiety and depression problems lead to higher rates of bullying or whether they are consequences of it. A number of studies confirm both possibilities (Boivin et al. 1995; Bond et al. 2001; Hodges et al. 1997; Hodges and Perry 1999; Schwartz et al. 1993, 1999). On one hand, some may misdirect their anger and other psychological issues and in turn become bullies (Lam and Liu 2007). On the other, it may have been the act of bullying that leads to psychological maladjustment. Studies have found active bullying to be associated with higher levels of depression and emotional and behavioral disorders (Rigby 1998; van der Wal et al. 2003).

Bystanders

Bystanders, too, are impacted. Students who have observed bullying report feeling helpless, uneasy, and distressed. They often harbor guilt for not having helped the victim, anger toward themselves and the bully, and fear of becoming targets themselves (Kohut 2007; Whitted and Dupper 2005). They may also feel insecure at school and become inattentive in class as their attention is directed toward the avoidance of bullying (Kohut 2007). These effects can also carry over into adulthood, leading to an inability to solve problems assertively, distorted views of personal responsibility, desensitization toward antisocial acts, and diffusion of boundaries on acceptable behavior (Kohut 2007).

Risk and Protective Factors

A number of variables have been found to correlate with victim and bullying behavior (for a review, see Hong and Espelage 2012). These variables shape the individuals at various levels. For instance, students' psychosocial functioning and their accessibility to violent values are found to be related to school bullying (Bosworth et al. 1999; Espelage et al. 2003; Lee 2011; Rigby 2007; Wong et al. 2008). Students, who have unstable emotions, unsatisfactory school performance, and poor relationships with their family members, teachers, and peers, are more likely to be victimized (Wong et al. 2008). Those who are exposed to violent values, such as growing up in an aggressive background (Baldry 2003; Lee 2011), having frequent contact with deviant peers (Haynie et al. 2001), and being exposed to violence messages through the media (Kuntsche et al. 2006; Zimmerman et al. 2005), are more likely to engage in disturbed violent behavior, either as passive victims or as ruthless bullies.

In the past, literature generally showed that boys are more likely to engage in bullying than girls (Espelage et al. 2000; Nansel et al. 2001; Rigby 1998). However, more recent research pointed out that gender may not necessarily be a significant predictor for bullying behavior (Espelage et al. 2004). Bullying occurs more frequently among gay, lesbian, bisexual, and transgender individuals (Clarke et al. 2004; Rivers 2004; van Wormer and McKinney 2003). Obese adolescents in British schools were found to be significantly more likely to be both victims and perpetrators of bullying, while obese girls had a high propensity to become victims (Griffith et al. 2005). Youth with learning and developmental disabilities are at risk of being targeted (Baumeister et al. 2008; Saylor and Leach 2009). Likewise, academically high-achieving students are at an elevated risk of experiencing social exclusion from their peers (Woods and Wolke 2004). Bullying victimization has been found to correlate with lack of parental support (Holt and Espelage 2007), negative family interactions (Duncan 2004), and interparental violence at home (Baldry 2003).

Bullying behavior is greatly influenced by the social context as well (Espelage and Swearer 2003). Because bullying is a group process, peer acceptance, popularity, quality of friendship, and social support are all important factors against peer victimization (Espelage 2002; Hong and Espelage 2012). Likewise, a sense of connectedness and belonging to school can reduce the risk of aggression (Brookmeyer et al. 2006). Teachers' involvement in students' social lives may improve the perception of the school environment, help students feel more safe at school (Hong and Eamon 2011), and influence students' relationships with their peers (Lee 2009). Students are at a greater risk of engaging in bullying acts if there are often conflicts in their school or low morale among students and teachers. On the contrary, schools with a positive climate have less bullying-related problems, and students are more likely to engage in altruistic behavior (James et al. 2008; Lee 2011; Orpinas and Horne 2006; Smith et al. 2003; Whitted and Dupper 2005). These research findings point to the significance of promoting a harmonious school culture as a means of preventing school bullying.

Bullying Intervention Approaches

Since the turn of the century, school bullying has attracted extensive research interests in Hong Kong (Fung et al. 2007, 2009; Law and Fung 2013). Paralleling this is the development of a number of programs for bullies and victims (Chang et al. 2004; Field 2007; Fung and Wong 2007; Hong Kong Children and Youth Services 2002; Wong 2003). In school guidance, there have been three major approaches to dealing with student problems, including school bullying, namely, remedial, preventive, and developmental guidance (Chang et al. 2004).

Remedial guidance focuses on offering interventions and therapies to students experiencing emotional, psychological, or behavioral difficulties. In the case of school bullying, a remedial guidance approach focuses on the individual student level, victims, as well as bullies. Such an approach is a responsive and curative one. On the other hand, preventive guidance takes on a proactive approach, which stresses anticipation of problems like bullying, enhancing students' awareness of bullying and victimization, as well as their skills and strategies to handle bullying. Finally, developmental guidance is a positive approach to facilitate students' whole person development, including their personal, social, and moral self-formation. Developmental guidance addresses issues such as self-knowledge, self-responsibility, interpersonal relationships, and bonding. These are delivered through a guidance curriculum at classroom level and in school-wide programs. Through education on the need for respect for self and for others, tolerance of individual differences, self-determination, and responsible decision-making, students will attain positive self- and interpersonal development. Among these three approaches, developmental guidance contributes the most to the holistic development of students and is considered one of the most effective measures in promoting students' healthy development and preventing juvenile delinquency. Developmental guidance has been the guidance approach and focus of schools in Hong Kong and elsewhere (Field 2007; Hui et al. 2011).

School bullying is a systemic and complex process of social interactions that involves bullies, victims, peers, adults, parents, school, as well as home environments (Fekkes et al. 2005; Hong Kong Children and Youth Services 2002). A review of bullying intervention programs suggests that intervention may target the individual student level, for example, teaching the victims self-assertion skills, helping the victims to deal with their negative emotions arising from being bullied, helping the bullies to develop empathy for their victims, and forming a support group involving the victims and bystanders (Wong 2003). Such an approach is a remedial guidance approach in combating school bullying. Meanwhile, some interventions target the classroom level, for example, through classroom discussion to enhance students' awareness of and developing rules to deal with bullying. Other interventions target the whole-school level, such as devising a whole-school anti-bullying policy that is communicated to the whole-school community (Wong 2003). These interventions usually target all school members including staff, pupils, and parents to enhance their knowledge and responses to bullying (Smith and Ananiadou 2003). In addition, peer-led intervention utilizes peer support, such as peer counseling to improve students' communication and empathy skills and peer mediation to resolve conflicts. Other forms of peer-led intervention involve setting up cooperative work groups, thereby creating a circle of friends to support students at risk of victimization (Barton 2006; Salmivalli 1999).

Since bullying springs from factors external to individual child subsystems, bullying interventions need to involve different systems within the school community in order to have a significant, consistent impact. A whole-school approach to bullying that is directed at the entire school and involves a comprehensive, multilevel strategy then becomes pertinent (Hong Kong Children and Youth Services 2002; Stueve et al. 2006). Classroom intervention and whole-school anti-bullying programs illustrate the preventive guidance approach to school bullying. These programs usually aim at providing training in social skills, altering group norms, and increasing self-efficacy. A review of the effectiveness of anti-bullying interventions has shown that the incidence of bullying cannot be reduced by implementing the curriculum alone (Hong Kong Children and Youth Services 2002). Implementation of intervention across different levels within schools has a higher success rate (Davis and Davis 2007), and the intervention is most effective when the anti-bullying curriculum is integrated into the regular school curriculum (Barton 2006). School climate factors, such as interpersonal relationships and quality of communication, and important ecological factors influencing bullying, however, are not usually included in the whole-school intervention program (Twemlow et al. 2004). Developmental guidance precisely addresses building a positive school climate and a guidance-oriented community where each individual's rights are respected and valued.

Despite a number of anti-bullying programs or guidelines developed by the governmental authorities and practitioners both locally and internationally (Gini et al. 2008; Lodge and Frydenberg 2005; Schwartz et al. 1993; Wong 2004), most of them lack citywide, recognized initiatives (Olweus 1993), and their effectiveness is unknown due to a lack of evaluation. Anti-bullying intervention has focused on the individual student level, adopting a suppressive strategy. Such an approach is bully focused and blame driven. Measures such as withdrawal of privileges, meeting parents, school suspension, and expulsion have been adopted by schools to deter students from bullying. However, this strategy is considered punitive and may worsen the bully-victim relationship or even intensify the problem (Barton 2006; Olweus 1993). Such an approach is also very remedial and reactive in focus, falling short of teaching bullies and victims the skills for dealing with conflicts.

Another approach is a comprehensive anti-bullying strategy which aims to tackle risk factors contributing to bullying and to involve everyone in the school (Olweus 1993). Four useful tactics underlying this strategy are (1) encouraging victims to tell the truth and develop a strong character; (2) educating bullies who lack social skills; (3) shaming bullies who intend to do harm or who have done harm, in a reintegrative manner; and (4) promoting a peaceful environment by using restorative practices (Olweus 1993, p. 546). This approach focuses on prevention of the problem and functions more like preventive guidance in schools. So far, there has been insufficient integration of anti-bullying initiatives into schools' policy from a developmental guidance perspective as a means of strengthening students' personal and social development. There is also a lack of intervention at the classroom level, such as incorporating an anti-bullying curriculum into the school's regular guidance curriculum, and a similar lack of intervention at the whole-school level through promoting a harmonious school culture. Therefore, a guidance curriculum which focuses on developing students' strengths will help address the problem of bullying from a developmental guidance perspective and fill in the gap in existing interventions.

Finally, even though it is obvious that school bullying typically occurs in social contexts, existing studies often assume a bully-victim (dyadic) rather than a bully-victim-bystander (triadic) perspective. Bystanders are often taken as mere "passersby," "observers," or "onlookers" as if they are transparent and immobile. In fact, bystanders warrant research attention because, in the social context of school bullying (Barton 2006; Salmivalli 1999), all people present are inevitably engaged in the process, whether explicitly or implicitly. Bystanders who witness the bullying as it develops, occurs, and ends cannot possibly be inactive in the process – whether they act or refrain, they have already added energy to either the bully or the victim. Understanding bystanders is also important because (a) they typically outnumber the bullies and victims and (b) they experience intrapsychic struggles, which are amenable to adjustment through psychoeducation. Thus, an effective anti-bullying program should give enough attention to the role of bystanders in the understanding and management of school bullying.

References

Baldry, A. C. (2003). Bullying in school and exposure to domestic violence. *Child Abuse & Neglect, 27*, 713–732.

Barton, E. A. (2006). *Bully prevention: Tips and strategies for school leaders and classroom teachers*. Thousand Oaks: Corwin Press.

Bauman, S., & Hurley, C. (2005). Teachers' attitudes and beliefs about bullying: Two exploratory studies. *Journal of School Violence, 4*(3), 49–61.

Baumeister, A. L., Storch, E. A., & Geffken, G. R. (2008). Peer victimization in children with learning disabilities. *Child and Adolescent Social Work Journal, 25*, 11–23.

Boivin, M., Vitaro, F., & McCord, J. (1995). The impact of peer relationships on aggression in childhood: Inhibition through coercion or promotion through peer support. In J. McCord (Ed.), *Coercion and punishment in long-term perspectives* (pp. 183–197). New York: Cambridge University Press.

Bond, L., Carlin, J. B., Thomas, L., Rubin, K., & Patton, G. (2001). Does bullying cause emotional problems? A prospective study of young teenagers. *British Medical Journal, 323*, 480–484.

Bosworth, K., Espelage, D. L., & Simon, T. R. (1999). Factors associated with bullying behavior in middle school students. *Journal of Early Adolescence, 19*, 341–362.

Brookmeyer, K. A., Fanti, K. A., & Henrich, C. C. (2006). Schools, parents, and youth violence: A multilevel, ecological analysis. *Journal of Clinical Child and Adolescent Psychology, 35*, 504–514.

Chang, L., Fung, Y. F. K., & Wang, Y. (2004). *Social emotional development of schooling: Preventing school bullying and helping social withdrawn children*. Hong Kong: The Chinese University Press.

Cheng, Y., Newman, I. M., Qu, M., Mbulo, L., Chai, Y., Chen, Y., & Shell, D. F. (2010). Being bullied and psychosocial adjustment among middle school students in China. *Journal of School Health, 80*(4), 193–199.

Clarke, V., Kitzinger, C., & Potter, J. (2004). "Kids are just cruel anyway": Lesbian and gay parents' talk about homophobic bullying. *British Journal of Social Psychology, 43*(4), 531–550.

Cleary, S. D. (2000). Adolescent victimization and associated suicidal and violent behaviors. *Adolescence, 35*(140), 671–682.

Davis, S., & Davis, J. (2007). *Schools where everyone belongs: Practical strategies for reducing bullying*. Campaign: Research Press

Duncan, R. D. (2004). The impact of family relationships on school bullies and victim. In D. L. Espelage & S. M. Swearer (Eds.), *Bullying in American schools: A social-ecological perspective on prevention and intervention* (pp. 227–244). Mahwah: Lawrence Erlbaum Associates.

Egan, L. A., & Todorov, N. (2009). Forgiveness as a coping strategy to allow school students to deal with the effects of being bullied: Theoretical and empirical discussion. *Journal of Social and Clinical Psychology, 28*(2), 198–222.

Espelage, D. L. (2002). *Bullying in early adolescence: The role of the peer group (Report No. EDO-PS-02-16)*. Champaign: Clearinghouse on Elementary and Early Childhood Education (ERIC Document Reproduction Service No. ED-99-CO-0020).

Espelage, D. L., & Swearer, S. M. (2003). Research on school bullying and victimization: What have we learned and where do we go from here? *School Psychology Review, 32*, 365–383.

Espelage, D. L., Bosworth, K., & Simon, T. R. (2000). Examining the social context of bullying behaviors in early adolescence. *Journal of Counseling and Development, 78*(3), 326–333.

Espelage, D. L., Holt, M. K., & Henkel, R. R. (2003). Examination of peer-group contextual effects on aggression during early adolescence. *Child Development, 74*(1), 205–220.

Espelage, D. L., Mebane, S. E., & Swearer, S. M. (2004). Gender differences in bullying: Moving beyond mean level differences. In D. L. Espelage & S. M. Swearer (Eds.), *Bullying in American schools: A social-ecological perspective on prevention and intervention* (pp. 15–35). Mahwah: Lawrence Erlbaum Associates.

Fekkes, M., Pijpers, F. I., & Verloove-Vanhorick, S. P. (2005). Bullying: Who does what, when and where? Involvement of children, teachers and parents in bullying behavior. *Health Education Research, 20*(1), 81–91.

Field, E. M. (2007). *Bully blocking: Six secrets to help children deal with teasing and bullying*. London: Jessica Kingsley Publishers.

Fung, A. L. C., & Wong, J. L. P. (2007). *Project C.A.R.E.: Children and adolescents at risk education*. Hong Kong: Hong Kong Christian Service.

Fung, A. L. C., Wong, J. L. P., & Chak, Y. T. C. (2007). School bullying: Risk factors, cognitive distortion and intervention for reactive aggressors. *Journal of Youth Studies, 10*(1), 3–13.

Fung, A. L. C., Raine, A., & Gao, Y. (2009). Differentiation between proactive and reactive aggression in age, gender, and factor structure: A cross-section study of 11 to 15-year-old schoolchildren. *Journal of Adolescence, 91*(5), 473–479.

Gini, G., Albiero, P., Benelli, B., & Altoe, G. (2008). Determinants of adolescents' active defending and passive by standing behavior in bullying. *Journal of Adolescence, 31*(1), 93–105.

Griffith, L. J., Wolke, D., Page., A. S., Horwood, J. P., & ALSPAC Study Team. (2005). Obesity and bullying: Different effects for boys and girls. *Archives of Disease in Childhood, 91*, 121–125.

Haynie, D. L., Nansel, T., Eitel, P., Crump, A. D., Saylor, K., Yu, K., & Simons-Morton, B. (2001). Bullies, victims, and bully/victims: Distinct groups of at-risk youth. *The Journal of Early Adolescence, 21*(1), 29–49.

Hodges, E. V., & Perry, D. G. (1999). Personal and interpersonal antecedents and consequences of victimization by peers. *Journal of Personality and Social Psychology, 76*, 677–685.

Hodges, E. V., Malone, M. J., & Perry, D. G. (1997). Individual risk and social risk as interacting determinants of victimization in the peer group. *Developmental Psychology, 33*, 1032–1099.

Holt, M. K., & Espelage, D. L. (2007). Perceived social support among bullies, victims, and bully-victims. *Journal of Youth and Adolescence, 36*, 984–994.

Hong Kong Children & Youth Services. (2002). *Peace campaign*. Hong Kong: Hong Kong Children & Youth Services.

Hong Kong Family Welfare Society. (2012). *Survey report on interpersonal relationship and conflict among youth*. (In Chinese). Retrieved from http://www.hkfws.org.hk/b5_report_detail. aspx?id=2&aaa=3

Hong Kong Playground Association, & União Geral das Associações dos Moradores de Macau. (2008). *Survey report on bullying in Hong Kong and Macau*. (In Chinese). Retrieved from http://hq.hkpa.hk/upload/bullying_press_200408.pdf

Hong, J. S., & Eamon, M. K. (2011). Students' perceptions of unsafe schools: An ecological systems analysis. *Journal of Child and Family Studies, 21*(3), 428–438.

Hong, J. S., & Espelage, D. L. (2012). A review of research on bullying and peer victimization in school: An ecological system analysis. *Aggression and Violent Behavior, 17*(4), 311–322.

Hui, E. K., Tsang, S. K., & Law, B. C. (2011). Combating school bullying through development guidance for positive youth development and promoting harmonious school culture. *The Scientific World Journal, 11*, 2266–2277.

James, D. J., Lawlor, M., Courtney, P., Flynn, A., Henry, B., & Murphy, N. (2008). Bullying behaviour in secondary schools: What roles do teachers play? *Child Abuse Review, 17*(3), 160–173.

Kaltiala-Heino, R., Rimpelä, M., Marttunen, M., Rimpelä, A., & Rantanen, P. (1999). Bullying, depression, and suicidal ideation in Finnish adolescents: School survey. *BMJ, 319*(7206), 348–351.

Kohut, M. R. (2007). *The complete guide to understanding, controlling, and stopping bullies & bullying: A complete guide for teachers & parents*. Ocala: Atlantic Publishing Company.

Kuntsche, E., Pickett, W., Overpeck, M., Craig, W., Boyce, W., & de Matos, M. G. (2006). Television viewing and forms of bullying among adolescents from eight countries. *Journal of Adolescent Health, 39*(6), 908–915.

Lam, D. O., & Liu, A. W. (2007). The path through bullying – A process model from the inside story of bullies in Hong Kong secondary schools. *Child and Adolescent Social Work Journal, 24*(1), 53–75.

Law, A. K. Y., & Fung, A. L. C. (2013). Different forms of online and face-to-face victimization among schoolchildren with pure and co-occurring dimensions of reactive and proactive aggression. *Computers in Human Behavior, 29*, 1224–1233.

Lee, C. H. (2009). Personal and interpersonal correlates of bullying behaviors among Korean middle school students. *Journal of Interpersonal Violence, 25*, 152–176.

Lee, C. H. (2011). An ecological systems approach to bullying behaviors among middle school students in the United States. *Journal of Interpersonal Violence, 26*(8), 1664–1693.

Lodge, J., & Frydenberg, E. (2005). The role of peer bystanders in school bullying: Positive steps toward promoting peaceful schools. *Theory Into Practice, 44*(4), 329–336.

Ma, H. K. (2005a). An analysis of the nature and causes of bullying and the proposal of educare as its solution. In K. B. Yiu, C. Fong, W. L. Tsui Yip, & T. Y. Law (Eds.), *From bullying to caring* (pp. 82–106). Hong Kong: Educational Publisher.

Ma, H. K. (2005b). How to prevent and reduce school bullying: A whole-person education proposal. In K. B. Yiu, C. Fong, W. L. Tsui Yip, & T. Y. Law (Eds.), *From bullying to caring* (pp. 65–73). Hong Kong: Educational Publisher.

McCabe, R. E., Antony, M. M., Summerfeldt, L. J., Liss, A., & Swinson, R. P. (2003). Preliminary examination of the relationship between anxiety disorders in adults and self-reported history of teasing or bullying experiences. *Cognitive Behaviour Therapy, 32*(4), 187–193.

Nansel, T. R., Overpeck, M. D., Pilla, R. S., Ruan, W. J., Simons-Morton, B., & Scheidt, P. (2001). Bullying behaviours among U.S. youth: Prevalence and association with psychosocial adjustment. *Journal of the American Medical Association, 16*, 2094–2100.

Ng, J. W., & Tsang, S. K. (2008). School bullying and the mental health of junior secondary school students in Hong Kong. *Journal of School Violence, 7*(2), 3–20.

Olweus, D. (1993). *Bullying at school: What we know and what we can do.* Cambridge, MA: Blackwell.

Orpinas, P., & Horne, A. M. (2006). *Bullying prevention: Creating a positive school climate and developing social competence.* Washington, DC: American Psychological Association.

Rigby, K. (1998). The relationship between reported health and involvement in bully/victim problems among male and female secondary school children. *Journal of Health Psychology, 3*, 465–476.

Rigby, K. (1999). Peer victimisation at school and the health of secondary school students. *British Journal of Educational Psychology, 69*(1), 95–104.

Rigby, K. (2003). *Addressing bullying in schools: Theory and practice.* Canberra: Australian Institute of Criminology.

Rigby, K. (2007). *Bullying in schools and what to do about it: Revised and updated.* Victoria: Australian Council for Educational Research.

Rivers, I. (2004). Recollections of bullying at school and their long-term implications for lesbians, gay men, and bisexuals. *Crisis: The Journal of Crisis Intervention and Suicide Prevention, 25*(4), 169–175.

Roth, D. A., Coles, M. E., & Heimberg, R. G. (2002). The relationship between memories for childhood teasing and anxiety and depression in adulthood. *Journal of Anxiety Disorders, 16*(2), 149–164.

Salmivalli, C. (1999). Participant role approach to school bullying: Implications for interventions. *Journal of Adolescence, 22*(4), 453–459.

Salmon, G., James, A., & Smith, D. M. (1998). Bullying in schools: Self reported anxiety, depression, and self esteem in secondary school children. *British Medical Journal, 317*(7163), 924–925.

Saylor, C. F., & Leach, J. B. (2009). Perceived bullying and social support in students accessing special inclusion programming. *Journal of Developmental and Physical Disabilities, 21*, 69–80.

Schäfer, M., Korn, S., Smith, P. K., Hunter, S. C., Mora-Merchán, J. A., Singer, M. M., & Meulen, K. (2004). Lonely in the crowd: Recollections of bullying. *British Journal of Developmental Psychology, 22*(3), 379–394.

Schwartz, D., Dodge, K. A., & Coie, J. D. (1993). The emergence of chronic peer victimization in boys' play groups. *Child Development, 64*(6), 1755–1772.

Schwartz, D., McFadyen, K. S., Dodge, K. A., Pettit, G. S., & Bates, J. E. (1999). Early behavior problems as a predictor of later peer group victimization: Moderators and mediators in the pathways of social risk. *Journal of Abnormal Child Psychology, 27*, 191–201.

Shek, D. T. L., Ma, H. K., & Sun, R. C. F. (2011). A brief overview of adolescent developmental problems in Hong Kong. *The Scientific World Journal, 11*, 2243–2256.

Smith, P. K., & Ananiadou, K. (2003). The nature of school bullying and the effectiveness of school-based interventions. *Journal of Applied Psychoanalytic Studies, 5*(2), 189–209.

Smith, P. K., Ananiadou, K., & Cowie, H. (2003). Interventions to reduce school bullying. *Canadian Journal of Psychiatry, 48*(9), 591–599.

Stueve, A., Dash, K., O'Donnell, L., Tehranifar, P., Wilson-Simmons, R., Slaby, R. G., & Link, B. G. (2006). Rethinking the bystander role in school violence prevention. *Health Promotion Practice, 7*(1), 117–124.

The Hong Kong Federation of Youth Groups. (2010). *Youth study series 44: A study on cyber bullying of secondary school students.* Retrieved from http://yrc.hkfyg.org.hk/chi/ys44.html

Tsang, S. K., Hui, E. K., & Law, B. C. (2011). Bystander position taking in school bullying: The role of positive identity, self-efficacy, and self-determination. *The Scientific World Journal, 11*, 2278–2286.

Twemlow, S. W., Fonagy, P., & Sacco, F. C. (2004). The role of the bystander in the social architecture of bullying and violence in schools and communities. *Annals of the New York Academy of Sciences, 1036*(1), 215–232.

Van der Wal, M. F., de Wit, C. A., & Hirasing, R. A. (2003). Psychosocial health among young victims and offenders of direct and indirect bullying. *Pediatrics, 111*, 1312–1317.

Van Wormer, K., & McKinney, R. (2003). What schools can do to help gay/lesbian/bisexual youth: A harm reduction approach. *Adolescence, 38*(151), 409–420.

Whitted, K. S., & Dupper, D. R. (2005). Best practices for preventing or reducing bullying in schools. *Children and Schools, 27*(3), 167–175.

Williams, K., Chambers, M., Logan, S., & Robinson, D. (1996). Association of common health symptoms with bullying in primary school children. *British Medical Journal, 313*, 17–19.

Wong, D. S. W. (2002). *Helping pupils away from bullying*. Hong Kong: Centre for Restoration of Human Relationships.

Wong, D. S. W. (2003). *Research and countermeasures on student bullying: Life education as the direction*. Hong Kong: Arcadia Press.

Wong, D. S. W. (2004). School bullying and tackling strategies in Hong Kong. *International Journal of Offender Therapy and Comparative Criminology, 48*(5), 537–553.

Wong, D. S. W., Lok, D. P., Lo, T. W., & Ma, S. K. (2008). School bullying among Hong Kong Chinese primary schoolchildren. *Youth and Society, 40*(1), 35–54.

Woods, S., & Wolke, D. (2004). Direct and relational bullying among primary school children and academic achievement. *Journal of School Psychology, 42*, 135–155.

Wurf, G. (2010). *Reducing bullying in high schools: An evaluation of school-based initiatives for the prevention and management of bullying*. Retrieved from http://www.aare.edu.au/08pap/wur08639.pdf

Zimmerman, F. J., Glew, G. M., Christakis, D. A., & Katon, W. (2005). Early cognitive stimulation, emotional support, and television watching as predictors of subsequent bullying among grade-school children. *Archives of Pediatrics & Adolescent Medicine, 159*(4), 384–388.

Prevention of Cyberbullying: A Conceptual Review

Diego Busiol and Tak Yan Lee

Abstract Cyberbullying normally refers to Internet or mobile phone practices for deliberate, repeated, and inimical behavior to harm others by an individual or a group. Cyberbullying is a more complex phenomenon than traditional face-to-face bullying, and this has important implications for prevention and intervention approach. In this chapter, similarities and differences between bullying and cyberbullying will be examined. Basing on extensive literature research, risk and protective factors for cyberbullying in Hong Kong, as well as psychological consequences, will be presented. It is imperative to address cyberbullying because it occurs in the hidden online world of youth. As a consequence, students who are cyberbullied generally do not seek help because of fear of reprisal and embarrassment or because they assume that adults will not act; on the other hand, parents and teachers often underestimate cyberbullying because it has less physical consequences than traditional bullying.

Introduction

In the last few years, several cases of teenagers who committed suicide after being harassed on the Internet have garnered global attention. On 2 August 2013, Hannah Smith, 14, hanged herself in her bedroom in Lutterworth, Leicestershire, after being "cyberbullied" on the question-and-answer website ask.fm, which allows users to send messages without their identity being disclosed (The Guardian 2013). In September 2013, a 12-year-old Florida girl named Rebecca Ann Sedwick committed suicide after she was allegedly bullied online by more than a dozen other girls. Messages included phrases like "Go kill yourself" and "Why are you still alive?" (Aljazeera America 2013). Unfortunately, these stories are very much alike the stories of Ryan Halligan, Megan Meier, Jessica Logan, Hope Witsell, Tyler Clementi,

The preparation for this work and the Project P.A.T.H.S. were financially supported by The Hong Kong Jockey Club Charities Trust.

D. Busiol • T.Y. Lee (✉)
Department of Applied Social Sciences, City University of Hong Kong, Kowloon, Hong Kong, China
e-mail: ty.lee@cityu.edu.hk

© Springer Science+Business Media Singapore 2015   59
T.Y. Lee et al. (eds.), *Student Well-Being in Chinese Adolescents in Hong Kong*,
Quality of Life in Asia 7, DOI 10.1007/978-981-287-582-2_5

Amanda Todd, Audrie Pott, and many other teenagers who found themselves victims of cyberbullying and ended their lives. Suicide is the most extreme and tangible of the possible consequences of being cyberbullied. The phenomenon itself is complex and articulated and can happen in different ways.

In China, cyberbullying is very much related to the "human flesh search" (人肉 搜索; pinyin: Rénròu Sōusuǒ), a phenomenon that became popular from 2006 when a video showing a woman who stomped a cat to death with her high-heeled shoes was posted online; suddenly the lady was identified by many angered Internet users as a nurse in Heilongjiang province. Under the pressure, her hospital fired her, and she had to make an open apology for her misbehavior. This was one of the first and most popular cases to show the growing importance of the "human flesh search" as a tool by web surfers to expose and hunt for immoral and unethical individuals (Liang and Lu 2010). In October 2013, a video showing a 20-year-old Hong Kong girl slapping 14 times in the face her 23-year-old boyfriend who was kneeling went viral on the Internet, and it is believed to have been seen by more than 700,000 people. The video provoked the reaction of thousands of users. After a few days, another 18-year-old girl who looked very similar to the woman in the video was recognized in the MTR, and her pictures were uploaded to the Internet and even printed in a newspaper, mistakenly identifying her as the attacker. As a consequence, the girl was blamed by the public and had to report the case of her being cyberbullied to the police (South China Morning Post 2013). In November 2012, a Hong Kong lady was criticized for posting a Facebook status in which she wrote "I'm not opening a charity…. If you really only want to give me a HK$500 cash gift, then don't bother coming to my wedding." This status update was reported in online forums and provoked large-scale criticism by users, who raced to find details about the bride's identity and her online photos, including images of her friends and fiancé. Finally, people went on to search for the couple and their wedding information, and about a thousand even threatened to gate-crash the wedding ceremony of the young couple (Wall Street Journal China 2013).

What Is Cyberbullying?

Literature suggests that cyberbullying is a global phenomenon that must be addressed by international research (Aricak et al. 2008; Wong et al. 2013). Slonje and Smith (2008) asserted that cyberbullying rates were much higher for adolescents aged 12–15. Cyberbullying normally refers to Internet (including e-mail, social networking sites, instant messaging, chat rooms, blogs) or mobile phone practices that are (a) intended to hurt, (b) part of a repetitive pattern of negative offline or online actions, and (c) performed in a relationship characterized by a power imbalance, such as technological know-how and anonymity (Vandebosch and Van Cleemput 2008; Williams and Godfrey 2011). According to Belsey (2004), cyberbullying involves the use of communication and information technologies for deliberate, repeated, and inimical behavior to harm others by an individual or a group. "StopCyberbullying" was the first cyberbullying prevention program in North America, which described "Cyberbullying" as "when a child, preteen or teen is tormented, threatened, harassed, humiliated, embarrassed or otherwise targeted by another child, preteen or teen using the Internet, interactive and digital technologies or mobile phones. It has to have a minor on both sides, or at least have been instigated by a minor against another minor. Once adults become involved, it is plain and simple cyber-harassment or cyberstalking. Adult cyber-harassment or cyberstalking is NEVER called cyberbullying" (Stop Cyberbullying 2014). The Hong Kong Federation of Youth Groups (2010) generalized that bullying is composed of three elements: (1) repetition, bullying behavior occurs in a period of time repeatedly, instead of a single event; (2) intent, the bullies bully or harass others purposely; and (3) power imbalance, compared with those who are bullied, bullies usually have greater power. Furthermore, Willard (2005, pp. 1–2) sums up seven main ways in which cyberbullying may occur:

1. Flaming – sending angry, rude, vulgar messages directed at a person or persons, privately or to an online group.
2. Harassment – repeatedly sending a person offensive messages.
3. Cyberstalking – harassment that includes threats of harm or is highly intimidating.
4. Denigration (put-downs) – sending or posting harmful, untrue, or cruel statements about a person to other people.
5. Masquerading – pretending to be someone else and sending or posting material that makes that person look bad or places that person in potential danger.
6. Outing and Trickery – sending or posting material about a person that contains sensitive, private, or embarrassing information, including forwarding private messages or images and engaging in tricks to soliciting embarrassing information that is then made public.
7. Exclusion – actions that specifically and intentionally exclude a person from an online group, such as exclusion from an IM "buddies" list.

Differences Between Traditional Bullying and Cyberbullying

Face-to-face bullying and cyberbullying partially overlap. However, considering cyberbullying simply as the electronic form of face-to-face bullying may overlook the intricacies of this behavior. Even if in both cases aspects of repetition, power imbalance, and intentionality may be identified, they may find application in very different ways and may give rise to very different scenarios. The same can be said for the role of the group and the bystanders (for a review see Dooley et al. 2009). Olweus' (1993) classical definition of bullying included three dimensions: intentionality, repetition, and imbalance of power. Several studies have tried to assess if the same definition could apply to cyberbullying. These criteria, plus another two (anonymity and public vs. private), were tested in a study on cyberbullying across six European countries (Menesini et al. 2012). The results suggested a clear first dimension characterized by imbalance of power and a clear second dimension characterized by intentionality and, at a lower level, by anonymity. However, the role of repetition as a criterion for cyberbullying was questioned; indeed, in the virtual context, a single aggressive act can lead to an immense number of repetitions of the victimization, without the contribution of the perpetrator (Menesini et al. 2012). According to Slonje and Smith (2008, p. 148), bullying and cyberbullying differ because of (1) the difficulty of getting away from it. Bullying can continue at any time, unlike traditional bullying that is possible only face to face. (2) The breadth of the potential audience. Cyberbullying can reach particularly large audiences, for example, by uploading videos or pictures on the Internet. (3) The invisibility of those doing the bullying. Cyberbullying and rumor spreading provide some degree of invisibility or even anonymity to bullies. (4) The cyberbully may be less aware of the consequences caused by his or her actions. Distance may leave fewer opportunities for empathy or remorse, and there may also be less opportunity for bystander intervention. According to the Hong Kong Federation of Youth Groups (2010), other differences between cyberbullying and face-to-face bullying include (1) roles to play cyberbullies (the cyberbullied and witnesses may swap roles, i.e., today's bullies could be tomorrow's bullied, whereas this rarely happens in traditional bullying) and (2) problem solving (cyberbullying is a more complex problem due to its swift and widespread nature and the difficulty in finding the source, whereas face-to-face bullying is less complicated because fewer people are involved, its spread is limited, and both bullies and bullied can be brought together). For Patchin and Hinduja (2006), in cyberbullying situations, the power of bullies does not come from their physical advantage over the victims but from their competence in using the technology and their ability to hide their identity on the Internet. According to Leung and McBride-Chang (2013) in traditional school bullying, bullies usually know their victims, but this may not apply to the cyber world. Li (2007) suggested that 40 % of cyber victims did not know their cyberbullies. Furthermore, in cyberbullying, the perpetrator is less likely to see the victim or any direct response from him/her. This might reduce direct gratification but might also reduce any inhibition (Smith et al. 2008). Indeed, it was found (Aricak et al. 2008) that the most frequent behavior that students engaged in was saying things online that would not be said face to face, introducing oneself as someone else, and saying untrue things on the Internet. Traditional bullying occurs in a defined, physical space, from which the victim cannot easily escape. Instead, cyberbullying may be perpetrated on different websites at the same time and cannot be easily terminated, as there might be difficulties in removing messages or pictures from the Internet (Wolak et al. 2007). Younger adolescents are more likely than older youth to engage in physical bullying because the physical capacity to attack others generally precedes the development of the intellectual and social skills to harm by verbal aggression or social exclusion (Brame et al. 2001). Lastly, but not less important, Willard (2007) suggested that there is a concept of harmful bystanders in cyberbullying. Harmful bystanders are "those who encourage and support the bully or watch the bullying from the sidelines, but do nothing to intervene or help the target" (Willard 2007, p. 6).

Current Situation in Hong Kong

Cyberbullying is increasing (The Hong Kong Federation of Youth Groups 2010). In recent years, from the local news and survey reports, it has been shown that more and more teenagers are being cyberbullied in Hong Kong.

In 2009, a survey conducted among 908 primary 4 students to secondary F.6 students (The Hong Kong Christian Service 2009) showed that 18 % of respondents had been cyberbullied in the past year and 13 % had cyberbullied others in the same period of time. The methods of bullying included harassing, frightening, or threatening e-mail, uploading embarrassing photos or video clips online, and personal attacks on the Internet. The Church of United Brethren in Christ (2009) conducted another survey (viz., "The help seeking pattern among young cyber bullying victims") among 2,629 primary and secondary students, which showed that 10.9 % of the respondents had been bullied, and in most cases the victims were males. In the same year, the Hong Kong Federation of Youth Groups (2009) analyzed a sample of 559 youth aged 10–24 years old by phone interview and found that 22.7 % of youth had used crude language to ridicule or revile others. One year after, they surveyed 2,981 pupils in 18 secondary schools and conducted 18 in-depth interviews with students and 10 experts/academics (The Hong Kong Federation of Youth Groups 2010). The results showed that 30.2 % of interviewed secondary school students had been cyberbullied over the past year, while 22.0 % said that they had cyberbullied others. Furthermore, research results indicated that (a) cyberbullying is rising and it is a consequence of the unavoidable use of information technology, and (b) among secondary school students, male students are easier to be cyberbullies or cyberbullied. Furthermore, results showed five features of cyberbullying among Hong Kong secondary school students: (1) it generally takes the form of rumor spreading; (2) social network sites are the main platform; (3) it normally occurs after school and is based from home; (4) the people involved in cyberbullying usually are classmates; and (5) cyberbullying is treated as fun making rather than a problem. The Hong Kong Family Welfare Society commissioned the Social Work Department of the Chinese University of Hong Kong to investigate the cyberbullying of F.1 to F.7 students in the period from December 2009 to February 2010. Results showed that 30.9 % had suffered different levels of cyberbullying and 17.8 % had cyberbullied others. In 2013, the Hong Kong Playground Association, União Geral das Associações dos Moradores de Macau (澳門街坊會聯合總會), and Guangzhou Youth Cultural Palace (廣州市青年文化宮) conducted a survey among 2,460 youths in Hong Kong, Macau, and Guangzhou on cyberbullying. The results showed that (a) 73.7 % of the respondents had witnessed cyberbullying within 1 year, (b) 63.7 % of the respondents had been attacked by cyberbullying, and (c) 17 % of the respondents had bullied others. In research across 288 Hong Kong university students aged mainly (94 %) 18–25 years (Xiao and Wong 2013), it was found that (1) cyber-victimization had a strong positive impact on the likelihood to perform cyberbullying behavior (cyber victims are more likely to become cyberbullies); (2) Internet self-efficacy (expertise in using Internet applications) had a significant influence on cyberbullying behavior; (3) students had a greater tendency to engage in cyberbullying when they held positive normative beliefs about such behavior, meaning when they believed that their relevant others approved of such behavior; and (4) motivation was the strongest predictor of cyberbullying, meaning that students who desired power, attention, and/or peer approval were more likely to perpetrate cyberbullying behavior.

Types of Cyberbullying and Victimization

Internet use should not simply be understood as an alternative to or retiring from "real life" or as a rejection of real encounters. A number of studies suggested that children and adolescents can meet friends when they go online (Griffiths 2000). Building up online friendships in multiplayer online games (MMOGs) can be positive for teens. Indeed, findings from research across 626 Hong Kong Chinese fifth and sixth graders (Leung and McBride-Chang 2013) suggest that online friendship quality is positively related to children's social competence, friendship satisfaction, self-esteem, and life satisfaction.

Among all types of cyberbullying behavior among Hong Kong students, most participants who reported engaging in cyberbullying were involved in online social groups or forums in which a key objective was to tease or insult others (14.3 %) or which was followed up with online texts to cyberbully others (13.5 %). In Hong Kong, cyberbullying actions such as hacking into others' online accounts to alter personal information (6.6 %) and editing and posting others' photographs on the Internet for humiliation purposes (7.6 %) are not very prevalent. Victims of cyberbullying most frequently report having their own or family members' photographs or videos uploaded to the cyber world without their permission (12.5 %) or receiving annoying or vulgar online messages (12.1 %). The least frequent form of cyber-victimization was having one's personal information disclosed on the Internet (8 %) (Wong et al. 2013). Li (2008) conducted cross-cultural research comparing Canadian and Chinese students aged 11–15 and found that proportionally more Chinese students than Canadian students reported that adults in school tried to stop cyberbullying when notified. Another finding was that Chinese cyberbullying victims and bystanders were more likely to tell adults about the incidents than their Canadian counterparts. One possible explanation was that teachers in China often have more authoritative power over students than teachers in Canada. Findings from this research also suggest that cultural differences in cyberbullying exist and that effective prevention and intervention programs should take it into account.

Risk and Protective Factors and Psychological Consequences

Predictable risk factors for involvement in cyberbullying as a bully are traditional bullying, rule-breaking behavior, and frequency of online communication (Sticca et al. 2013). In a study focusing on students aged 11–16 years, Harman et al. (2005)

found that children who reported the most faking behavior on the Internet (e.g., pretending to be older) had poorer social skills, lower levels of self-esteem, higher levels of social anxiety, and higher levels of aggression. They suggest that a strong relationship exists between inflated self-esteem and violence. Youth victims of cyberbullying have been found to be more likely to show symptoms of depression and to have problems at school and psychological distress (Kowalski and Limber 2007; Wang et al. 2011). Perpetration of cyberbullying has been found to be associated with higher anxiety (Hawker and Boulton 2000) and lower self-esteem (Yang et al. 2013). Beran and Li (2008) found that students who were cyberbullied experienced difficulties at school such as low marks, poor concentration, and absenteeism. Findings from research across 1,917 secondary school adolescents in Hong Kong indicated that male adolescents were more likely than female adolescents to cyberbully others and to be cyber-victimized. Cyberbullying perpetration and victimization were found to be negatively associated with the adolescents' psychosocial health and sense of belonging to school. Cyberbullying and traditional bullying were positively correlated. Multivariate analyses indicated that being male, having a low sense of belonging to school, involvement in traditional bullying perpetration, and experiencing cyber-victimization were associated with an increased propensity to cyberbully others (Wong et al. 2013). Results from an online survey of 1,378 adolescent Internet users (Hinduja and Patchin 2008) showed that computer proficiency and time spent online were positively related to cyberbullying victimization. Additionally, cyberbullying experiences were also linked to respondents who reported school problems (including traditional bullying), assaultive behavior, and substance use. Cyberbullying was also found to be associated with an increase in suicide ideation and suicide attempts (Hinduja and Patchin 2008). In research across 2,215 Finnish adolescents aged 13–16 years, Sourander et al. (2010) identified a number of risk factors for (1) cyber victim only, living in a family with other than two biological parents, perceived difficulties, emotional and peer problems, headaches, recurrent abdominal pain, sleeping difficulties, and not feeling safe at school; (2) cyberbully only, perceived difficulties, hyperactivity, conduct problems, low prosocial behavior, frequent smoking and drunkenness, headaches, and not feeling safe at school; and (3) cyberbully-victim, all of the above risk factors. Furthermore, it was found that among cyber victims, being cyberbullied was associated with fear for safety, indicating possible trauma. Some scholars (Sutton and Smith 1999) suggest that bullies are skillful in understanding social cues and others' mental states and that they use this ability to their own advantage, acting as "skilled social manipulators." Instead, what they would lack is the empathic reactivity towards their mates' emotions and, in particular, towards victims' suffering. Indeed, low levels of empathic responsiveness were found to be associated with students' involvement in bullying others. In contrast, empathy was positively associated with actively helping victimized schoolmates (Gini et al. 2007). In research on 1,334 Korean children aged 12 (Yang et al. 2013), it was found that cyberbullying has different predictors from traditional bullying. For instance, in this sample, low academic level was associated with perpetration and victimization of cyberbullying, but not with traditional bullying.

According to Hoff and Mitchell (2009), cyberbullying emerges most commonly from relationship problems (breakups, envy, intolerance, and ganging up). There is growing evidence that children who are frequently involved in bullying are at an increased risk of social and emotional problems (for a review, see O'Brennan et al. 2009). Youth who bully or who are victims of bullying tend to lack appropriate social skills (Smokowski and Kopasz 2005). Children who are victims of bullying have reported feelings of insecurity and loneliness (Bond et al. 2001). In 2010, a study of 1,917 Hong Kong students aged between 12 and 15 years old (54.6 % were boys and 45.4 % were girls) revealed that being male, having a low sense of belonging to school, involvement in traditional bullying perpetration, and experiencing cyber-victimization were associated with an increased propensity to cyberbully others (Wong et al. 2013).

An important preventive factor is the feeling of "belongingness" or connectedness to others in school (Glew et al. 2005); youth who are aggressively victimized and perpetrate violent behavior are less likely to feel connected to others at their school (Wilson 2004). A study explored the influence of gender, religion, and parenting style on risky online behavior in a sample of 825 secondary 2 students in Hong Kong (Lau and Yuen 2013). Taken together, gender, religion, and parenting style predicted risky online behavior significantly. It was found that males tend to be involved in more risky behavior than females, which corroborates previous findings from the literature (Kim and Kim 2012). However, none of the parenting styles seemed to be effective in reducing risky online behavior; likewise, there was no statistically significant difference between Christians and non-Christians.

Necessity of Educational Programs

According to Willard (2005), it is imperative that adults begin to address cyberbullying because it occurs in the hidden online world of youth. Hoff and Mitchell (2009) claim that students who are cyberbullied generally do not seek help because of fear of reprisal or embarrassment or because they assume that adults will not act; instead, those who do take action often wait until the bullying reaches intolerable levels and then retaliate, so that the spiral of cyberbullying will continue. Students are generally reluctant to tell their families and teachers about cyberbullying and tend to prefer their friends as a better resource for advice (Aricak et al. 2008). For this reason, and because cyberbullying normally has less physical consequences than traditional bullying, parents and teachers see physical bullying as more serious and harmful than verbal and indirect (relational) bullying and are less likely to intervene when children experience indirect bullying (Aricak et al. 2008).

Leung and Lee (2012), in their study across 718 adolescents and teenagers, aged 9–19 in Hong Kong, found that (1) the stricter the parenting styles, the fewer Internet risks that adolescents will experience and the lower the likelihood that adolescents will be addicted to the Internet, and (2) the stricter and the more involved the parents, the less time adolescents will spend interacting on social networks and downloading audio/videos. However, results indicate that strict parental rules, involvement, and mediation had no or few effects on suffering from harassment and privacy risks: even if parents have the strictest rules against the use of the Internet at home, adolescents may still be targets. Neither parental supervision nor the use of filtering technology would decrease the solicitation risk, although parents who exercise strict rules and provide guidance and mediation at home were found to generally reduce the seductive influence of pornography and violent content online (Leung and Lee 2012). Interestingly, the strongest effects against cyberbullying were found to be due to prevention programs focused at the school level (Couvillon and Ilieva 2011). Whereas while rules are important, the primary focus of anti-bullying programs should be based on values (Willard 2005): (1) kindness and respect for others and self, (2) peaceful relations, (3) respecting and honoring differences, (4) improving the world and the Internet, and (5) learning to do what is right in accordance with one's own personal morals, regardless of the potential of detection and punishment imposed by an authority. Furthermore, specific educational strategies can strengthen students' empathy, and students should be taught effective decision-making strategies to assist in deciding what the right action is.

In line with these findings, the Hong Kong Federation of Youth Groups (2010) suggested that schools should strengthen training in media literacy for the students in order for them to learn about information technology and know more about online safety. In addition, they also provided guidelines for parents whose children have been cyberbullied as well as for parents whose children have cyberbullied others. Finally, the Hong Kong government created a website to provide general information about cyberbullying and how to prevent it (InfoSec 2012).

References

Aljazeera America (2013). *12-year-old cyber-bully victim commits suicide*. Retrieved from http://america.aljazeera.com/articles/2013/9/12/bullied-12-year-oldusgirlcommitssuicide.html

Aricak, T., Siyahhan, S., Uzunhasanoglu, A., Saribeyoglu, S., Ciplak, S., Yilmaz, N., & Memmedov, C. (2008). Cyberbullying among Turkish adolescents. *Cyberpsychology & Behavior, 11*(3), 253–261.

Belsey, B. (2004). *Cyberbullying an emerging threat to the always-on generation*. Retrieved February 2014, from www.cyberbullying.ca/pdf/Cyberbullying_Presentation_Description.pdf

Beran, T., & Li, Q. (2008). The relationship between cyberbullying and school bullying. *The Journal of Student Wellbeing, 1*(2), 16–33.

Bond, L., Carlin, J. B., Thomas, L., Rubin, K., & Patton, G. (2001). Does bullying cause emotional problems? A prospective study of young teenagers. *British Medical Journal, 323*, 480–484.

Brame, B., Nagin, D. S., & Tremblay, R. E. (2001). Developmental trajectories of physical aggression from school entry to late adolescence. *Journal of Child Psychology and Psychiatry, 42*(4), 503–512.

Couvillon, M. A., & Ilieva, V. (2011). Recommended practices: A review of schoolwide preventative programs and strategies on cyberbullying. *Preventing School Failure: Alternative Education for Children and Youth, 55*(2), 96–101.

Dooley, J. J., Pyżalski, J., & Cross, D. (2009). Cyberbullying versus face-to-face bullying. *Zeitschrift für Psychologie/Journal of Psychology, 217*(4), 182–188.

Gini, G., Albiero, P., Benelli, B., & Altoè, G. (2007). Does empathy predict adolescents' bullying and defending behavior? *Aggressive Behavior, 33*(5), 467–476.

Glew, G. M., Ming-Yu, F., Katon, W., Rivara, F. P., & Kernic, M. A. (2005). Bullying, psychosocial adjustment, and academic performance in elementary school. *Archives of Pediatric and Adolescent Medicine, 159*, 1026–1031.

Griffiths, M. D. (2000). Video game violence and aggression: Comments on "Video fame playing and its relations with aggressive and prosocial behavior" by O. Wiegman and E.G.M. van Schie. *British Journal of Social Psychology, 39*(Part 1), 147–149.

Harman, J. P., Hansen, C. E., Cochran, M. E., & Lindsey, C. R. (2005). Liar, liar: Internet faking but not frequency of use affects social skills, self-esteem, social anxiety, and aggression. *Cyberpsychology & Behavior, 8*(1), 1–6.

Hawker, D. S., & Boulton, M. J. (2000). Twenty years' research on peer victimization and psychosocial maladjustment: A meta-analytic review of cross-sectional studies. *Journal of Child Psychology and Psychiatry, 41*(4), 441–455.

Hinduja, S., & Patchin, J. W. (2008). Cyberbullying: An exploratory analysis of factors related to offending and victimization. *Deviant Behavior, 29*(2), 129–156.

Hoff, D. L., & Mitchell, S. N. (2009). Cyberbullying: Causes, effects, and remedies. *Journal of Educational Administration, 47*(5), 652–665.

Hong Kong Christian Service. (2009). *A survey on cyber bullying* (In Chinese). Retrieved from http://www.hkcs.org/commu/2009press/press20090509.html

Hong Kong Playground Association, & União Geral das Associações dos Moradores de Macau, and Guangzhou Youth Cultural Palace. (2013). *Survey report on cyber bullying in Guangzhou, Hong Kong and Macau* (In Chinese). Retrieved from http://hq.hkpa.hk/upload/(Report)2013CB(NOV)(5).pdf

InfoSec. (2012). *Cyber-bullying*. Retrieved from http://www.infosec.gov.hk/english/youngsters/cyberbullying.html

Kim, J. E., & Kim, J. (2012). *Determinants of online problematic behavior among teen users: Data from South Korea*. Retrieved February 2014, from www.consumerinterests.org

Kowalski, R. M., & Limber, S. P. (2007). Electronic bullying among middle school students. *Journal of Adolescent Health, 41*(6), S22–S30.

Lau, W. W. F., & Yuen, H. K. A. (2013). Adolescents' risky online behaviours: The influence of gender, religion, and parenting style. *Computers in Human Behavior, 29*(6), 2690–2696.

Leung, L., & Lee, P. S. (2012). The influences of information literacy, internet addiction and parenting styles on internet risks. *New Media & Society, 14*(1), 117–136.

Leung, A. N. M., & McBride-Chang, C. (2013). Game on? Online friendship, cyberbullying, and psychosocial adjustment in Hong Kong Chinese children. *Journal of Social and Clinical Psychology, 32*(2), 159–185.

Li, Q. (2007). New bottle but old wine: A research of cyberbullying in schools. *Computers in Human Behavior, 23*, 1777–1791.

Li, Q. (2008). A cross-cultural comparison of adolescents' experience related to cyberbullying. *Educational Research, 50*(3), 223–234.

Liang, B., & Lu, H. (2010). Internet development, censorship, and cyber crimes in China. *Journal of Contemporary Criminal Justice, 26*(1), 103–120.

Menesini, E., Nocentini, A., Palladino, B. E., Frisén, A., Berne, S., Ortega-Ruiz, R., & Smith, P. K. (2012). Cyberbullying definition among adolescents: A comparison across six European countries. *Cyberpsychology, Behavior and Social Networking, 15*(9), 455–463.

O'Brennan, L. M., Bradshaw, C. P., & Sawyer, A. L. (2009). Examining developmental differences in the social-emotional problems among frequent bullies, victims, and bully/victims. *Psychology in the Schools, 46*(2), 100–115.

Olweus, D. (1993). *Bullying at school: What we know and what we can do*. Cambridge, MA: Blackwell.

Patchin, J. W., & Hinduja, S. (2006). Bullies move beyond the schoolyard a preliminary look at cyberbullying. *Youth Violence and Juvenile Justice, 4*(2), 148–169.

Slonje, R., & Smith, P. K. (2008). Cyberbullying: Another main type of bullying? *Scandinavian Journal of Psychology, 49*, 147–154.

Smith, P. K., Mahdavi, J., Carvalho, M., Fisher, S., Russell, S., & Tippett, N. (2008). Cyberbullying: Its nature and impact in secondary school pupils. *Journal of Child Psychology and Psychiatry, 49*(4), 376–385.

Smokowski, P. R., & Kopasz, K. H. (2005). Bullying in school: An overview of types, effects, family characteristics, and intervention strategies. *Children & Schools, 27*, 101–110.

Sourander, A., Klomek, A. B., Ikonen, M., Lindroos, J., Luntamo, T., Koskelainen, M., Ristkari, T., & Helenius, H. (2010). Psychosocial risk factors associated with cyberbullying among adolescents: A population-based study. *Archives of General Psychiatry, 67*(7), 720–728.

South China Morning Post. (2013). *Mistaken identity.* Retrieved February 19, 2014, from http://www.yp.scmp.com/home/website/Article.aspx?id=5825

Sticca, F., Ruggieri, S., Alsaker, F., & Perren, S. (2013). Longitudinal risk factors for cyberbullying in adolescence. *Journal of Community & Applied Social Psychology, 23*(1), 52–67.

Stop Cyberbullying (2014). *What is cyberbullying, exactly?.* Retrieved February 2014, from http://stopcyberbullying.org/what_is_cyberbullying_exactly.html

Sutton, J., & Smith, P. K. (1999). Bullying as a group process: An adaptation of the participant role approach. *Aggressive Behavior, 25*, 97–111.

The Church of United Brethren in Christ Social Service Division. (2009). *The help seeking pattern among young cyber bullying victims* (In Chinese). Retrieved from http://www.cubc.org.hk/web/cyberbullying-report.pdf

The Guardian. (2013). *Teenager Hannah Smith killed herself because of online bullying, says father.* Retrieved from http://www.theguardian.com/society/2013/aug/06/hannah-smith-online-bullying

The Hong Kong Federation of Youth Groups. (2009). *What's wrong about web-surfing to children and youth?* (In Chinese). Retrieved from http://yrc.hkfyg.org.hk/chinese/yr-p186c.html

The Hong Kong Federation of Youth Groups. (2010). *A study on cyber bullying among secondary school students in Hong Kong* (In Chinese). Retrieved from http://benetwise.hk/download/cyberbully_research.pdf

Vandebosch, H., & Van Cleemput, K. (2008). Defining cyberbullying: A qualitative research into the perceptions of youngsters. *Cyberpsychology & Behavior, 11*(4), 499–503.

Wall Street Journal China. (2013). *How to attract protesters to your wedding.* Retrieved February 19, 2014, from http://blogs.wsj.com/chinarealtime/2012/11/14/how-to-attract-protesters-to-your-wedding/

Wang, J., Nansel, T. R., & Iannotti, R. J. (2011). Cyber and traditional bullying: Differential association with depression. *Journal of Adolescent Health, 48*(4), 415–417.

Willard, N. (2005). *Educator's guide to cyberbullying addressing the harm caused by online social cruelty.* Retrieved from http://cyberbully.org

Willard, W. (2007). *Educator's guide to cyberbullying and cyberthreats.* Retrieved from http://www.csriu.org/cyberbully/docs/cbcteducator.pdf

Williams, S. G., & Godfrey, A. J. (2011). What is cyberbullying and how can psychiatric-mental health nurses recognize it. *Journal of Psychosocial Nursing and Mental Health Service, 16*, 1–6.

Wilson, D. (2004). The interface of school climate and school connectedness and relationships with aggression and victimization. *Journal of School Health, 74*, 293–299.

Wolak, J., Mitchell, K. J., & Finkelhor, D. (2007). Does online harassment constitute bullying? An exploration of online harassment by known peers and online-only contacts. *Journal of Adolescent Health, 41*, S51–S58.

Wong, D. S., Chan, H. C. O., & Cheng, C. H. (2013). Cyberbullying perpetration and victimization among adolescents in Hong Kong. *Children and Youth Services Review, 36*, 133–140.

Xiao, B. S., & Wong, Y. M. (2013). Cyber-bullying among university students: An empirical investigation from the social cognitive perspective. *International Journal of Business and Information, 8*(1), 34–69.

Yang, S. J., Stewart, R., Kim, J. M., Kim, S. W., Shin, I. S., Dewey, M. E., …, & Yoon, J. S. (2013). Differences in predictors of traditional and cyber-bullying: A 2-year longitudinal study in Korean school children. *European Child & Adolescent Psychiatry, 22*(5), 309–318.

Preventing and Combating Internet Addiction: A Concept Review

Daniel T.L. Shek, Lu Yu, and Diego Busiol

Abstract The use of the Internet has brought a variety of conveniences to our modern life. Nonetheless, negative impacts are also created by addictive behavior to the Internet pervasively affecting one's academic and working performance, family life, social relationships, physical health, and psychological well-being. Internet addiction is becoming a serious problem across the world, especially for adolescents. In the past years, several studies have examined the prevalence of youth Internet addiction across cultures and will be presented in this chapter. Some studies suggest that Internet addictive behavior is not a transient phenomenon that naturally disappears as adolescents grow up; this implies that prevention might be essential for addressing this issue. Finally, it is difficult to say whether Internet addiction is a stand-alone problem or not, given that it does not exist independently but is associated with other manifestations, as presented here.

Introduction

The use of the Internet has brought a variety of conveniences to our modern life. Nonetheless, negative impacts are also created by addictive behavior to the Internet pervasively affecting one's academic and working performance, family life, social relationships, physical health, and psychological well-being (Kaltiala-Heino et al. 2004; Yen et al. 2007; Young and Rogers 1998). Although there are different views

The preparation for this work and the Project P.A.T.H.S. were financially supported by The Hong Kong Jockey Club Charities Trust.

This paper is based on an article originally published by The Scientific World Journal: Shek, D. T. L., & Yu, L. (2012). Internet addiction phenomenon in early adolescents in Hong Kong. *The Scientific World Journal, 2012.*

D.T.L. Shek (✉) • L. Yu
Department of Applied Social Sciences, The Hong Kong Polytechnic University,
11 Yuk Choi Road, Hung Hom, Kowloon, Hong Kong, China
e-mail: daniel.shek@polyu.edu.hk

D. Busiol
Department of Applied Social Sciences, City University of Hong Kong,
Kowloon, Hong Kong, China

© Springer Science+Business Media Singapore 2015   71
T.Y. Lee et al. (eds.), *Student Well-Being in Chinese Adolescents in Hong Kong,*
Quality of Life in Asia 7, DOI 10.1007/978-981-287-582-2_6

on the term, "Internet addiction" or "pathological use of the Internet" usually refers to the phenomenon that an individual is unable to control his or her use of the Internet (including any online-related, compulsive behavior) which eventually causes one's marked distress and functional impairment in daily life (Young 1999). Young (2009) identified five subtypes of Internet addiction:

1. Cybersexual Addiction: the most likely form of Internet abuse seen among clinics, especially with high relapse rates among sexual compulsives. Individuals typically are engaged in viewing, downloading, and trading online pornography or are involved in adult fantasy role-play chat rooms.
2. Cyber-Relational Addiction: online friends quickly become more important to the individual often at the expense of real-life relationships with family and friends. In many instances, this will lead to marital discord and family instability.
3. Net Compulsions: including obsessive online gambling, shopping, or stock trading behavior. Individuals will lose excessive amounts of money and even other job-related duties or significant relationships can be disrupted.
4. Information Overload: individuals will spend greater amounts of time searching for and collecting data from the web and organizing information. Obsessive-compulsive tendencies and reduced work productivity are typically associated with this behavior.
5. Computer Addiction: obsessive computer game playing.

With the soaring number of Internet users, it has been reported that Internet addiction is becoming a serious problem across the world, especially for adolescents. Scholars have also warned that Internet addiction could bring substantial loss of productivity in schools and companies where no Internet governance policies are implemented (Yellowlees and Marks 2007; Young and de Abreu 2010).

In the past years, several studies have examined the prevalence of youth Internet addiction, with the reported data varying across different areas of the world (Beard 2005). Lee et al. (2006) reported that 4 % of 627 Korean adolescent respondents could be classified as high-risk Internet users and 20.4 % potential risk Internet users. Furthermore, 28 % of adolescents from the high-risk user group did not recognize the degree of severity of Internet addiction, and another 24 % of them could not properly manage the amount of time playing online games. Another study conducted in Korea among high school students (Kim et al. 2006) found 1.6 % and 37.9 % of the 1,573 respondents to be Internet addicts and possible Internet addicts, respectively.

Even in different Chinese communities, prevalence findings of Internet addiction were inconsistent. For example, in Chou and Hsiao's study, 5.9 % of Taiwan college students were classified as having Internet addiction (2000), whereas Wu and Zhu reported that 10.6 % of university students in Mainland China could be identified as Internet addicts (2004). Whereas a study of high school students in Changsha showed a prevalence rate of 2.4 % (Cao and Su 2007), another study in Shanxi revealed that 6.44 % of first-year university students were addicted to the Internet. In Hong Kong, using Young's 20-item questionnaire to examine Internet addiction among youth, 61.4 % of senior primary school students, 35.2 % of Secondary 1–3 students, 18.8 % of Secondary 4–5 students, 35.8 % of Secondary 6–7 students, and 37.0 % of college students were identified as highly at risk of Internet addiction. There were also findings (Yang and Tung 2007) showing that 13.8 % of a sample of high school adolescents in Taiwan met the criterion of Internet addiction and were also found to have lower self-esteem, higher levels of depressed mood and feelings of sadness, poorer interpersonal relationships, and more negative self-concepts when compared with their nonaddicted counterparts. Another study conducted by Ko et al. (2007) in Taiwan reported that 18.18 % of 517 adolescent respondents were Internet addicts.

In Hong Kong, comparing results from two studies based on Young's eight-item questionnaire, Chan (2004) found that the prevalence of Internet addiction had increased from 3.0 % in 2000 to 14.7 % in 2002. One year later, Yip and Kwok (2005) using the modified Young's eight-item questionnaire found that 5.4 % of 1,182 adolescents were online game addicts. Leung (2004) investigated 699 adolescents and identified 37.9 % of them as Internet addicts. In another study, Shek and Tang (2008) estimated that approximately 20 % of the respondents from Hong Kong could be classified as Internet addicts. Surprisingly, using the same instrument and the same cut-off point (five or more than five symptoms), Fu et al. (2010) found a prevalence rate of Internet addiction of only 6.7 % among a population of 208 Hong Kong secondary school students (age 15–19). The authors suggest that such differences in findings might be attributable to a non-standardized instrument as well as the differences in respondents' demographic profiles or the mode of data collection and sampling method.

These inconsistent findings may be explained by several factors at the conceptual and methodological levels. First, various instruments for assessing Internet addiction were used. In Taiwan, researchers tended to use a 40-item Chinese Internet-Related Addictive Behavior Inventory to assess Internet addiction in adolescents (Tsuen Wan Centre 2004). However, Young's questionnaires were usually adopted by scholars in Mainland China and Hong Kong (Ni et al. 2009; Yang and Tung 2007). Second, inconsistent diagnostic criteria and cut-off scores were employed in different studies. Although most researchers followed Young's proposed cut-off (i.e., having four out of ten symptoms as the threshold of being classified as Internet addiction), other researchers used a higher cut-off score. Third, some prevalence studies were based on small and unrepresentative samples which limited the generalizability of the findings. Fourth, most of the existing studies utilized cross-sectional designs and thus cannot provide a complete understanding of how Internet addiction develops over time. These problems point to the urgent need to conduct methodologically sound research on youth Internet addiction, particularly in Chinese contexts, where few validated measures exist (Shek et al. 2008).

It has to be said that initially the Internet was a new phenomenon unknown to many clinicians, and its incidence and use was underestimated. Many practitioners simply could not understand the seduction of the Internet, tending to underestimate its growing importance, whereas others started considering the overuse of the Internet as necessarily pathological and a reflection of some inner psychological problem, a sign of incapacity/immaturity, a defense from the "outer" world, an alternative to "real life," or even an escape from negative evaluations and possible stress of interpersonal relationships (Chou et al. 1998; Young 2004). Internet addiction was found to be associated with subjective distress and social impairment (Shapira et al. 2000). Pratarelli et al. (1999) argued that increased Internet use was associated with feelings of isolation, which were mutually reinforcing. This first interpretation of the Internet was likely superficial and shortsighted. As the Internet is becoming more and more common and even pervasive, it is always more difficult to distinguish the time we spend being connected. Modern phones and tablets every day are becoming more powerful and more similar to small portable computers, so that we do not need to be at home or in the office to be connected. Particularly in cities like Hong Kong, we are always connected. So, the use of the Internet has deeply changed over the years, and it is hard to compare data from a few years ago with findings from the most up-to-date research, because technology and its use have changed dramatically. This can also explain the large variability that has been found in the occurrence rate (from 1.98 % to 35.8 %; see Aboujaoude et al. 2006; Niemz et al. 2005; Johansson and Götestam 2004) of Internet addiction among adolescents in Western and Eastern societies thought these years.

Persistence of the Addiction Over Time

Another important puzzle in Internet addiction research is whether an individual's tendency of displaying Internet addictive behavior remains the same or changes over time. On the one hand, some researchers claimed that Internet addiction is a short-term phenomenon, which gradually diminishes as time passes (Widyanto and McMurran 2004; Kraut et al. 1998). For example, Widyanto and McMurran (2004) proposed that Internet addiction is "a temporary phenomenon for some individuals, likely related to the initial novelty of the Internet and wearing off with increased familiarity" (p. 444). Young reported that over half of those self-identified as "Internet dependent" had been online for less than 1 year, suggesting that new users may be more inclined to develop addictive behavior associated with Internet use (Young 1998). In fact, more than two-thirds of "non-Internet-dependent" subjects in Young's study had been online for over a year, which seems to indicate that excessive use of the Internet could be a transient phenomenon that wears off over time in most individuals. There are also perspectives suggesting that real-life difficulties may contribute to Internet addiction because the Internet provides an escape for the individual from stressful life events (Armstrong et al. 2000). Once the problems in reality are solved, Internet addictive behavior would gradually taper off.

On the other hand, another school of thought and empirical studies support the stability and persistence of Internet addiction where pathological use of the Internet is believed to be associated with personality factors and other problems. In one study, individuals who were self-reliant, emotionally sensitive, reactive, vigilant, and nonconformist with low self-disclosure were found to be more likely to become

Internet dependent (Young and Rogers 1998). Amiel and Sargent found that the use of the Internet gave highly neurotic subjects a sense of belonging and made them feel informed, while extraverts tended to use the Internet for instrumental purposes (Amiel and Sargent 2004). The comorbidity of Internet addiction and other psychosocial problems provides extra support to expect stability in Internet addiction, although there is no consensus regarding whether Internet addiction should be considered a cause or effect. It was found that lonely individuals use the Internet more frequently and are more likely to use the Internet for emotional support than non-lonely people (Morahan-Martin and Schumacher 2003). All these findings seem to indicate the stability of Internet addiction tendency. However, the studies are severely limited by their cross-sectional design, which collected data only once and/or examined the stability of Internet addiction through retrospective recall techniques. Hence, such an approach can only provide a snapshot of Internet addiction. To determine whether Internet addictive behavior is temporary or stable among adolescents, longitudinal studies examining data across different time points are necessary.

Against the above background, a 3-year study on youth Internet addiction was conducted in Hong Kong (Yu and Shek 2013). There was found an occurrence rate of Internet addiction higher than previously reported prevalence data on Hong Kong adolescents by other researchers (Shek et al. 2008; Chan 2004). Although the percentage of students who were identified as having Internet addiction according to Young's criterion had reduced by roughly 4 % from Wave 1 to Wave 3 (26.4 %, 26.7 %, and 22.5 %), the authors concluded that still little behavior appeared to be stable over time and that Internet addictive behavior is not a transient phenomenon that naturally disappears as adolescents grow up.

Risk and Protective Factors and Psychological Consequences

It is difficult to say whether Internet addiction is a stand-alone problem or not, given that it does not exist independently but is associated with other manifestations like depressive symptoms (Ko et al. 2008), depression and insomnia (Cheung and Wong 2011), suicidal ideation (Fu et al. 2010), shyness (Chak and Leung 2004), low self-esteem (Steinfield et al. 2008), anxiety disorder (Caplan 2006), attention deficit disorder (Young 2008; Biederman 2005), and impulsivity (Cao et al. 2007). As such, a focus on a so-called Internet addiction only would hinder an understanding of the undergoing cause that provokes this behavior. According to Block (2008), about 86 % of Internet addiction cases have some other DSM-IV diagnosis.

Research of 2,433 First-year university students in Hong Kong (Kim et al. 2010) showed that heavy Internet use was significantly associated with being male, being an engineering student, being nonreligious, having lower parental educational attainment and younger age of residence in Hong Kong, and not having a romantic partner. In a study of 3,480 Taiwanese high school students (Yen et al. 2007), it was found that Internet addiction could be predicted by higher parent-adolescent conflict, habitual alcohol use by siblings, perceived parents' positive attitude to adolescents' substance use, and lower family function. Furthermore, results showed that the former three factors were also able to predict substance use, indicating a close similarity with Internet addiction. Another study of the same sample (Ko et al. 2006) confirmed similarities between the two groups of Internet-addicted and substance users; both groups were found to be high in regard to "novelty seeking" and low in relation to reward dependence (to social approval and sentiment), but interestingly, Internet addicts scored high for "harm avoidance" and drug users scored low.

In a study to test the validity and reliability of Young's Internet Addiction Test (IAT) for use with Hong Kong students in grades 5–9 (Ngai 2007), factor analysis revealed four factors: interference with family relationships, silence and withdrawal, overindulgence in online relationships, and tolerance and neglect of daily routines.

In several cases, adolescents were found to be aware of the negative impact of Internet addiction. A study of 1,716 secondary 1–3 students (Against Child Abuse 2004) showed that 37 % of the respondents "could not resist the attraction from being online" and 28.5 % of the respondents agreed that "online activities largely affected their normal daily lives." In another study (Akin 2012), highly Internet-addicted students were found to be low in subjective vitality and subjective happiness.

Youth Internet addictions reflect on their families and might generate further burdens. For example, it was found (Choi et al. 2005) that 14.5 % of 677 pairs of parent-child often had conflicts regarding the child's online problems. The same study highlighted that 17.1 % of adolescents who spent more than 6 hours online daily had difficulty in controlling their unstable emotions. Also the findings from Yu and Shek (2013) indicate that the characteristics of family relationships, communication, and mutuality among family members profoundly influence the development of youth's Internet addiction.

It has been noted that a great component of Internet usage is about making social relationships, particularly when speaking of massive multiuser online role-playing games or chat-rooms and messaging services (Young 2008). So, it is difficult to clearly differentiate when the Internet can be a resource and when it becomes a limitation for an individual.

References

Aboujaoude, E., Koran, L. M., Gamel, N., Large, M. D., & Serpe, R. T. (2006). Potential markers for problematic internet use: A telephone survey of 2,513 adults. *CNS Spectrums, 11*(10), 750–755.

Against Child Abuse. (2004). *The impacts of internet on junior secondary school students: A research report*. Hong Kong: Against Child Abuse.

Akın, A. (2012). The relationships between internet addiction, subjective vitality, and subjective happiness. *Cyberpsychology, Behavior, and Social Networking, 15*(8), 404–410.

Amiel, T., & Sargent, S. L. (2004). Individual differences in internet usage motives. *Computers in Human Behavior, 20*(6), 711–726.

Armstrong, L., Phillips, J. G., & Saling, L. L. (2000). Potential determinants of heavier internet usage. *International Journal of Human-Computer Studies, 53*(4), 537–550.

Beard, K. W. (2005). Internet addiction: A review of current assessment techniques and potential assessment questions. *Cyberpsychology & Behavior, 8*(1), 7–14.

Biederman, J. (2005). Attention-deficit/hyperactivity disorder: A selective overview. *Biological Psychiatry, 57*(11), 1215–1220.

Block, J. (2008). Issues for DSM-V: Internet addiction. *American Journal of Psychiatry, 165*(3), 306–307.

Cao, F., & Su, L. (2007). Internet addiction among Chinese adolescents: Prevalence and psychological features. *Child: Care, Health and Development, 33*(3), 275–281.

Cao, F. L., Su, L. Y., Liu, T., & Gao, X. (2007). The relationship between impulsivity and internet addiction in a sample of Chinese adolescents. *European Psychiatry, 22*(7), 466–471.

Caplan, S. E. (2006). Relations among loneliness, social anxiety, and problematic internet use. *Cyberpsychology & Behavior, 10*(2), 234–242.

Chak, K., & Leung, L. (2004). Shyness and locus of control as predictors of internet addiction and internet use. *Cyberpsychology & Behavior, 7*(5), 559–570.

Chan, T. C. F. (2004). Cyber risk of Hong Kong youngsters. *Journal of Youth Studies, 7*(2), 155–168.

Cheung, L. M., & Wong, W. S. (2011). The effects of insomnia and internet addiction on depression in Hong Kong Chinese adolescents: An exploratory cross sectional analysis. *Journal of Sleep Research, 20*(2), 311–317.

Choi, C. W., Wu, K. T., Zah, K. K., & Ying, C. W. (2005). *The impacts of internet on adolescents' family relationships and mental health: A research report*. Hong Kong: Hong Kong Family Welfare Society.

Chou, C., & Hsiao, M. C. (2000). Internet addiction, usage, gratification, and pleasure experience: The Taiwan college students' case. *Computers & Education, 35*(1), 65–80.

Chou, C., Chou, J., & Tyan, N. C. N. (1998). An exploratory study of internet addiction, usage and communication pleasure: The Taiwan's case. *International Journal of Educational Telecommunication, 5*(1), 47–64.

Fu, K. W., Chan, W. S., Wong, P. W., & Yip, P. S. (2010). Internet addiction: Prevalence, discriminant validity and correlates among adolescents in Hong Kong. *The British Journal of Psychiatry, 196*(6), 486–492.

Johansson, A., & Götestam, K. G. (2004). Internet addiction: Characteristics of a questionnaire and prevalence in Norwegian youth (12–18 years). *Scandinavian Journal of Psychology, 45*(3), 223–229.

Kaltiala-Heino, R., Lintonen, T., & Rimpelä, A. (2004). Internet addiction? Potentially problematic use of the internet in a population of 12–18 year-old adolescents. *Addiction Research & Theory, 12*(1), 89–96.

Kim, K., Ryu, E., Chon, M. Y., Yeun, E. J., Choi, S. Y., Seo, J. S., & Nam, B. W. (2006). Internet addiction in Korean adolescents and its relation to depression and suicidal ideation: A questionnaire survey. *International Journal of Nursing Studies, 43*(2), 185–192.

Kim, J. H., Lau, C. H., Cheuk, K. K., Kan, P., Hui, H. L., & Griffiths, S. M. (2010). Brief report: Predictors of heavy internet use and associations with health-promoting and health risk behaviors among Hong Kong university students. *Journal of Adolescence, 33*(1), 215–220.

Ko, C. H., Yen, J. Y., Chen, C. C., Chen, S. H., Wu, K., & Yen, C. F. (2006). Tridimensional personality of adolescents with internet addiction and substance use experience. *Canadian Journal of Psychiatry. Revue Canadienne de Psychiatrie, 51*(14), 887–894.

Ko, C. H., Yen, J. Y., Yen, C. F., Lin, H. C., & Yang, M. J. (2007). Factors predictive for incidence and remission of internet addiction in young adolescents: A prospective study. *Cyberpsychology & Behavior, 10*(4), 545–551.

Ko, C. H., Yen, J. Y., Chen, C. S., Chen, C. C., & Yen, C. F. (2008). Psychiatric comorbidity of internet addiction in college students: An interview study. CNS spectrums. *The International Journal of Neuropsychiatric Medicine, 13*(2), 147–153.

Kraut, R., Patterson, M., Lundmark, V., Kiesler, S., Mukophadhyay, T., & Scherlis, W. (1998). Internet paradox: A social technology that reduces social involvement and psychological well-being? *American Psychologist, 53*(9), 1017–1031.

Lee, M. S., Ko, Y. H., Song, H. S., Kwon, K. H., Lee, H. S., Nam, M., & Jung, I. K. (2006). Characteristics of internet use in relation to game genre in Korean adolescents. *Cyberpsychology & Behavior, 10*(2), 278–285.

Leung, L. (2004). Net-generation attributes and seductive properties of the internet as predictors of online activities and internet addiction. *Cyberpsychology & Behavior, 7*(3), 333–348.

Morahan-Martin, J., & Schumacher, P. (2003). Loneliness and social uses of the internet. *Computers in Human Behavior, 19*(6), 659–671.

Ngai, S. S. Y. (2007). Exploring the validity of the internet addiction test for students in grades 5–9 in Hong Kong. *International Journal of Adolescence and Youth, 13*(3), 221–237.

Ni, X., Yan, H., Chen, S., & Liu, Z. (2009). Factors influencing internet addiction in a sample of freshmen university students in China. *Cyberpsychology & Behavior, 12*(3), 327–330.

Niemz, K., Griffiths, M., & Banyard, P. (2005). Prevalence of pathological internet use among university students and correlations with self-esteem, the General Health Questionnaire (GHQ), and disinhibition. *Cyberpsychology & Behavior, 8*(6), 562–570.

Pratarelli, M. E., Browne, B. L., & Johnson, K. (1999). The bits and bytes of computer/internet addiction: A factor analytic approach. *Behavior Research Methods, Instruments, & Computers, 31*(2), 305–314.

Shapira, N. A., Goldsmith, T. D., Keck, P. E., Jr., Khosla, U. M., & McElroy, S. L. (2000). Psychiatric features of individuals with problematic internet use. *Journal of Affective Disorders, 57*(1), 267–272.

Shek, D. T. L., & Tang, M. Y. (2008). *Working group of @er.com: Youngster internet addiction prevention and counseling service: An evaluation study*. Hong Kong: Hong Kong Jockey Club.

Shek, D. T. L., Tang, V. M., & Lo, C. Y. (2008). Internet addiction in Chinese adolescents in Hong Kong: Assessment, profiles, and psychosocial correlates. *The Scientific World Journal, 8*, 776–787.

Steinfield, C., Ellison, N. B., & Lampe, C. (2008). Social capital, self-esteem, and use of online social network sites: A longitudinal analysis. *Journal of Applied Developmental Psychology, 29*(6), 434–445.

Tsuen Wan Centre. (2004). *Chinese YMCA of Hong Kong study on adolescents' internet using behaviors*. Hong Kong: Tsuen Wan Centre, Chinese YMCA of Hong Kong.

Widyanto, L., & McMurran, M. (2004). The psychometric properties of the internet addiction test. *Cyberpsychology & Behavior, 7*(4), 443–450.

Wu, H. R., & Zhu, K. J. (2004). Path analysis on related factors causing internet addiction disorder in college students. *Chinese Journal of Public Health, 20*(1363), 1363–1366.

Yang, S. C., & Tung, C. J. (2007). Comparison of internet addicts and non-addicts in Taiwanese high school. *Computers in Human Behavior, 23*(1), 79–96.

Yellowlees, P. M., & Marks, S. (2007). Problematic internet use or internet addiction? *Computers in Human Behavior, 23*(3), 1447–1453.

Yen, J. Y., Ko, C. H., Yen, C. F., Wu, H. Y., & Yang, M. J. (2007). The comorbid psychiatric symptoms of Internet addiction: Attention deficit and hyperactivity disorder (ADHD), depression, social phobia, and hostility. *Journal of Adolescent Health, 41*(1), 93–98.

Yip, W. S., & Kwok, Y. K. (2005). *Adolescents' computer using phenomena*. Hong Kong: Hong Kong Christian Service.

Young, K. S. (1998). Internet addiction: The emergence of a new clinical disorder. *Cyberpsychology & Behavior, 1*(3), 237–244.

Young, K. S. (1999). Internet addiction: Symptoms, evaluation and treatment. In L. Van de Creek & T. Jackson (Eds.), *Innovations in clinical practice: A source book* (Vol. 17, pp. 19–31). Sarasota: Professional Resource Press.

Young, K. S. (2004). Internet addiction: The consequences of a new clinical phenomena. In K. Doyle (Ed.), *Psychology and the new media* (pp. 1–14). Thousand Oaks: Sage.

Young, J. (2008). Common comorbidities seen in adolescents with attention-deficit/hyperactivity disorder. *Adolescent Medicine: State of the Art Reviews, 19*(2), 216–228.

Young, K. S. (2009). Internet addiction: Diagnosis and treatment considerations. *Journal of Contemporary Psychotherapy, 39*(4), 241–246.

Young, K. S., & de Abreu, C. N. (Eds.). (2010). *Internet addiction: A handbook and guide to evaluation and treatment*. New York: Wiley.

Young, K. S., & Rogers, R. C. (1998). The relationship between depression and internet addiction. *Cyberpsychology & Behavior, 1*(1), 25–28.

Yu, L., & Shek, D. T. L. (2013). Internet addiction in Hong Kong adolescents: A three-year longitudinal study. *Journal of Pediatric and Adolescent Gynecology, 26*(3), S10–S17.

Construction of a Conceptual Framework on Money Literacy

Tak Yan Lee, Ben M.F. Law, and Diego Busiol

Abstract The cultivation of a positive concept of money and success among adolescents is of paramount concern to parents, teachers, helping professionals, and policymakers. Indeed, recent research in Hong Kong showed that a large number of adolescents would consider using unethical or even unlawful means to get money. Young people's value judgments toward money are affected by the relationships between money and self-image, family relationships, one's life mission, and the social environment; these issues are critical for the development of measures that help prevent the phenomenon of an excessive materialistic orientation among adolescents and should be considered prior to the implementation of a money literacy program. In this chapter, the notion of financial education is reviewed in order to develop a conceptual framework for guiding preventive actions.

Materialistic Orientation as a Developmental Issue

Economic and social environments are changing at an ever-increasing pace in modern cities around the world. The money problems of any society range from generating enough work opportunities for various classes of people, providing access to opportunities to accumulate wealth, and helping our younger generations face other challenging issues involving money. With the rise of globalization, especially over

---

The preparation for this work and the Project P.A.T.H.S. were financially supported by The Hong Kong Jockey Club Charities Trust.

This paper is based on an article originally published by The Scientific World Journal: Lee, T. Y., & Law, M. F. (2011). Teaching money literacy in a positive youth development program: The project P.A.T.H.S. in Hong Kong. *The Scientific World Journal, 11*, 2287–2298.

T.Y. Lee (✉) • D. Busiol
Department of Applied Social Sciences, City University of Hong Kong,
Kowloon, Hong Kong, China
e-mail: ty.lee@cityu.edu.hk

B.M.F. Law
Department of Social Work and Social Administration,
The University of Hong Kong, Pok Fu Lam, Hong Kong, China

© Springer Science+Business Media Singapore 2015   81
T.Y. Lee et al. (eds.), *Student Well-Being in Chinese Adolescents in Hong Kong*,
Quality of Life in Asia 7, DOI 10.1007/978-981-287-582-2_7

the last two decades, aspects of the money problem appear as (i) gaining money for survival, (ii) equitable distribution among different classes, and (iii) materialism or hyperconsumption. For example, a national poll in the United States found that 53 % of teens said that buying certain products makes them feel better about themselves (New American Dream 2002).

The Trend of the Money Problem

Apart from studying adolescents' and youth's financial knowledge – studies in Hong Kong focused on investigating their value judgments toward money and success, covering topics on the relationships between money and self-image, family relationships, clarifying one's life mission, and so forth – Law (1985) stated that young people's value judgments toward money were affected by the social environment. Studies have also confirmed that the less conservative saving habits of adolescents have roots in their parents' behavior (Chinese Young Men's Christian Association 2002; Hong Kong Federation of Youth Groups 1995). A survey found that as high as 34.3 % of Grade 7–9 students wished to find quick ways to get money to the extent that they would ignore the negative consequences of the way they chose to earn the money (Hong Kong Federation of Youth Groups 2007). Most worrisome is that one third of the adolescents would consider using unethical or even unlawful means to get money. In a survey of 586 children and youth aged 12–20, 34 % of the respondents indicated that they would consider offering compensated dating (serving as a companion of whoever who will give them money or luxury gifts), and 57 % of these respondents opined that they would do it in order to earn quick money (Hong Kong Christian Service 2009). A recent study of 98 young people under the age of 18 who had engaged in compensated dating showed that 16.8 % of them had engaged in prostitution or compensated dating involving sexual relationships (Cheung et al. 2011).

The Concept of Success

According to the Encyclopedia Britannica (2011), the definitions of success are (1) outcome and result; (2) a degree or measure of succeeding: favorable or desired outcome and the attainment of wealth, favor, or eminence; and (3) one that succeeds. Chinese parents usually expect their children to show obedience, proper behavior, and good academic results (Ho 1986) because they believe that outstanding examination results will lead to better job opportunities and better pay. Their concept of success is quite instrumental and often materialistic. Parental influences on the development of the concept of money and success in adolescents are reflected in a number of surveys on the most desired outcomes of youths. Good academic results, outstanding sports performance, and harmonious family relationships receive the top rankings (Hong Kong Federation of Youth Groups 1997, 2000, 2009; Law 1985). Although about half (Law 1985) to 77 % (Hong Kong Federation of Youth Groups 2009) of teenage respondents do not agree, about 20–30 % of the respondents view money as the only criterion for measuring success.

Results from a recent survey among students from six secondary schools showed that half of the teenage respondents agreed that "with money, they will have a better future" and "money can buy happiness." Only about 80 % of respondents agreed that they will not break the law for money (H.K.S.K.H. Kowloon City Children and Youth Integrated Service – Jockey Club Youth Express 2007). Another survey found that 11 % of teenagers opined that success depends on luck instead of personal efforts (Hong Kong Federation of Youth Groups and Hong Kong Independent Commission against Corruption 2000). This disturbing figure was attributed to the sudden growth of gambling through the internet in that period of time.

Adolescents' conception of success can change as a result of social change. For example, after the financial tsunami in 2008, over 77.4 % of youths opined that earning quick money does not mean success (Hong Kong Federation of Youth Groups 2009). The above studies showed that teenagers' view toward money and success may change depending on the social and economic environment. Therefore, education and preventive measures are important for adolescents, helping them to form responsible values and independent thinking on issues related to money and success.

To most adolescents living in modern cities, one of the challenges is how to cultivate proper attitudes toward money and success and to make responsible decisions to guide their behavior regarding money. A pressing question arising from the rapid changes in the global economy is how to ensure that children and adolescents are prepared in terms of having the competencies to survive and develop in the pervasive transformations of the information or network society (Al-Hawamdeh and Hart 2002; Castells 2011; Hassan 2008; Webster 2006). The cultivation of a positive concept of money and success is of paramount concern to parents, teachers, helping professionals, and policymakers. Against this background, the notion of financial education is reviewed in order to develop a conceptual framework for guiding preventive actions.

Money Literacy: A Framework for Action

Bannister and Monsma (1982) suggest that financial education aims at enhancing people's knowledge in financial matters and their ability to make wise financial decisions. The US Financial Literacy and Education Commission (United States Financial Literacy and Education Commission 2006) adopted a similar definition of financial education. Brenneke (1981) focused on other concerns, such as understanding real needs, social participation, social responsibilities, being responsible for the natural environment, and the solidarity of consumers. Recent efforts in financial education in schools generally adopt a combination of these two different views. The Ministry of Finance of the Czech Republic (2007) defines financial literacy as a necessary competency for dealing with money in both its cash and noncash forms, monetary transactions, and the instruments used with money (e.g., bank accounts, payment tools, etc.). Financial education, according to Mandell (2008), moves beyond a narrow definition of financial knowledge to financial capability. Law (1985) studied the subjective ways by which young people give meaning to the concept of money, coming up with eight dimensions using factor analysis: (a) money as a symbolic meaning of power, (b) money as a symbolic meaning of good or bad, (c) exchange power of money, (d) cautious use of money, (e) trouble encountered due to money, (f) desire to gain money, (g) money as the criterion to determine success or failure, and (h) sense of satisfaction arising from money. Such a comprehensive view of the concepts of money and success offers a systematic way of understanding and analysis, avoids overly technical conceptualizations, and fits the need for value clarification in relation to money and success among children and adolescents in the local cultural context.

A narrow definition of financial education should be adopted when introducing money issues to adolescents. The term money literacy should be chosen in order to exclude the more complicated financial knowledge, skills, and strategies that young adults should later also possess. As a result of the review, a working definition of money literacy for adolescents is proposed. It incorporates a set of perspectives that adolescents actively use to expose themselves to the world and to interpret the meaning and values behind money-related messages that they encounter.

The concept of money literacy is multidimensional and can be grouped into cognitive, value judgment, affective, and behavioral domains (Magnavita 2002; Nucci 2001). The cognitive domain emphasizes knowledge and critical thinking related to money. It covers the exchange power of money, the desire to gain money, and money as the criterion to determine success or failure. The value judgment domain emphasizes one's personal value judgment of money based on personal experiences. It includes money as a symbolic meaning of power and money as a symbolic meaning of good or bad. The affective domain covers all the emotional responses prompted by money and success. It contains troubles encountered due to money and a sense of satisfaction arising from money. Finally, the behavioral domain involves actual behavior in relation to money and the notion of success. The only dimension is cautious use of money.

A Typology of Money Literacy

Money literacy is not a category; it is best regarded as a continuum. There is no point below which we could say that someone has no literacy, and there is no point at the high end where we can claim that we are fully literate. Inspired by Potter's (2011) work on media literacy and taking into consideration the developmental and cultural characteristics, the following six components are proposed in the typology of money literacy. They are (i) narrative acquisition, (ii) cultivation of traditional values, (iii) developing skepticism, (iv) experiential exploring, (v) critical appreciation, and (vi) social responsibility. The first three components can be classified as a foundation level and the rest as an advanced level. While the foundation level involves largely the cognitive and value judgment domains, the advanced level requires continual use of practical knowledge and skills in the cognitive, value judgment, affective, and behavioral domains (see Table 1). Descriptions of these six components are provided below.

Narrative acquisition aims at helping children and adolescents develop an understanding of the differences between wants and needs. The desire to gain money is the major component, and it involves mainly the cognitive domain. It helps differentiate their "feelings" from "reality."

Table 1 Framework on money literacy for children and adolescents

Levels of components	Name of components	Major contents	Relevant dimensions
Foundation level	Narrative acquisition	Develop an understanding of the differences between needs and wants; learn the biopsychosocial needs of human beings at different stages	Desire to gain money (cognitive domain); money as a symbolic meaning of power (cognitive domain)
	Cultivation of traditional values	Differentiate values of money, success, wealth, beauty, power, sex, self-worth, and self-esteem	Money as a symbolic meaning of good or bad (value judgment domain)
	Developing skepticism	Discount claims made in ads and assertions; dispute beliefs about hedonism and materialism	Exchange power of money (cognitive domain)
Advanced level	Experiential exploring	Search for gratification and fulfillment from new emotional, moral, aesthetic, and sports experiences	Trouble encountered due to money (cognitive and affective domains); sense of satisfaction arising from money (affective domain)
	Critical appreciation	Develop the ability to make subtle comparisons and contrasts among different beliefs and behavior about money, wealth, success, beauty, power, sex, self-worth, and self-esteem; develop a moral perspective that certain beliefs and behavior are more constructive to society than others	Money as the criterion to determine success or failure (cognitive and affective domains)
	Social responsibility	Recognize that one's own individual decisions and behavior affect oneself, peers, family, and society; recognize that there are actions that an individual can take to make a more constructive impact on society	Cautious use of money (cognitive domain, value judgment domain, affective and behavioral domains)

Cultivation of traditional values helps adolescents understand the biopsychosocial needs of human beings at different developmental stages and clarify their own values about money, success, wealth, beauty, power, sex, self-worth, and self-esteem. Two dimensions are involved in this component. They are money as a symbolic meaning of power and as a symbolic meaning of good or bad. Both involve the value judgment domain. This component also helps adolescents clarify their personal values with regard to money and success.

Developing skepticism functions by generating disputes in relation to the beliefs of hedonism and materialism. The exchange power of money is the relevant component engaged from the cognitive domain. This helps children and adolescents think critically about the concepts of money and success.

Experiential exploring focuses on exploring new gratification experiences. A sense of satisfaction arising from money and difficulties encountered due to money are the two components which involve both the cognitive and affective domains. Children and adolescents are encouraged to examine the satisfaction brought by the use of money and compare these to the gratifications brought by new experiences including emotional, moral, aesthetic, and sports experiences.

Critical appreciation aims to develop adolescents' ability to make comparisons among different beliefs and behavior about money, success, beauty, power, sex, self-worth, and self-esteem. The component of "money as the criterion to determine success or failure" is involved, and it requires both skills and knowledge from the cognitive and affective domains.

The component of *social responsibility* aims to help adolescents develop a moral perspective in relation to beliefs and behavior that are more constructive to society. It also helps adolescents recognize that their own decisions and behavior affect self, peers, family, and society. Their actions can have a constructive impact on society. Cautious use of money is the component, and it involves all of the four domains.

Toward the Operationalization of the Money Literacy Framework

Several issues are critical for the development of measures that help prevent the phenomenon of an excessive materialistic orientation among adolescents and should be considered prior to the implementation of a money literacy program.

First of all, children and adolescents are routinely exposed to materialistic and hedonistic ideas, concepts, goods, values, and beliefs through the mass media, information and communication technologies (ICTs), interactions with peers, and even from their own families. However, although we may design and promote financial education among children and adolescents through all sorts of educational and prevention programs, such programs cannot usually reach every child.

Secondly, even though the inclusion of money literacy components in the extensive phase of the project is deemed necessary, the program is unlikely to influence parents with excessively materialistic and hedonistic orientations. The effects of parental influence cannot be tackled or reduced in the curriculum units designed for students, since students usually cannot change their parents' attitudes. Special training in teaching skills will have to be provided for teachers who may encounter students who come from such families and feel puzzled about the conflict in values.

Thirdly, one common strategy for financial education among children is learning to make decisions about products, but its effect is uncertain because this kind of comparative analysis requires a proper conceptual framework. For example, Schor (2004) disputes the argument that this will empower children. She wrote "If a kid buys a pair of Nike shoes and feels better about himself or herself because of them, then Nike's ads may enhance self-esteem. But the messages are a double-edged sword because they also do the reverse, undermining self-worth" (p. 179).

Fourthly, research findings have shown that there are age and gender differences in relation to the concepts of money and success. For age differences, higher-grade students place a higher value on money than do lower-grade students (Law 1985; Leung and Cheung 2000). They also have a higher tendency to use credit cards and money in advance, engaging in impulsive buying and value finding a job with higher status (Hong Kong Federation of Youth Groups 1999; Lin and Lin 2004; Lupart et al. 2004). For gender differences, studies have found that males more frequently excessively value money, rating "to be paid well" and "earn a great deal of money" highly compared to females. On the other hand, females show more concern for human relationships and contributions to society than males (Hong Kong Federation of Youth Groups 1999). In designing the units for money literacy, age and gender differences should be taken into consideration.

References

Al-Hawamdeh, S., & Hart, T. L. (2002). *Information and knowledge society*. Singapore: McGraw-Hill.

Bannister, R., & Monsma, C. (1982). *The classification of concepts in consumer education* [Monograph 137]. Cincinnati: South-Western Publishing.

Brenneke, J. S. (1981). *Integrating consumer and economic education into the school curriculum*. New York: Joint Council on Economic Education.

Castells, M. (2011). *The rise of the network society*. Cambridge, MA: Blackwell Publishers.

Cheung, J. C. K., Lee, T. Y., & Li, J. C. M. (2011). *Family-Centered prevention of adolescent girls' and boys' prostitution*. Final Report Submitted to the Central Policy Unit, Government of the Hong Kong Special Administrative Region. H.K. Social Capital and Impact Assessment Research Unit and Department of Applied Social Studies, City University of Hong Kong, Hong Kong.

Chinese Young Men's Christian Association. (2002). *Youngsters' consumption behavior: a comparative study of Guangzhou, Hong Kong, and Macau* (in Chinese). Retrieved from http://www.ymca.org.hk/eng/images/research/20020400.pdf

Encyclopedia Britannica. (2011). *Definition of success*. Retrieved from http://www.merriam-webster.com/dictionary/success?show=0&t=1306808861

H.K.S.K.H. Kowloon City Children and Youth Integrated Service – Jockey Club Youth Express. (2007). Adolescents' money management and consumption behavior. In K. Chan (Ed.), *Youth and consumption* (pp. 17–19). Hong Kong: City University Press.

Hassan, R. (2008). *The information society: Cyber dreams and digital nightmares*. Malden: Polity.

Ho, D. Y. (1986). Chinese patterns of socialization: A critical review. In M. H. Bond (Ed.), *The psychology of the Chinese people* (pp. 1–37). New York: Oxford University Press.

Hong Kong Christian Service. (2009). *Press release on youth's opinion of the "compensated dating" survey*. Retrieved from http://www.hkcs.org

Hong Kong Federation of Youth Groups. (1995). *How do adolescents and youth view about saving?* (in Chinese). Retrieved from http://yrc.hkfyg.org.hk/eng/p30.html

Hong Kong Federation of Youth Groups. (1997). *Young people's outlook on life*. Retrieved from http://yrc.hkfyg.org.hk/eng/p41.html

Hong Kong Federation of Youth Groups. (1999). *How youths' view on spending money in advance?* Retrieved from http://yrc.hkfyg.org.hk/eng/p70.html

Hong Kong Federation of Youth Groups. (2000). *The views of teenagers on success and failure*. Retrieved from http://yrc.hkfyg.org.hk/eng/p83.html

Hong Kong Federation of Youth Groups. (2007). *How do adolescents and youth view about "quick money"?* Retrieved from http://yrc.hkfyg.org.hk/eng/p159.html

Hong Kong Federation of Youth Groups. (2009). *The effects of the financial tsunami on young people's views towards money and career*. Retrieved from http://yrc.hkfyg.org.hk/eng/p183.html

Hong Kong Federation of Youth Groups and Hong Kong Independent Commission against Corruption. (2000). *Young people's outlook on life (II)*. Retrieved from http://yrc.hkfyg.org.hk/eng/p78.html

Law, C. K. (1985). *Money and life: Survey research report*. Hong Kong: Federation of Youth Groups.

Leung, S. Y., & Cheung, S. K. (2000). *Opinion survey on the view of money among grade 1 to 10 students in Hong Kong*. Retrieved from http://www.breakthrough.org.hk/ir/youthdatabank/cv/cv03.htm#E3-324

Lin, C. H., & Lin, H. M. (2004). An exploration of Taiwanese adolescents' impulsive buying tendency. *Adolescence, 40*(157), 215–223.

Lupart, J. L., Cannon, E., & Telfer, J. A. (2004). Gender differences in adolescent academic achievement, interests, values and life-role expectations. *High Ability Studies, 15*(1), 25–42.

Magnavita, J. J. (2002). *Theories of personality: Contemporary approaches to the science of personality*. New York: Wiley.

Mandell, L. (2008). Financial education in high school. In A. Lusardi (Ed.), *Overcoming the saving slump: How to increase the effectiveness of financial education and saving programs* (pp. 257–279). Chicago: University of Chicago Press.

Ministry of Finance of the Czech Republic. (2007). *Financial education strategy: In keeping with the conceptual material created by the ministry of finance*. Retrieved from http://www.mfcr.cz/cps/rde/xbcr/mfcr/Financial Education Strategy.pdf

New American Dream. (2002). Thanks to ads, kids won't take no, no, no, no, no, no, no, no, no, for an answer. http://www.newdream.org/kids/poll.php.

Nucci, L. P. (2001). *Education in the moral domain*. Cambridge, UK: Cambridge University Press.

Potter, W. J. (2011). *Media literacy*. Thousand Oaks: Sage.

Schor, J. (2004). *Born to buy: The commercialized child and the new consumer culture*. New York: Simon and Schuster.

United States Financial Literacy and Education Commission. (2006). *Taking ownership of the future: The national strategy for financial literacy*. Retrieved from http://205.168.45.52/sites/default/files/downloads/ownership.pdf

Webster, F. (2006). *Theories of the information society*. New York: Routledge.

Promotion of Bonding Among Peers

Diego Busiol and Tak Yan Lee

Abstract Bonding is the emotional attachment and commitment an individual makes to social relationships with parents, siblings, peers, school, teachers, schoolmates, partners, community, and culture. The quality of bonding greatly affects one's self-esteem/self-efficacy, academic achievements, and life satisfaction. Promotion of bonding and development of healthy relations have proven to be an effective intervention for adolescents at risk. However, even though the need for bonding among peers might be universal, nevertheless it is likely influenced by social, cultural, and historical factors and thus might change over time and across cultures and societies. Some differences about the conception of friendship among Chinese and Western cultures will be highlighted in this chapter, as well as the clinical relevance of this concept.

Introduction

Bonding is the emotional attachment and commitment an individual makes to social relationships with parents, siblings, peers, school, teachers, schoolmates, partners, community, and culture (Catalano et al. 2004a; Lee and Lok 2012). The first interaction of a child is normally with his/her mother, father, and caregivers. How a child establishes bonds in these early relations will affect the manner in which she/he later bonds to others, his/her sense of trust in self and others, and the overall quality of his/her development. Thus, the importance of bonding goes far beyond the family (Catalano et al. 2004a); as Mesch (2009) writes, "acceptance of social norms and the development of social consciousness depend on attachment to significant others, in particular family and school, which are seen as central social institutions" (p. 605). The quality of bonding greatly affects self-esteem/self-efficacy, academic achievements, and life satisfaction (Catalano et al. 2004b; Maddox and Prinz 2003). Promotion of bonding has proven to be an effective intervention for adolescents at

The preparation for this work and the Project P.A.T.H.S. were financially supported by The Hong Kong Jockey Club Charities Trust.

D. Busiol • T.Y. Lee (✉)
Department of Applied Social Sciences, City University of Hong Kong,
Kowloon, Hong Kong, China
e-mail: ty.lee@cityu.edu.hk

© Springer Science+Business Media Singapore 2015   89
T.Y. Lee et al. (eds.), *Student Well-Being in Chinese Adolescents in Hong Kong*,
Quality of Life in Asia 7, DOI 10.1007/978-981-287-582-2_8

risk of antisocial behavior (Caplan et al. 1992; Simons-Morton et al. 1999), pornography consumption (Mesch 2009), and substance abuse (Maddox and Prinz 2003; Akers and Lee 1999).

Friendship describes just one kind of bonding that normally occurs among peers. Healthy relations can have a positive impact on one's life; however, friendship is more complex than it seems, and it is not always easy to distinguish it from kinship and loving relationships. In addition, bonding among peers is likely influenced by social, cultural, and historical factors and thus might change over time and across cultures and societies.

What Is Friendship?

In his *Nicomachean Ethics*, Aristotle (384–322 BC) stated that people are social beings, and thus they require friends in order to be happy. He defines genuine friendship as that in which two people have mutual goodwill toward each other, are aware of it, and appreciate the goodwill of the other. Then, he distinguishes three types of friendship, "wherein affection for the other is based on (a) *utility* of the other to oneself, (b) *pleasure* that the other provides to oneself, and (c) *virtuous caring* for the other in a more enduring sense" (Prus 2007, p. 29). For Aristotle, the latter is the best kind of friendship, the more genuine, and likely the longer lasting. He also speculated that friendship normally occurs among equals and that among the young is more likely based on pleasure, whereas friendship among the elderly is often based on utility. For Montaigne (1533–1592), friendship is characterized by two essential criteria: forgiveness and generosity (Thompson 1998). Friends normally tend not to condemn the other for his/her faults; a friend is one who gives to the other in a way that nobody else is willing or able to, without expecting anything back. A well-known saying states that "you can choose your friends, but you can't choose your family." However, Grey and Sturdy (2007) observe that it would be too naive to understand friendship merely in terms of an individual choice. Instead, they suggest that friendship is based on some sort of shared interests. For instance, two persons might share some hobby, and this might lead them to find some affinity (they identify in one another), or they can share some common goal or a set of concerns and aims (identification of an external and higher scope). In the latter case, the relation has a more structural accent.

Is Friendship the Same Everywhere?

According to the literature (Krappmann 1996), despite differences in societies in terms of how individuals relate to each other (more or less interdependent, more self-oriented, or more other oriented), children from different places tend to consider friendship in a similar way, as a supportive and intimate relationship. Results from a comparative study on Canadian and Taiwanese school students (Benjamin et al. 2001) showed no significant differences in the positive features of friendships (help, security, and closeness) between the two groups. However, the authors noted that in Taiwan, the presence of conflict significantly predicted less positive friendship quality, and they concluded that this reflected a more general cultural inhibition to express conflict in Chinese culture. Not only did Taiwanese children display less conflict in their relations than the Canadian sample, but they also reported higher agreement regarding the presence of conflict in the friendship relationship. Knapp (1978) suggested a model of interpersonal relationship development in five stages: (a) initiating, (b) experimenting, (c) intensifying, (d) integrating, and (e) bonding. Cross-cultural research on children and young adults (Keller 2004a) showed that both Western and Chinese respondents generally follow a similar path to friendship, which can be divided into four levels: (1) playing and sharing, (2) helping and supporting, (3) trust and intimacy, and (4) autonomy and integration. However, it was found that the Chinese emphasized the moral quality of close friendship and the connection of friendship and society more than Westerners, who instead focused more on interaction qualities, promise keeping, and relationship intimacy (Keller 2004b).

Culture, societal structure, and communication largely reflect on development of bonding. Chinese have been described as high context, collectivistic, interdependent, and homogeneous, whereas, for example, Americans have been referred to as low context, individualistic, independent, and heterogeneous (Gudykunst et al. 1988; Yang et al. 2011). Hong Kong Chinese culture is traditionally other oriented, although economic development, modernization, and exposure to Western values might have altered such disposition. Social relationships are essential in the Chinese context, more than communication. Preserving harmony is more important than expressing oneself, so that much can remain untold. This is why, contrary to Western cultures, in Hong Kong, communication can be meaningless outside the context of social relationships; when speaking, appropriateness is more important than effectiveness (Yeh 2010). The Chinese generally have a negative understanding of communication, as persuasive behavior finalized to establish utilitarian relations (Yeh 2010). The ritual of gift giving occurs in all societies and serves to promote ties and bonding between individuals. The act of gift giving reflects one's self- and other orientation, and thus it varies largely across cultures. Observing gift giving behavior in Hong Kong, Joy (2001) could provide some significant hints on bonding in different interpersonal relationships. She distinguished five categories: (1) family relations, which are asymmetrical and not based on reciprocity; the hierarchy is maintained; (2) romantic relationships; (3) close friends (*yihhei*), who are in most cases treated as family members, so that gift giving is not driven by feelings of obligation; (4) good friends and *renqing*, where the obligation to repay and not be in debt prevail, and reciprocity and equivalence are sought; and (5) just friends/hi-bye friends and *guanxi*, which are relations driven mainly by calculation and intention of developing networks. Further evidence suggests that family and friends are two qualitatively different groups that should be examined separately. Li (2002) compared Anglo-Canadians and Mainland Chinese regarding how they build relationships with family members and friends. Results reported strong cultural differences in self-family connectedness, but not in self-friends connectedness; Chinese were closer to their family members than Canadians (no gender difference was found), whereas the latter were as close to their friends as Chinese. Furthermore, Chinese males were found to be closer to their friends than females, whereas Canadian males reported a more independent relationship with their best friend than Canadian females. Javidi and Javidi (1991) compared Western (mainly referring to the United States) and Eastern (mainly Chinese and Japanese) cultures and suggested that "the direction of interpersonal communication in the process of forming interpersonal bonding is distinctly unique in each of these two cultures" (p. 130). For instance, in most Western cultures, interpersonal communication occurs on the horizontal axis, whereas in Chinese cultures it occurs on the vertical axis. Furthermore, they identified several categories of values that concur in developing interpersonal bonding and friendship:

1. *Self-concept* versus *group concept*: Americans emphasize their self-concept in terms of self-awareness, self-image, self-esteem, self-identity, self-reliance, self-actualization, self-expression, and self-determination; people are assumed to be more independent and to be relatively freer to decide who they want to become. Instead, in Chinese culture people are more interdependent and the self-concept is not as significant in the process of interpersonal bonding; people's goals and behavior are congenial to maintaining affiliations in the group and developing social relations.
2. *Doing* versus *being*: Chinese culture is more hierarchical than many European and American cultures. In such "vertical" society, "who a person is" (where a person comes from, what his/her background is) is more important than "what a person does."
3. *Equality* versus *inequality*: In horizontal cultures, people believe that all are created equal. In contrast, in vertical cultures interpersonal relations and communication are structured according to status; individuals are concerned with whom to talk to, when, and how. Interestingly, in vertical cultures individuals are more likely attracted to same-sex friendships.
4. *Uncertainty reduction*: In cultures that are horizontal, heterogeneous, individualistic, and loose, low-context communication is more likely to occur. On the contrary, in cultures that are vertical, homogeneous, collectivistic, and tight, high-context communication is the standard. Different cultures have different strategies for reducing uncertainty in communication and increase the predictability of others' behavior: (1) Members of low-context cultures reduce their uncertainties by utilizing more oral (explicit) means than members of high-context cultures; (2) members of high-context cultures are interested in gathering background information (hometown, school attended, occupation, income) because this increases the accuracy in predicting others' future behavior. The same does not happen in Western cultures, where instead people might be more interested in gathering information about attitudes and values (about food, hobbies, political orientation, favorite movies, etc.), and (3) people from low-context

cultures tend to value at most and encourage self-disclosure, whereas people from Eastern cultures tend to keep their self private.

5. *Common interest* versus *acceptance*: In Western cultures, relationships are formed primarily around activities (work, school, leisure) and thus remain relatively more compartmentalized and impermanent; a relation is healthy when it serves the expected activity for each party. Instead, friendships in most Eastern cultures are relatively more stable over time; rather than on activities, relationships are based on mutual liking and a full acceptance of the other person (close friends become brothers or sisters) and are often expected to last for life.

Because social values inherent in Chinese societies are different, and sometimes opposite, to social values in European and North American countries, it is likely that the socialization of Chinese children differs greatly. For instance, Chinese children are normally required to learn self-control, to develop an interdependent sense of sense, and to engage in cooperative and prosocial behavior (Chen et al. 2000). This might explain why shyness sensitivity in primary school kids is often associated with acceptance by peers in China, whereas inhibited children are frequently victimized in Western societies. Schwartz et al. (2001) found that peer victimization among Chinese children was associated with poor academic functioning, submissive-withdrawal behavior, aggression, and low levels of assertive-prosocial behavior. Although this partially overlaps previous findings from Western cultural settings, the authors claim that some form of behavioral inhibition might be adaptive in a Chinese context. For example, they notice that "a shy disposition could function to facilitate interdependent functioning within the group social context. In contrast, more overtly withdrawn behaviors, by definition, decrease interaction with peers and might be incompatible with a collectivistic orientation" (p. 528). Similar findings were reported by Chang et al. (2005), who examined a sample of 377 Hong Kong secondary school students and found that, as observed in Western cultural settings, social withdrawal negatively predicted peer acceptance and self-perceived social competency. Furthermore, because communication avoidance in Western contexts is sometimes interpreted as an unwillingness to communicate, the authors tested how this attitude could affect socialization in Hong Kong. Usually, communication avoidance is negatively related to peer acceptance in Western societies that base communication primarily on oral means. However, findings from this research showed that communication avoidance in Hong Kong was predictive only of self-perceived social competence but not of peer acceptance.

Friendship in Hong Kong

It is often reported that Chinese limit their social sharing of personal experiences to family members (Chow et al. 2007); although this might be true in Mainland China, it might not be the case of Hong Kong. Results from a study of 292 respondents from Hong Kong (Chow et al. 2007) showed that 90 % did share their bereavement experiences with others, and in most cases these persons were best friends, siblings, and professionals. In another studies on counseling preferences among Hong Kong university students (Busiol 2015), non-family members like close friends and professionals were often indicated as a first choice when seeking help. The influence of peers and parents on youth life satisfaction was assessed based on data from 1,906 secondary school students in Hong Kong (Man 1991). The results showed that parent orientation was the better predictor of youth's life satisfaction, surpassing peer orientation. Furthermore, it was found that adolescents with lower peer orientation reported higher satisfaction with family life, whereas those with higher peer orientation gained more satisfaction from school, media, and acceptance by others. These findings were interpreted as adolescents with higher levels of peer identification not necessarily being happy with every aspect of their lives. Friend intimacy is an important variable that affects some aspects of psychosocial adjustment. In a study of 289 Hong Kong students between 16 and 19 years of age (Chou 2000), consistent with previous findings in Western societies, it was found that friend intimacy was positively associated with self-esteem and purpose in life; however, friend intimacy was negatively correlated with deviant behavior. Self-esteem among Hong Kong students was positively related to three dimensions of friend intimacy: giving/sharing (giving support to a friend), imposition (obligations imposed on a friend), and common activities (participating in common activities with a friend). On the contrary, deviant behavior was negatively associated with frankness/spontaneity, giving/sharing, and trust/loyalty. Researchers investigated the characteristics of the ideal best friends in a sample of 215 girls and 215 boys from Hong Kong (Cheng et al. 1995). The dimensions considered in the study included emotional stability, extraversion, application, openness to experience, assertiveness, restraint, helpfulness, and intellect. The results showed that ideal female best friends were rated higher on helpfulness, whereas ideal male best friends were rated higher on extraversion, assertiveness, and application. Furthermore, ideal best friends were expected to be similar in openness to experience and complimentary in assertiveness. The researchers interpreted this as proof that Hong Kong Chinese adolescents are particularly sensitive to matching attitudes (thus maintaining harmony) and avoiding conflicts of opinion. This might also help to understand why the social networks are gaining so much relevance in Hong Kong and why several youth are partially withdrawing from socializing. Research conducted in Hong Kong among 162 Internet users compared the qualities of online and offline friendships. Offline friendships involved more interdependence, breadth, depth, code change, understanding, commitment, and network convergence than online friendships (Chan and Cheng 2004).

Clinical Relevance of Bonding with Peers

On one hand peers provide companionship, stimulation, physical support, ego support, and intimacy (Gottman and Parker 1987; Parker and Gottman 1989). Adolescents having friendships with more positive features reported having greater involvement in school and higher self-perceived social acceptance (Berndt 2002).

On the other hand, some studies reported the negative aspects of "peer pressure" or peer influence on adolescents (Berndt 1996; Millstein et al. 1993), including being excluded or rejected by peers, victimized by bullies, dumped by romantic partners, and detested by enemies. Social learning theory and primary socialization theory, as summarized by Kobus (2003), suggest that peer relationships can be negative if the adolescent learns and acquires negative behavior from their friends, for example, smoking and substance abuse. However, Bauman and Ennett (1996) concluded that the peer influence on drug use is exaggerated. Instead, attachment to a peer group can help adolescents avoid the problem of alienation (Hurrelmann and Engel 1992), and interventions have successfully used the positive aspects of peer relationships to benefit delinquent youth (Kuchuck 1993). Crosnoe and Needham (2004) also found that adolescents with high-achieving friends in schools and high levels of bonding had the least behavioral problems. They add "in the adolescence stage, friendships enable adolescents to meet a key developmental task establishing their own lives independent from their families by helping them develop identities, test conventional boundaries, and gain autonomy" (p. 265). In conclusion, peers may push each other toward risks and delinquent behavior or help each other develop positively (Brown et al. 1986; Giordano et al. 1986).

References

Akers, R. L., & Lee, G. (1999). Age, social learning, and social bonding in adolescent substance use. *Deviant Behavior, 20*(1), 1–25.

Bauman, K. E., & Ennett, S. T. (1996). On the importance of peer influence for adolescent drug use: Commonly neglected considerations. *Addiction, 91*(2), 185–198.

Benjamin, W. J. J., Schneider, B. H., Greenman, P. S., & Hum, M. (2001). Conflict and childhood friendship in Taiwan and Canada. *Canadian Journal of Behavioural Science/Revue Canadienne des Sciences du Comportement, 33*(3), 203–211.

Berndt, T. J. (1996). Transitions in friendship and friends' influence. In J. A. Graber, J. Brooks-Gunn, & A. C. Petersen (Eds.), *Transitions through adolescence: Interpersonal domains and context* (pp. 55–84). Mahwah: Lawrence Erlbaum Associates.

Berndt, T. J. (2002). Friendship quality and social development. *Current Directions in Psychological Science, 11*(1), 7–10.

Brown, B. B., Clasen, D. R., & Eicher, S. A. (1986). Perceptions of peer pressure, peer conformity dispositions, and self-reported behavior among adolescents. *Developmental Psychology, 22*(4), 521–530.

Busiol, D. (2015). Cultural mediators in help-seeking behaviors and attitudes towards counseling: A qualitative study among Hong Kong Chinese University students. *British Journal of Guidance and Counselling.* In press.

Caplan, M., Weissberg, R. P., Grober, J. S., Sivo, P. J., Grady, K., & Jacoby, C. (1992). Social competence promotion with inner-city and suburban young adolescents: Effects on social adjustment and alcohol use. *Journal of Consulting and Clinical Psychology, 60*(1), 56–63.

Catalano, R. F., Berglund, M. L., Ryan, J. A., Lonczak, H. S., & Hawkins, J. D. (2004a). Positive youth development in the United States: Research findings on evaluations of positive youth development programs. *The Annals of the American Academy of Political and Social Science, 591*(1), 98–124.

Catalano, R. F., Oesterle, S., Fleming, C. B., & Hawkins, J. D. (2004b). The importance of bonding to school for healthy development: Findings from the social development research group. *Journal of School Health, 74*(7), 252–261.

Chan, D. K. S., & Cheng, G. H. L. (2004). A comparison of offline and online friendship qualities at different stages of relationship development. *Journal of Social and Personal Relationships, 21*(3), 305–320.

Chang, L., Lei, L., Li, K. K., Liu, H., Guo, B., Wang, Y., & Fung, K. (2005). Peer acceptance and self-perceptions of verbal and behavioural aggression and social withdrawal. *International Journal of Behavioral Development, 29*(1), 48–57.

Chen, X., Li, D., Li, Z. Y., Li, B. S., & Liu, M. (2000). Sociable and prosocial dimensions of social competence in Chinese children: Common and unique contributions to social, academic, and psychological adjustment. *Developmental Psychology, 36*(3), 302–314.

Cheng, C., Bond, M. H., & Chan, S. C. (1995). The perception of ideal best friends by Chinese adolescents. *International Journal of Psychology, 30*(1), 91–108.

Chou, K. L. (2000). Intimacy and psychosocial adjustment in Hong Kong Chinese adolescents. *The Journal of Genetic Psychology, 161*(2), 141–151.

Chow, A. Y., Chan, C. L., & Ho, S. M. (2007). Social sharing of bereavement experience by Chinese bereaved persons in Hong Kong. *Death Studies, 31*(7), 601–618.

Crosnoe, R., & Needham, B. (2004). Holism, contextual variability, and the study of friendships in adolescent development. *Child Development, 75*(1), 264–279.

Giordano, P. C., Cernkovich, S. A., & Pugh, M. D. (1986). Friendships and delinquency. *American Journal of Sociology, 91*(5), 1170–1202.

Gottman, J. M., & Parker, J. G. (1987). *Conversations of friends: Speculations on affective development*. New York: Cambridge University Press.

Grey, C., & Sturdy, A. (2007). Friendship and organizational analysis toward a research agenda. *Journal of Management Inquiry, 16*(2), 157–172.

Gudykunst, W. B., Ting-Toomey, S., & Chua, E. (1988). *Culture and interpersonal communication*. Newbury Park: Sage.

Hurrelmann, K., & Engel, U. (1992). Delinquency as a symptom of adolescents' orientation toward status and success. *Journal of Youth and Adolescence, 21*(1), 119–138.

Javidi, A., & Javidi, M. (1991). Cross-cultural analysis of interpersonal bonding: A look at East and West. *Howard Journal of Communications, 3*(1–2), 129–138.

Joy, A. (2001). Gift giving in Hong Kong and the continuum of social ties. *Journal of Consumer Research, 28*(2), 239–256.

Keller, M. (2004a). Self in relationship. In D. K. Lapsley & D. Narvez (Eds.), *Moral development, self, and identity* (pp. 269–300). Mahwah: Lawrence Erlbaum Associates.

Keller, M. (2004b). A cross-cultural perspective on friendship research. *Newsletter of the International Society for the Study of Behavioral Development, 46*(2), 10–11. 14.

Knapp, M. L. (1978). *Social intercourse: From greeting to goodbye*. Boston: Allyn and Bacon.

Kobus, K. (2003). Peers and adolescent smoking. *Addiction, 98*(s1), 37–55.

Krappmann, L. (1996). Amicitia, Drujba, Shin-yu, Philia, Freundschaft, friendship: On the cultural diversity of human relationship. In W. M. Bukowski, A. F. Newcomb, & W. W. Hartup (Eds.), *The company they keep: Friendship in childhood and adolescence* (pp. 19–40). New York: Cambridge University Press.

Kuchuck, S. (1993). Understanding and modifying identifications in an adolescent boys therapy group. *Journal of Child and Adolescent Group Therapy, 3*(4), 189–201.

Lee, T. Y., & Lok, D. P. (2012). Bonding as a positive youth development construct: A conceptual review. *The Scientific World Journal, 2012*, 1–11.

Li, H. Z. (2002). Culture, gender and self–close-other(s) connectedness in Canadian and Chinese samples. *European Journal of Social Psychology, 32*(1), 93–104.

Maddox, S. J., & Prinz, R. J. (2003). School bonding in children and adolescents: Conceptualization, assessment, and associated variables. *Clinical Child and Family Psychology Review, 6*(1), 31–49.

Man, P. (1991). The influence of peers and parents on youth life satisfaction in Hong Kong. *Social Indicators Research, 24*(4), 347–365.

Mesch, G. S. (2009). Social bonds and Internet pornographic exposure among adolescents. *Journal of Adolescence, 32*(3), 601–618.

Millstein, S. G., Petersen, A. C., & Nightingale, E. O. (Eds.). (1993). *Promoting the health of adolescents: New directions for the twenty-first century*. New York: Oxford University Press.

Parker, J. G., & Gottman, J. M. (1989). Social and emotional development in a relational context: Friendship interaction from early childhood to adolescence. In T. J. Berndt & G. W. Ladd (Eds.), *Peer relationships in child development* (pp. 95–131). New York: Wiley.

Prus, R. (2007). Aristotle's Nicomachean ethics: Laying the foundations for a pragmatist consideration of human knowing and acting. *Qualitative Sociology Review, 3*(2), 5–45.

Schwartz, D., Chang, L., & Farver, J. M. (2001). Correlates of victimization in Chinese children's peer groups. *Developmental Psychology, 37*(4), 520–532.

Simons-Morton, B. G., Crump, A. D., Haynie, D. L., & Saylor, K. E. (1999). Student-school bonding and adolescent problem behavior. *Health Education Research, 14*(1), 99–107.

Thompson, M. G. (1998). Manifestations of transference: Love, friendship, rapport. *Contemporary Psychoanalysis, 34*(4), 543–561.

Yang, J., Morris, M. R., Teevan, J., Adamic, L., & Ackerman, M. (2011). *Culture matters: A survey study of social Q&A behavior*. International AAAI conference on weblogs and social media, pp. 409–416.

Yeh, J. H. B. (2010). Relations matter: Redefining communication competence from a Chinese perspective. *Chinese Journal of Communication, 3*(1), 64–75.

Bonding as a Cornerstone for Positive Youth Development

Tak Yan Lee and Diego Busiol

Abstract Attachment describes how parent-child bonding serves as an internal model that affects the child's future relationship with others. The development of attachment would seem to be a necessary, universal biopsychosocial requirement to be found in all cultures under normal circumstances as a species-specific consequence of our phylogenetic heritage. However, there are cultural differences since the biological system of attachment is interwoven with cultural practices. In this chapter, different perspectives and theories on attachment will be presented. Particularly, development of adolescents' bonding will be examined in relation to parents, romantic partners, and teachers. Finally, results from cross-cultural studies on attachment are critically examined; not only differences across cultures exist, but also wide variation within a given culture is sometimes reported.

Introduction

Extensive literature and research indicate that bonding is crucial for adolescents' healthy development. Theorists and empirical studies (Carter et al. 2005; Resnick et al. 1997; Schofield 2002) indicate that social and emotional support from the family is essential for adolescents who are in a transitional developmental period. In a study based on interviews of a randomized sample of 10,000 US youth across social classes (Resnick et al. 1997), bonding to parents and school was identified as protective factors mitigating the numerous developmental risks faced by adolescents.

The preparation for this work and the Project P.A.T.H.S. were financially supported by The Hong Kong Jockey Club Charities Trust.

This paper is based on an article originally published by The Scientific World Journal: Lee, T. Y., & Lok, D. P. (2012). Bonding as a positive youth development construct: A conceptual review. *The Scientific World Journal*, 11 pages.

T.Y. Lee (✉) • D. Busiol
Department of Applied Social Sciences, City University of Hong Kong,
Kowloon, Hong Kong, China
e-mail: ty.lee@cityu.edu.hk

© Springer Science+Business Media Singapore 2015
T.Y. Lee et al. (eds.), *Student Well-Being in Chinese Adolescents in Hong Kong*,
Quality of Life in Asia 7, DOI 10.1007/978-981-287-582-2_9

Besides, bonding with healthy adults is also positively related to adolescents' psychological health and acts as a protective factor for the adolescent (Ainsworth 1991; Catalano et al. 2002, 2004; Hawkins et al. 1992). The development of attachment would seem to be a necessary, universal biopsychosocial requirement to be found in all cultures under normal circumstances as a species-specific consequence of our phylogenetic heritage (Cole and Packer 2011). However, even if the attachment system is universal, there are cultural differences since the biological system of attachment is interwoven with cultural practices (Van Ijzendoorn and Sagi 1999).

Attachment Perspectives

Attachment perspectives emphasize the strong emotional ties between parents and adolescents and describe how parent-child bonding serves as an internal model that affects the child's future relationship with others. Bowlby (1979) asserted that "attachment behavior is held to characterize human beings from the cradle to the grave" (p. 129). His meaning is that the effect of bonding is lifelong and will transfer among different kinds of relationships (Bowlby 1969; Carter et al. 2005; Noller et al. 2013). Ainsworth (1991) listed six types of affectional bonds throughout the life span: (1) mother to infant, (2) father to child, (3) friendship, (4) companionship, (5) bonds between siblings and other kin, and (6) bonding with a romantic partner. Bowlby argued that the fundamental need to establish contact and connection has adaptive roots in biological survival, and his attachment theory emerged as a major paradigm for empirical study of the mother-child relationship (1979). Even though attachment with significant others during infancy and childhood has important consequences for a child's later development, Bowlby (1969) believed that the attachment from adolescents to their parents still remains strong, although they may also have developed important bonding with peers and significant others. Thus, parent-adolescent bonding is both essential and significant during adolescence (Collins and Sroufe 1999). Many studies have suggested that having a secure relationship with their parents would have positive influences on adolescents' subsequent adjustment and healthy development (Armsden and Greenberg 1987; Collins and Sroufe 1999). A key implication of attachment perspectives is that when children grow up in a social environment that provides sensitive and responsive interactions with strong emotional ties, this facilitates well-adjusted adaptation during the transitions of adolescence.

Social-Psychological Perspectives

During the transition from childhood to adulthood, multiple adaptations are required to respond to age-related changes in expectations, tasks, and settings (Bandura 1964). Three major sources of impact on interpersonal relationships have been identified (Collins and Steinberg 2006). The first is the increase in anxiety arising from adapting to the multiple changes of early adolescence. The second is parent-child conflict as a result of the changes in the adolescent in adapting to the outside world (Youniss 1980). The third is the pressure to reduce dependence on the family when adapting to extrafamilial contexts (Youniss 1980). Such pressures affect adolescents' self-esteem, perceived independence, valuing of independence, methods of control, and overt behavior (Collins 1995). Subsequently, these changes will affect the quality of bonding. A key implication of the social-psychological viewpoint is that adolescents will go through an increase and then a decrease in relationship difficulties from early to late adolescence (Collins and Laursen 2004a), and the course of their development may encounter more accidental influences than implied by other theories.

Bonding and Positive Adolescence

While infants need a secure attachment with caregivers, adolescents also need a sense of security and the encouragement to explore as they develop toward independent and autonomous individuals (Scharf et al. 2004) through building both social and nonsocial bonds, including culturally based beliefs, traditions, values, and institutions. These bonds formed later in life provide benefits similar to infant attachment and parental bonding, such as a sense of security, comfort in stressful situations, guidance and support in decision-making, physiological regulation, as well as long-term mental and physical health benefits (Carter et al. 2005). Certain specific bonds may be more likely to develop at different stages, including peer bonding in latency, commitment to social/cultural values during adolescence, and bonding to romantic partners after puberty. At the adolescent stage, peers, cultural belief systems, traditions, values, and associated institutions are important socialization agents where youngsters turn for emotional support and conformity (Ainsworth 1991; Carter et al. 2005; Choi et al. 2003; Hong Kong Federation of Youth Groups 1996). Owing to the changing environment and the development of adolescents' social and cognitive skills, bonding with peers and teachers may begin to substitute for bonding with parents (Collins 1995; Noller et al. 2013). On the other hand, adolescents still look for full support from their parents (Collins and Laursen 2004b; Noller et al. 2013). Therefore, simultaneously supporting adolescents to build and maintain bonds with parents, friends, teachers, and mature adults in the community can facilitate their whole-person development.

Bonding with Parents

Theorists and researchers have indicated that the types of parent-child bonding (the first bonding) will affect one's development of interpersonal relationships as one grows (Carter et al. 2005; Giordano 2003; Schneider et al. 2001). For instance, children having a secure attachment with parents are more likely to become healthy and functional adults (Bowlby 1988; Schofield 2002). They will grow up with high self-esteem, self-confidence, self-understanding, self-regulation, social competence, and better skills in problem solving and in building quality friendships (Bowlby 1988; Carter et al. 2005; Schofield 2002). Although adolescents probably will change their attachment object from their parents to peers or teachers, they still want full support from their parents (Noller et al. 2013). Thus, it is vital to promote their bonding with parents. The importance of the attachment relationship with parents or caregivers is well documented. Based on a comprehensive study of 90,000 American teenagers, Blum and Rinehart (1997) concluded "across all the health outcomes examined, the results points to the importance of family and the home environment for protecting adolescents from harm. What emerges most consistently as protective is the teenager's feeling of connectedness with parents and family" (p. 31). In addition, research studies have shown that family relationships during the adolescent period have important follow-on effects in a number of domains, such as autonomy and later independence of the individual (Coleman and Hendry 1999), adolescent personality (Heaven 1997), individual pathology (Scott and Scott 1987), and problem behavior (Pettit et al. 1997). While parenting styles influence the social and emotional development of adolescents, parents transmit their values and morals to their children which include beliefs about acceptable behavior. Finally, parents are a vital source of information on a range of topics (Jaccard and Dittus 1991). Litovsky and Dusek (1985) also pointed out that adolescents who view their parents as warm, accepting, and providing them autonomy feel better about themselves and have more opportunity to practice social skills than those adolescents who perceive their parents as controlling, cold, and rejecting. Studies have also found that college students who are securely attached to their parents show better psychological and social adjustment and academic performance during their transition to college than students who are insecurely attached (Lapsley et al. 1990; Larose et al. 2005). In short, positive outcomes from secure bonding to parents include a stronger sense of identity, higher self-esteem, greater social competence, better emotional adjustment, and fewer behavioral problems than less securely attached peers. On the other hand, maladaptive bonding with parents may lead to negative consequences such as parent-child conflicts when the parent-child dyad cannot strike a balance between the adolescents' need for autonomy and the parents' perception of connectedness. This is because when adolescents express their own individuality, parents with maladaptive bonding may take it as a sign of rejection and a weakening relationship (Laursen and Collins 2009). Although conflict management processes vary across parent-child dyads, the significance of a disagreement depends on the perceived quality of the relationship. Hauser and his colleagues (1991) suggested that feelings of positive bonding promote the use of alternatives in a nonthreatening way whereas disagreement may be interpreted as a hostile attack that justifies an antagonistic response in maladaptive bonding. Furthermore, it was found that adolescents whose parents use a great deal of enabling and little psychological and behavioral control show a higher level of individuality and score higher on measures of psychological competence and ego development (Allen et al. 1994; Hauser et al. 1991).

Bonding with Romantic Partners

Hazan and Shaver (1987) suggested that attachment patterns between romantic partners are similar to the secure, anxious/ambivalent, and avoidant classification deriving from infant observation. The nature of the link between infant attachment style and bonding with romantic partners needs to be further investigated – it cannot be ignored. For instance, in psychoanalysis (Weiss 1991) the term transference indicates the tendency to "transfer" in present-day relationship qualities of other relevant figures of our early life (parents, caregivers, siblings). We tend to "project" on others beliefs and expectations that we unconsciously formed during early years; this is particularly evident in intimate relationships which lead to greater emotional involvement. Bonding with romantic partners may reflect early bonding with parents; thus, improving adolescents' quality of family bonding can have important reflections on the latter as well.

Carter and colleagues (2005) concluded that emotionally close relationships developed during later childhood, adolescence, and adulthood are generally more mutual. These include "dyadic bonds" (individual to individual bonds), such as "love between parents and their older/adult children," "sibling bonds," "friendships in childhood and adulthood," "bonds between sexual partners," and "love between other biological relatives" (p. 387). Psychologists suggest that a romantic relationship may emerge as an individual grows through adolescence (Noller et al. 2013). Early romantic experiences play a crucial role in the development of the self and the ability to build up and maintain intimate relationships with significant others in the future. Interaction and relationships in the adolescent period with the opposite sex are believed to influence future romantic involvements and marriage in adulthood (Erikson 1968; Sullivan 1953; Bowlby 1988). According to Brown (1999), adolescent romantic relationships develop through four stages: (1) initiation, (2) status, (3) affection, and (4) bonding. The focus of the first stage is on testing oneself as a person capable of relating to the opposite sex in a romantic way. During the second stage, peer approval is needed in order to maintain or raise one's status in a large peer group. In the third stage, romantic relationships become more personal and caring. In the bonding phase, together with a long-term commitment, the emotional intimacy achieved helps create a lasting attachment. Sternberg (1986) proposed that love consists of three basic ingredients: intimacy, passion, and decision/commitment. The intimacy component refers to feelings that promote closeness, bonding, and connectedness. The passion component refers to sources of arousal that promote the experience of passion, such as sexual needs, needs for self-esteem, affiliation, and submission, while the decision/commitment component refers to the decision that one is in love with another and the commitment to maintain that love. In short, adolescent dating serves multiple purposes, including recreation, autonomy seeking, status seeking, sexual experimentation, social skills development, and courtship (Hansen and Hicks 1980). Studies suggest that dating at an early age may have more negative than positive outcomes. This may be either because troubled adolescents start dating early or because they get hurt in dating or they become involved in teenage problem behavior (Collins 2003; Compian et al. 2004). However, both secure bonding with parents and same-gender peers can protect young adolescents from the negative effects of early dating (Brendgen et al. 2002). In general, dating typically has more positive than negative developmental outcomes. Involvement and commitment in a steady relationship promote self-esteem and better overall adjustment (Collins 2003). Securely attached college students who were able to keep a close and caring bond with their parents were found to be able to form new relationships with romantic partners. On the contrary, resistantly attached college students experienced more difficulties when entering into romantic relationships (Mayseless et al. 1996).

Bonding with Teachers

Teachers too are often perceived by youth as parental substitutes (Baker and Baker 1987), and as such they can easily become friends or rivals (Brunori 1998). Students in a supportive school environment (in which teachers are helpful but firm and maintain high, clearly defined standards for academic work and behavior) develop stronger bonds to teachers and the school and show higher achievement motivation. This bonding, in turn, helps adolescents have fewer problems, higher attendance, fewer incidents of delinquency, more supportive friendships, and higher academic performance (Eccles 2004; Ryan and Patrick 2001). Another study by Howes and Aikins (2002) found that a teacher who serves as an alternative attachment figure provides a secure base for new thoughts, promotes self-regulation, and leads to better friendship quality for adolescents. Moreover, Catalano and colleagues (2004) provide empirical support for the theoretical propositions on the influence of school bonding, demonstrating the effectiveness of interventions to improve school connectedness and reduce a variety of health and safety problems, promote positive behavior, and attain academic success for children and adolescents. They concluded, "school bonding appears to promote healthy development and to prevent problem behaviors" (p. 252). Adolescent-teacher relationships are critical for the healthy development of the adolescent. Studies have shown that exposure to positive classroom climates and sensitive teachers is related to adolescents' greater self-regulation (Skinner et al. 1998) and greater teacher-rated social competence (Murraya and Malmgrenb 2005). Teachers exert influences on both prosocial and antisocial behavior of adolescents; thus, teachers play a crucial role in the positive development of the adolescent (Ma et al. 2000). Blum and Rinehart (1997) concluded "school policies, classroom sizes, and teacher training appear unrelated to the emotional health and behaviors of students. Instead, what matters is the students' sense of connection to the school they attend: if students feel they are a part of the school, are treated fairly by teachers, and feel close to people at school, they have better emotional health and lower levels of involvement in risky behavior" (p. 32).

Cultural Issues

The development of attachment would seem to be a necessary, universal biological requirement to be found in all cultures under normal circumstances as a species-specific consequence of our phylogenetic heritage. Ainsworth et al. (1978) identified three kinds of attachment in infants: insecure-avoidant (type A), secure (type B), and insecure-ambivalent (type C). They demonstrated that 70 % of infants are secure, 20 % are insecure-avoidant, and 10 % are insecure-ambivalent. Ainsworth (1979) also claimed that attachment styles were universal across cultures. Cross-cultural studies showed that secure attachment patterns are prevalent. However, even if the attachment system is biologically based and universal, this in no way contradicts the principal of cultural mediation. The biological system of attachment is interwoven with cultural practices (Cole and Packer 2011). Research has initially suggested significant variation in the proportion of infants showing each pattern of attachment-related behavior. For example, when at the age of 11–14 months communally reared Israeli children were placed in the strange situation, many became very upset; half were classified as anxious resistant and only 37 % appeared to be securely attached (Sagi et al. 1985). Researchers suspect that cultural differences in the opportunities for sensitive caregiving account for differences in attachment quality. Moreover, attachment behavior will differ in distinct cultures and in different epochs depending on differences in customs of child care, family or social structure, devastating or benign living conditions, and similar environmental circumstances (Grossmann and Grossmann 2005). In a study on ethnic differences in the contribution of parents (Lopez et al. 2000), measures of parent-child bonds were more efficient and consistent predictors of adult attachment orientations among White participants than among Hispanic/Latino and Black participants. Among White college students, parental bonds explained variance in both adult avoidance and anxiety scores; instead, among Hispanic/Latino and Black participants, parental bonds only accounted for anxiety but not avoidance. The authors observed that the link between qualities of early bonds and later attachment was more evident within their White sample, and they suggested that race/ethnicity might have an impact on the adult attachment orientation.

Similarly, in the Chinese context the link between early parental bonding and adult attachment quality was not supported. For instance, among Chinese students, the perception of closeness with both parents was not associated with students' romantic attachment quality, whereas an association existed among American participants (Shi 2010). Similarly, Sun et al. (2010) tested the link between early parental bonding experiences and adult attachment in 565 graduate students in China. The results failed to support such links in both genders. However, securely attached females reported significantly higher levels of paternal care than fearfully attached females, and securely attached males reported significantly higher levels of parental care and lower levels of parental overprotection than the other three insecurely attached groups of males (preoccupied, fearful, and dismissing).

On the other hand, a comparison of the behavior of mother-child pairs observed in their homes in the United States and Uganda by Ainsworth (1967) found that children in both cultural groups exhibited similar patterns of attachment-related behavior although the Ugandan children seemed to express these behavior patterns more readily and intensely than did the American children. Most studies show that, across a variety of cultural settings, about two-thirds of the attachments to either parent are rated secure (Van Ijzendoorn and Sagi 1999). Across many cultures, secure attachments (type B) are the most common. However, in places like Israel, Japan, Indonesia, and China, insecure-ambivalent attachments (type C) appear more often than in other places. Children in interdependent societies show a higher percentage of anxious-resistant patterns, whereas children in independent societies report more anxious-avoidant patterns (Ainsworth et al. 1978; Li 2013; Trnavsky 1998; Van Ijzendoorn and Kroonenberg 1988). This also results from cultural differences in parenting styles (Van IJzendoorn and Sagi-Schnartz 2008). These could mean that parents in some countries are more or less sensitive than American parents, but this ethnocentric interpretation seems incorrect. The strange situation would not be psychologically similar for these babies and American babies (the psychological meaning of the procedure for infants from each culture may differ). A low percentage of securely attached babies have also been observed among northern German children. Researchers in one study found that 49 % of the 1-year-olds tested were anxious avoidant and only 35 % were securely attached (Grossmann et al. 1985). The researchers rejected the possibility that a large proportion of northern German parents were insensitive or indifferent to their children. They suggested that northern German parents were adhering to a cultural value that calls for the maintenance of a relatively large interpersonal distance and to a cultural belief that babies should be weaned from parental bodily contact as soon as they become mobile. In Japan, Miyake and his colleagues found a large proportion of anxious-resistant infants among traditional Japanese families and no anxious-avoidant infants at all (Miyake et al. 1985; Nakagawa et al. 1992). They explained this pattern by pointing out that traditional Japanese mothers rarely leave their children in the care of anyone else, and they behave toward them in ways that foster a strong sense of dependence. Consequently, the experience of being left alone with a stranger is unusual and upsetting to these children. In general, Western industrialized cultures tend to be viewed as individualistic with an emphasis on self-actualization, whereas Eastern cultures and those that are less industrialized tend to be viewed as collectivistic with an emphasis on interdependence (Goodwin and Pillay 2006; Kagitcibasi 1996).

Chi Kuan Mak et al. (2010) tested the link between anxious and avoidant attachment styles and depressive symptoms in 367 participants from Hong Kong and the USA and found these associations to be stronger in Hong Kong. Particularly, they found that avoidance in Hong Kong was linked more strongly to perception of less support, and they suggested that this might be due to a clash with values of a more collectivistic culture. Indeed, they speculated that partners of highly avoidant persons in interdependent cultures may feel distressed by the attitude of their lovers. Similar findings were reported by Friedman et al. (2010), who examined individual differences in avoidant-romantic attachment style in the cultures of Hong Kong, Mexico, and the USA. The results showed that attachment avoidance, which emphasizes emotional distance and independence, was more strongly associated with relationship problems in more interdependent cultures like Hong Kong and Mexico. For instance, greater attachment avoidance was more strongly related to less investment, less perceived support, greater conflict, and poorer relationship satisfaction for participants in Hong Kong than in the USA. Indeed, the authors suggested a "cultural fit" hypothesis, meaning that individual differences in personality might be associated with relationship problems if they encourage behavior that is incongruent with cultural norms. On the one hand, the authors interpreted these results as evidence that attachment processes and mechanisms operate in a relatively consistent manner in different cultures; on the other hand they suggested that culture affects the way in which highly anxious and avoidant attachment translate into important relational outcomes. Li (2013) examined adult attachment in Chinese and Germans subjects; despite significant cultural differences in the distribution of attachment patterns, the results supported the universality argument and findings from previous studies (Ainsworth et al. 1978; Van Ijzendoorn and Kroonenberg 1988). The author suggests that because "of the collectivistic background, Chinese are more dependent and have higher level of preoccupied attachment, while German individuals are more individualistic, which resulting in higher level of dismissing attachment" (p. 75).

Chinese are comparatively more concerned with interpersonal harmony and are more likely to have close relationships within the family. However, the individualism collectivism dimension does not provide a general theoretical model for distinguishing among cultural groups (Levitt and Cici-Gokaltun 2010). The evidence of cultural variation has been brought into question and balanced by evidence that there is a general tendency in all societies for children to become attached to their caregivers. An influential review of research on attachment in different cultures conducted by van Ijzendoorn and Sagi reported that although the proportion of children displaying one or another pattern of attachment behavior may vary in a small number of cases, the overall pattern of results is remarkably consistent with Ainsworth's initial findings (Van Ijzendoorn and Sagi 1999). The global distribution was found to be 21 % type A (anxious avoidant), 65 % type B (securely attached), and 14 % type C (anxious resistant), with greater variation within countries than between them. When Behrens et al. (2007) replicated Miyake's research with older Japanese children, they found a distribution of A, B, and C categories similar to worldwide norms.

Concluding Remarks

Assessing culture divergence in social attachment is nearly impossible. As described by Gjerde (2004), culture is a rapidly moving target, continually changing in a context of economic, political, and historical forces. Secondly, individuals within a given cultural group are heterogeneous, and there are often greater differences within cultures than across cultures. Furthermore, cultural effects are confounded with other cultural variables, such as social class, economic conditions, and geographic locations. Therefore, it is expected that wide variation can exist within a given culture. Longitudinal studies have documented both continuity in attachment relationships' quality from infancy to early adulthood and also discontinuity, with the latter being meaningfully related to changes in the lives of individuals and their family environments (Hamilton 2000; Waters et al. 2000b; Weinfield et al. 2000). Specifically, evidence supports the notion that negative life events (e.g., loss of a parent, parental divorce, life-threatening illness of parent or child, and parental psychiatric disorder) could bear on the caregiver's availability and responsiveness, which impacts child-parent interactions and in turn affects children's security (Waters et al. 2000a). The patterning of past interactions, present exchanges, and the ecology of the dyad all seem at play in helping account for individual differences in child-parent attachment relationships (Posada and Lu 2011).

References

Ainsworth, M. D. S. (1967). *Infancy in Uganda*. Baltimore: John Hopkins University Press.

Ainsworth, M. D. S. (1979). Attachment as related to mother-infant interaction. *Advances in the Study of Behavior, 9*, 1–51.

Ainsworth, M. D. S. (1991). Attachments and other affectional bonds across the life cycle. In C. M. Parkes, J. Stevenson-Hinde, & P. Marais (Eds.), *Attachment across the life cycle* (pp. 33–51). London: Tavistock.

Ainsworth, M. D. S., Blehar, M., Waters, E., & Wall, S. (1978). *Patterns of attachment: A psychological study of the strange situation*. Hillsdale: Erlbaum.

Allen, J. P., Hauser, S. T., Eickholt, C., Bell, K. L., & O'Connor, T. G. (1994). Autonomy and relatedness in family interactions as predictors of expressions of negative adolescent affect. *Journal of Research on Adolescence, 4*(4), 535–552.

Armsden, G. C., & Greenberg, M. T. (1987). The inventory of parent and peer attachment: Individual differences and their relationship to psychological well-being in adolescence. *Journal of Youth and Adolescence, 16*(5), 427–454.

Baker, H. S., & Baker, M. N. (1987). Heinz Kohut's self psychology: An overview. *American Journal of Psychiatry, 144*(1), 1–9.

Bandura, A. (1964). The stormy decade: Fact or fiction? *Psychology in the Schools, 1*(3), 224–231.

Behrens, K. Y., Hesse, E., & Main, M. (2007). Mothers' attachment status as determined by the adult attachment interview predicts their 6-year-olds' reunion responses: A study conducted in Japan. *Developmental Psychology, 43*(6), 1553–1567.

Blum, R. W., & Rinehart, P. M. (1997). *Reducing the risk: Connections that make a difference in the lives of youth*. Minneapolis: University of Minnesota, Division of General Pediatrics and Adolescent Health.

Bowlby, J. (1969). *Attachment and loss*. New York: Basic Books.

Bowlby, J. (1979). *The making and breaking of affectional bonds*. London: Tavistock.

Bowlby, J. (1988). *A secure base: Parent-child attachment and healthy human development*. New York: Basic Books.

Brendgen, M., Vitaro, F., Doyle, A. B., Markiewicz, D., & Bukowski, W. M. (2002). Same-sex peer relations and romantic relationships during early adolescence: Interactive links to emotional, behavioral, and academic adjustment. *Merrill-Palmer Quarterly, 48*(1), 77–103.

Brown, B. B. (1999). "You're going out with who?": Peer group influences on adolescent romantic relationships. In W. Furman, B. B. Brown, & C. Feiring (Eds.), *The development of romantic relationships in adolescence*. New York: Cambridge University Press.

Brunori, L. (1998). Siblings. *Group Analysis, 31*(3), 307–314.

Carter, C. S., Ahnert, L., Grossmann, K. E., Hrdy, S. B., Lamb, M. E., Porges, S. W., & Sachser, N. (2005). *Attachment and bonding: A new synthesis*, 92nd Dahlem workshop report. Cambridge, MA: MIT Press.

Catalano, R. F., Berglund, M. L., Ryan, J. A., Lonczak, H. S., & Hawkins, J. D. (2002). Positive youth development in the United States: Research findings on evaluations of positive youth development programs. *Prevention & Treatment, 5*(1), 15a.

Catalano, R. F., Oesterle, S., Fleming, C. B., & Hawkins, J. D. (2004). The importance of bonding to school for healthy development: Findings from the Social Development Research Group. *Journal of School Health, 74*(7), 252–261.

Chi Kuan Mak, M., Bond, M. H., Simpson, J. A., & Rholes, W. S. (2010). Adult attachment, perceived support, and depressive symptoms in Chinese and American cultures. *Journal of Social and Clinical Psychology, 29*(2), 144–165.

Choi, P. Y. W., Au, C. K., Tang, C. W., Shum, S. M., Tang, S. Y., Choi, F. M., & Lee, T. C. (2003). *Making young tumblers: A manual of promoting resilience in schools and families*. Hong Kong: Breakthrough.

Cole, M., & Packer, M. (2011). Culture in development. In M. H. Bornstein & M. E. Lamb (Eds.), *Developmental science: An advanced textbook* (6th ed., pp. 51–107). New York: Psychology Press.

Coleman, J. C., & Hendry, L. B. (1999). *The nature of adolescence* (3rd ed.). London: Routledge.

Collins, W. A. (1995). *Relationships and development: Family adaptation to individual change*. New York: Alex.

Collins, W. A. (2003). More than myth: The developmental significance of romantic relationships during adolescence. *Journal of Research on Adolescence, 13*(1), 1–24.

Collins, W. A., & Laursen, B. (2004a). Changing relationships, changing youth interpersonal contexts of adolescent development. *The Journal of Early Adolescence, 24*(1), 55–62.

Collins, W. A., & Laursen, B. (2004b). Parent-adolescent relationships and influences. In R. M. Lerner & L. Steinberg (Eds.), *Handbook of adolescent psychology* (pp. 331–361). New York: Wiley.

Collins, W. A., & Sroufe, L. A. (1999). Capacity for intimate relationships: A developmental construction. In W. Furman, C. Feiring, & B. B. Brown (Eds.), *Contemporary perspectives on adolescent romantic relationships* (pp. 123–147). New York: Cambridge University Press.

Collins, W. A., & Steinberg, L. (2006). Adolescent development in interpersonal context. In W. Damon & R. M. Lerner (Eds.), *Handbook of child psychology: Social, emotional, and personality development* (6th ed., Vol. 3, pp. 1003–1067). Hoboken: Wiley.

Compian, L., Gowen, L. K., & Hayward, C. (2004). Peripubertal girls' romantic and platonic involvement with boys: Associations with body image and depression symptoms. *Journal of Research on Adolescence, 14*(1), 23–47.

Eccles, J. S. (2004). Schools, academic motivation, and stage-environment fit. In R. M. Lerner & L. Steinberg (Eds.), *Handbook of adolescent psychology* (pp. 125–153). New York: Wiley.

Erikson, E. H. (1968). *Identity: Youth and crisis* (Vol. 7). New York: Norton.

Friedman, M., Rholes, W. S., Simpson, J., Bond, M., Diaz-Loving, R., & Chan, C. (2010). Attachment avoidance and the cultural fit hypothesis: A cross-cultural investigation. *Personal Relationships, 17*(1), 107–126.

Giordano, P. C. (2003). Relationships in adolescence. *Annual Review of Sociology, 29*, 257–281.

Gjerde, P. F. (2004). Culture, power, and experience: Toward a person-centered cultural psychology. *Human Development, 47*(3), 138–157.

Goodwin, R., & Pillay, U. (2006). Relationships, culture, and social change. In A. L. Vangelisti & D. Perlman (Eds.), *The Cambridge handbook of personal relationships* (pp. 695–708). New York: Cambridge University Press.

Grossmann, K. E., & Grossmann, K. (2005). Universality of human social attachment as an adaptive process. In C. S. Carter, L. Ahnert, K. E. Grossmann, S. B. Hardy, M. E. Lamb, & S. W. Porges (Eds.), *Attachment and bonding: A new synthesis*. Cambridge: MIT Press.

Grossmann, K., Grossmann, K. E., Spangler, G., Suess, G., & Unzner, L. (1985). Maternal sensitivity and newborns' orientation responses as related to quality of attachment in northern Germany. In I. Bretherton, & K. Waters (Eds.), Growing points of attachment theory and research. *Monographs of the Society for Research in Child Development, 50*, 233–256.

Hamilton, C. E. (2000). Continuity and discontinuity of attachment from infancy through adolescence. *Child Development, 71*(3), 690–694.

Hansen, S. L., & Hicks, M. W. (1980). Sex role attitudes and perceived dating-mating choices of youth. *Adolescence, 15*(57), 83–90.

Hauser, S., Powers, S. I., & Noam, G. G. (1991). *Adolescents and their families: Paths of ego development*. New York: Free Press.

Hawkins, J. D., Catalano, R. F., & Miller, J. Y. (1992). Risk and protective factors for alcohol and other drug problems in adolescence and early adulthood: Implications for substance abuse prevention. *Psychological Bulletin, 112*(1), 64–105.

Hazan, C., & Shaver, P. (1987). Romantic love conceptualized as an attachment process. *Journal of Personality and Social Psychology, 52*(3), 511–524.

Heaven, P. C. (1997). Perceptions of family influences, self-esteem and psychoticism: A two-year longitudinal analysis. *Personality and Individual Differences, 23*(4), 569–574.

Hong Kong Federation of Youth Groups. (1996). *Parent-child communication: From both perspectives* (Adolescent and youth opinion survey series, Vol. 33). Hong Kong: Federation of Youth Groups.

Howes, C., & Aikins, J. W. (2002). Peer relations in the transition to adolescence. *Advances in Child Development and Behavior, 29*, 195–230.

Jaccard, J., & Dittus, P. (1991). *Parent-teen communication: Toward the prevention of unintended pregnancies*. New York: Springer.

Kagitcibasi, C. (1996). The autonomous-relational self. *European Psychologist, 1*(3), 180–186.

Lapsley, D. K., Rice, K. G., & FitzGerald, D. P. (1990). Adolescent attachment, identity, and adjustment to college: Implications for the continuity of adaptation hypothesis. *Journal of Counseling & Development, 68*(5), 561–565.

Larose, S., Bernier, A., & Tarabulsy, G. M. (2005). Attachment state of mind, learning dispositions, and academic performance during the college transition. *Developmental Psychology, 41*(1), 281–289.

Laursen, B., & Collins, W. A. (2009). Parent-child relationships during adolescence. In R. M. Lerner & L. Steinberg (Eds.), *Handbook of adolescent psychology* (pp. 3–42). New York: Wiley.

Levitt, M. J., & Cici-Gokaltun, A. (2010). Close relationships across the life span. In C. A. Berg, J. Smith, & T. C. Antonucci (Eds.), *Handbook of life-span development* (pp. 457–486). New York: Springer.

Li, H. (2013). *Cultural differences in adult attachment and facial emotion recognition*. Doctoral dissertation, Universität Ulm. Medizinische Fakultät.

Litovsky, V. G., & Dusek, J. B. (1985). Perceptions of child rearing and self-concept development during the early adolescent years. *Journal of Youth and Adolescence, 14*(5), 373–387.

Lopez, F. G., Melendez, M. C., & Rice, K. G. (2000). Parental divorce, parent-child bonds, and adult attachment orientations among college students: A comparison of three racial/ethnic groups. *Journal of Counseling Psychology, 47*(2), 177–186.

Ma, H. K., Shek, D. T., Cheung, P. C., & Lam, C. O. B. (2000). Parental, peer, and teacher influences on the social behavior of Hong Kong Chinese adolescents. *The Journal of Genetic Psychology, 161*(1), 65–78.

Mayseless, O., Danieli, R., & Sharabany, R. (1996). Adults' attachment patterns: Coping with separations. *Journal of Youth and Adolescence, 25*(5), 667–690.

Miyake, K., Chen, S. J., & Campos, J. J. (1985). Infant temperament, mother's mode of interaction, and attachment in Japan: An interim report. In I. Bretherton, & K. Waters (Eds.), Growing points of attachment theory and research. *Monographs of the Society for Research in Child Development, 50*, 276–297.

Murraya, C., & Malmgrenb, K. (2005). Implementing a teacher-student relationship program in a high-poverty urban school: Effects on social, emotional, and academic adjustment and lessons learned. *The Journal of School Psychology, 43*(2), 137–152.

Nakagawa, M., Lamb, E., & Miyake, K. (1992). Antecedents and correlates of the strange situation behavior of Japanese infants. *Journal of Cross-Cultural Psychology, 23*, 300–310.

Noller, P., Feeney, J., & Peterson, C. (2013). *Personal relationships across the lifespan*. London: Routledge.

Pettit, G. S., Bates, J. E., & Dodge, K. A. (1997). Supportive parenting, ecological context, and children's adjustment: A seven-year longitudinal study. *Child Development, 68*(5), 908–923.

Posada, G., & Lu, T. (2011). Child-parent attachment relationships: A life-span phenomenon. In C. A. Berg, J. Smith, & T. C. Antonucci (Eds.), *Handbook of life-span development* (pp. 87–115). New York: Springer.

Resnick, M. D., Bearman, P. S., Blum, R. W., Bauman, K. E., Harris, K. M., Jones, J., Tabor, J., Beuhring, T., Sieving, R. E., Shew, M., Ireland, M., Bearinger, L. H., & Udry, J. R. (1997). Protecting adolescents from harm: Findings from the national longitudinal study on adolescent health. *The Journal of the American Medical Association, 278*(10), 823–832.

Ryan, A. M., & Patrick, H. (2001). The classroom social environment and changes in adolescents' motivation and engagement during middle school. *American Educational Research Journal, 38*(2), 437–460.

Sagi, A., Lamb, M. E., Lewkowicz, K. S., Shoham, R., Dvir, R., & Estes, D. (1985). Security of infant-mother, -father, and -metapelet attachments among kibbutz-reared Israeli children. In I. Bretherton, & K.Waters (Eds.), Growing points of attachment theory and research. *Monographs of the Society for Research in Child Development, 50*, 257–275.

Scharf, M., Mayseless, O., & Kivenson-Baron, I. (2004). Adolescents' attachment representations and developmental tasks in emerging adulthood. *Developmental Psychology, 40*(3), 430–444.

Schneider, B. H., Atkinson, L., & Tardif, C. (2001). Child-parent attachment and children's peer relations: A quantitative review. *Developmental Psychology, 37*(1), 86–100.

Schofield, G. (2002). *Attachment theory: An introduction for social workers*. Norwich: University of East Anglia, School of Social Work and Psychosocial Studies.

Scott, W. A., & Scott, R. (1987). Individual pathology and family pathology. *Australian Journal of Psychology, 39*(2), 183–205.

Shi, L. (2010). Adult attachment and their consequences in romantic relationships: A comparison between China and the United States. In P. Erdman & K. Ng (Eds.), *Attachment: Expanding the cultural connections* (pp. 259–277). New York: Routledge/Taylor and Francis.

Skinner, E. A., Zimmer-Gembeck, M. J., & Connell, J. P. (1998). Individual differences and the development of perceived control. *Monographs of the Society for Research in Child Development, 63*(2–3), 1–220.

Sternberg, R. J. (1986). A triangular theory of love. *Psychological Review, 93*(2), 119–135.

Sullivan, H. S. (1953). *The interpersonal theory of psychiatry*. New York: Norton.

Sun, Q. W., Ng, K. M., & Guo, L. (2010). The link between parental bonding and adult attachment in Chinese graduate students: Gender differences. *The Family Journal, 18*(4), 386–394.

Trnavsky, P. (1998). Strange situation behaviors in Chinese infants. *Child Study Journal, 28*, 69–88.

Van Ijzendoorn, M. H., & Kroonenberg, P. M. (1988). Cross-cultural patterns of attachment: A meta-analysis of the strange situation. *Child Development, 59*, 147–156.

Van Ijzendoorn, M. H., & Sagi, A. (1999). Cross-cultural patterns of attachment: Universal and contextual dimensions. In J. Cassidy & P. R. Shaver (Eds.), *Handbook of attachment: Theory, research, and clinical application* (pp. 713–734). New York: Guilford Press.

Van IJzendoorn, M. H., & Sagi-Schnartz, A. (2008). *Handbook of attachment: Theory, research, and clinical application*. New York: Guilford Press.

Waters, E., Hamilton, C. E., & Weinfield, N. S. (2000a). The stability of attachment security from infancy to adolescence and early adulthood: General introduction. *Child Development, 71*(3), 678–683.

Waters, E., Merrick, S., Treboux, D., Crowell, J., & Albersheim, L. (2000b). Attachment security in infancy and early adulthood: A twenty-year longitudinal study. *Child Development, 71*(3), 684–689.

Weinfield, N. S., Sroufe, L. A., & Egeland, B. (2000). Attachment from infancy to early adulthood in a high-risk sample: Continuity, discontinuity, and their correlates. *Child Development, 71*(3), 695–702.

Weiss, R. S. (1991). The attachment bond in childhood and adulthood. *Attachment Across the Life Cycle, 8*, 66–76.

Youniss, J. (1980). *Parents and peers in the social environment: A Sullivan Piaget perspective.* Chicago: University of Chicago Press.

Review of the Relationships Between Resilience and Positive Youth Development

Chau Kiu Cheung, Tak Yan Lee, Wai Man Kwong, and Diego Busiol

Abstract Resilience is the process of, capacity for, or outcome of successful adaptation despite challenging or threatening circumstances. There is a growing consensus from child and adolescent research on important protective factors, such as (1) bonding, (2) competence, (3) optimism, and (4) environment (organized home environment, authoritative parenting (high on warmth, structure/monitoring, and expectations), socioeconomic advantages, effective schools). According to various theories or models, there are eight possible relationships between resilience and positive youth development. Four of the relationships take resilience as a forerunner of positive youth development, and four others regard resilience as a result of positive youth development. These eight possible relationships between resilience and positive youth development are not necessarily mutually exclusive, since they can operate at the same time in an additive way. Evidence supporting the contribution of resilience to positive youth development will be discussed.

Introduction

Research on resilience has been a major theme in developmental psychopathology focusing on the question why some children and adolescents maintain positive adaptation (Rutter 1987) despite experiences of "distressing life conditions and demanding societal conditions" (Gitterman 1991, p. 1) such as violence, poverty, stress, trauma, deprivation, and oppression. Despite concerted efforts in research on the concept of resilience over three decades, there are still different definitions of the term.

The preparation for this work and the Project P.A.T.H.S. were financially supported by The Hong Kong Jockey Club Charities Trust.

This paper is based on an article originally published by *The Scientific World Journal*: Lee, T. Y., Cheung, C. K., & Kwong, W. M. (2012). Resilience as a positive youth development construct: a conceptual review. *The Scientific World Journal, 2012*.

C.K. Cheung (✉) • T.Y. Lee • W.M. Kwong • D. Busiol
Department of Applied Social Sciences, City University of Hong Kong,
Kowloon, Hong Kong, China
e-mail: ssjacky@cityu.edu.hk

Although resilience has connected with positive youth development (Catalano et al. 2004), there is a wide range of theories about the relationships between resilience and positive youth development. It is essential to answer the following questions: What is the theoretical conception of resilience? What are the relationships between resilience and positive youth development? What are the antecedents of resilience? And then, what are the ways of enhancing adolescents' resilience that are pertinent to positive development?

Definitions of Resilience

In studying resilience, there are three critical conditions: (i) growing up in distressing life conditions and demanding societal conditions that are considered significant threats or severe adversities; (ii) the availability of protective factors, including internal assets and external resources that may be associated with counteracting the effects of risk factors; and (iii) the achievement of positive adaptation despite experiences of significant adversity (Windle 2011; Luthar and Zigler 1991). A broad definition regards resilience as the process of, capacity for, or outcome of successful adaptation despite challenging or threatening circumstances (Masten et al. 1990). Since then, difficulties in defining resilience have become widely noticeable (Haskett et al. 2006; Kaplan 1999; Masten 2007; Windle 2011).

In explaining why some children and adolescents maintain positive adaptation even though they grow up in deprived, troubled, and threatening environments, differences in measuring the significance, quality, and quantity of adversities as well as positive adjustment are commonly found. The American Psychological Association also uses a broad definition: "the process of adapting well in the face of adversity, trauma, tragedy, threats, or even significant sources of stress – such as family and relationship problems, serious health problems, or workplace and financial stressors." "It means, 'bouncing back' from difficult experiences" (American Psychological Association n.d.). However, a review of existing studies indicates that the proportions of "resilient" youth varied from 25 % to 84 % (Vanderbilt-Adriance and Shaw 2008). This finding supports the adoption of a *narrow* definition of resilience focusing on specific development outcomes at different specific points in life (Vanderbilt-Adriance and Shaw 2008).

Benson (1997) postulated that the term "resilience" indicates a paradigm shift from the identification of the risk factors of an individual (i.e., a pathological view) to the identification of the strengths of an individual. A "resilient" individual is stress resistant and vulnerable despite the experiences of significant adversity (Garmezy 1996).

To sum up, resilience can be defined in terms of an individual's capacity, the process he or she goes through, and the result (Masten et al. 1990). Resilience as a *capacity* refers to an individual's capacity for adapting to changes and stressful events in a healthy way (Catalano et al. 2004). Resilience as a *process* is regarded as a reintegration process and a return to normal functioning with the support of protective factors after encountering a severe stressor (Richardson 2002). Resilience as a *result* is defined as positive and beneficial outcomes resulting from successfully navigating stressful events (Masten et al. 1990). Resilience has referred to a multidimensional construct in its operational characteristics and a key variable in predicting positive outcomes in the face of adversity. Therefore, an operational definition of resilience must encompass all of the key characteristics of resilience and include the components of the capacity, process, and result. Therefore, resilience can be defined as the process of effectively mobilizing internal and external resources in adapting to or managing significant sources of stress or trauma. Cultivation of resilience means fostering adolescents' capacity, flexibility, and coping strategies when they face developmental changes and life stresses in order to "bounce back" from difficult life experiences and achieve positive outcomes (Catalano et al. 2004; Choi et al. 2003; Wong and Lee 2005).

Research on Resilience

Differences in the definition of resilience lead to different understandings of the nature of potential risk and protective processes (Kaplan 1999; Haskett et al. 2006). Despite this, and despite various studies that use different measurement strategies, researchers have been able to identify many correlates of resilience (protective factors). Masten and Obradovic (Masten 2007; Masten and Obradović 2006) have summarized the first three waves of resilience research: (i) identifying the correlates and characteristics of good adaptation among children and adolescents who appear to develop well despite genetic or environmental risks, (ii) uncovering the processes and regulatory systems that explain how potential assets or protective factors work, and (iii) promoting resilience through prevention, intervention, and policy as a result of the concomitant rise of prevention science, which emphasizes the importance of promoting competence as a strategy. Furthermore, they have identified the following fundamental adaptive systems to play a crucial role in resilience: (i) learning systems of the human brain (problem-solving, information processing), (ii) attachment system (affective processes), (iii) mastery motivation system (self-efficacy processes), (iv) stress response systems (alarm and recovery processes), and (v) self-regulation systems (emotion and behavior regulation) and other systems including family, school, peer, and cultural and societal systems. Among them, research on psychological stress and ways of coping with stress attracts a lot of attention because these factors are crucial in the models of resilience for children and adolescents (Nolte et al. 2011; Cicchetti 2010). The psychological and biological processes of reaction to and recovery from stress play a central role in understanding how prolonged exposure to chronic stress exacts physical and emotional tolls. In a review of the psychobiological processes of stress and coping, Compas (2006) summarized substantial evidence suggesting that automatic responses to stress, including emotional and physiological arousal, impulsive action, intrusive thoughts, and some forms of escapist behavior, may spring from the triggering of the amygdala in response to threats in the environment. Researchers use advanced methods to examine the structure and function of the brain and central nervous system in order to illuminate the neurobiological structure and processes of human coping and adaptation to stress. Compas (2006) pointed out that recent research findings also provide evidence to support that "coping is a part of the overall set of executive functions that are regulated by the prefrontal cortex" (p. 230).

Protective Factors for Psychosocial Resilience in Children and Adolescents

Studies have shown that protective factors lead individuals to adapt in the face of risks. Thus, enhancing both internal and external protective factors of adolescents may help them adapt to stressful and risky life situations. For *internal protective factors*, Smith (Smith and Zautra 2008) summarized research findings and found that optimism, perceptions of control, self-efficacy, and active coping are associated with better health. Grotberg (1999) cited longitudinal studies to show that about half to two-thirds of children with resilience could overcome their initial traumatic life experiences, such as growing up in families with a mentally ill member, suffering from child abuse, or having criminally involved parents. Thus, cultivating resilience is an important way to promote the psychological and social development of adolescents. For *external protective factors*, theorists (Hepworth et al. 2006) have suggested that people who do not have a functional social support system are vulnerable to external stresses. Therefore, it is important to strengthen an individual's ability to recognize and utilize social support systems in his or her surroundings. There is a growing consensus from child and adolescent research on important protective factors (Masten 2007; Masten and Reed 2002). These factors represent four main groups as follows. Remarkably, the salience of these factors may vary across the life span.

Bonding

It consists in emotional attachment and commitment to parents or caregivers (particularly those who maintain a positive family climate, experience a low level of conflict, and are involved in the child's education), close relationships with mature and supportive adults, connections to prosocial and rule-abiding friends, and bonding to people in prosocial organizations.

Competence

Five core individual competencies are involved: (i) cognitive competence, that is, good cognitive abilities; (ii) emotional competence in terms of good self-regulation of emotions and impulses; (iii) moral competence, that is, positive self-perceptions;

(iv) behavioral competence, that is, talents valued by the self and society; and (v) social competence, that is, general appeal or attractiveness to others.

Optimism

This is manifested self-efficacy, spirituality, which is, faith and a sense of meaning in life and a clear and positive identity.

Environment

For example, organized home environment, authoritative parenting (high on warmth, structure/monitoring, and expectations), socioeconomic advantages, effective schools, neighborhoods with high "collective efficacy," high level of public safety, good emergency social services, as well as good public health and healthcare availability – the above list is not exhaustive. A growing body of literature supports the notion that resilience can also be enhanced by an ethnic family's cultural values and provision of mutual psychological support (Genero 1995; Lee et al. 2010). Furthermore, some internal assets may require two or more of the above protective factors. For example, research findings have suggested that a sense of humor, combining cognitive competence with an optimistic outlook, is an internal protective factor that alleviates an individual's focus on personal failure (Fonagy et al. 1994; Masten 1986). Humor is therapeutic for managing anxiety and creates a buffer for individuals against the negative effects of stress (Moran and Massam 1999). A good sense of humor is also positively associated with a healthy self-concept (Ruch and Köhler 1998). Dixon (1980) also pointed out that humor helps restructure the cognitive perception of a threatening situation. Thus, it allows the adolescent to explore cognitive alternatives and develop conflict management strategies in response to stressful and threatening situations. It is expected that these skills are better managed by adolescents who have gained certain social and cognitive competencies (Noller et al. 2001).

Theoretical Relationships Between Resilience and Positive Youth Development

Resilience researchers have conceptualized the relationship between adversity and competence differently (Luthar et al. 2000), and these different conceptual models have led to differing analytic strategies. Some have used person-based data analytic approaches, which involve identifying individuals with high risk and high competence and comparing them with low risk and high competence. Others have used variable-based analyses and found either main effects or interaction effects. This diversity in analytic structure and measurement reflects the need for both a clarification of different definitions of resilience and a critical examination of the conceptualized relationships between resilience and positive youth development. According to various theories or models, there are eight possible relationships between resilience and positive youth development. Four of the relationships take resilience as a forerunner of positive youth development, and four others regard resilience as a result of positive youth development. The distinction between the forerunner and the result represents a dimension of role. Alternatively, the eight relationships reflect four modes of conditionality, pertaining to the sufficient, necessary, probabilistic, and spurious conditions (Hage and Meeker 1988). A sufficient condition is able to invoke something solely. In contrast, a necessary condition is something that must be present. A probabilistic condition is likely to invoke something, usually contingent on other conditions. This represents neither a sufficient nor a necessary condition. A spurious condition does not invoke something and may merely represent coincidence. Combining the dimensions of role and conditionality thereby identifies eight possible relationships such that resilience is a (1) constituent, (2) determinant, (3) contributor, (4) concomitant, (5) indicator, (6) derivative of positive youth development, (7) collateral of positive youth development due to a common effect, and (8) collateral of positive youth development due to a common cause (see Table 1).

Resilience as a *constituent* maintains that it is a sufficient forerunner to define positive youth development. As such, resilience is a defining condition for positive youth development, and alternatively positive youth development must follow resilience. This is the view of the asset-building model and the inclusiveness model of positive youth development. Firstly, the asset-building model posits that resilience is one of youth's internal assets for constituting positive youth development, and as such, the development refers to the process of asset building (Larson 2006). In this connection, resilience would have an association with similar assets such as the optimism, controllability, conflict resolution, and problem-solving aspects of positive youth development (Roth et al. 1998; Sun and Stewart 2007). In this model, all these assets are constituent or sufficient conditions for positive youth development. Moreover, positive youth development also hinges on external assets.

Table 1 Models relating to resilience and positive youth development

Conditionality	Resilience as a forerunner	Resilience as a follower
Sufficient	*Constituent* Asset-building model Inclusiveness model	*Concomitant* Solution-focused model
Necessary	*Determinant* or substantial predictor Courage model Problem-avoidance model	*Indicator* Adaptation model Competence model
Probabilistic	*Contributor* or weak predictor Developmental systems model	*Derivative* Self-regulation theory
Spurious	*Collateral due to a common effect* Citizenship model	*Collateral due to a common cause* Control theory

A notable instance of asset building happens in the caring school, which provides opportunities or challenges for realizing resilience (Gomez and Ang 2007). Secondly, the inclusiveness model, which incorporates the asset-building approach, holds that resilience is particularly a constituent of positive youth development in an inclusive or comprehensive way (Bradshaw et al. 2008). As such, the inclusiveness model regards resilience as the key to relationship building and engagement of social support, which defines the inclusiveness required for positive youth development. Essentially, the inclusiveness model states that personal strength such as resilience is a constituent of social inclusiveness, and this inclusiveness is then a component of positive youth development. Both the asset-building model and the inclusiveness model thereby define positive youth development in terms of the use of strengths or assets such as resilience in the developmental process. Notably, positive youth development in this case refers to the process of asset building and inclusiveness. It is, therefore, an emergent or induced variable contingent on resilience (Cohen et al. 1990; Heise 1972). Essentially, resilience constitutes asset building and inclusiveness, which are tantamount to positive youth development according to the models.

Resilience as a *determinant* or strong predictor means that it is a necessary forerunner – giving rise to positive youth development. As a necessary forerunner, resilience is not something to define positive youth development. Instead, resilience only functions as a very important predictor of positive youth development. Hence, resilience and positive youth development is distinguishable such that the former does not necessarily create the latter. Despite that, positive youth development would be a distinctive outcome highly dependent on resilience. This is the view of both the courage model of resilience and the problem-avoidance model of positive youth development. The courage model maintains that resilience embodies courage for positive youth development through the manifestations of belonging, mastery, independence, and generosity. These characteristics then satisfy needs for attachment, achievement, autonomy, and altruism (Brendtro and Larson 2004). Therefore, resilience represents a mental force to engender positive youth development through need fulfillment. The problem-avoidance model, alternatively, posits that resilience is a necessary condition for positive youth development (Bradshaw et al. 2008). As such, positive youth development is only possible in the absence of problems, as problems are usually impediments to learning and growth. Essentially, this model contrasts with the inclusiveness model, which regards resilience as a sufficient condition for positive youth development.

Resilience as a *contributor* to or probabilistic condition for positive youth development means that it is likely to induce the development or resilience, but the likelihood is neither compelling nor straightforward. This role of resilience is inherent in the developmental systems theory of positive youth development (Balsano et al. 2009). This theory maintains that positive youth development results from the alignment of personal strengths with community assets. As such, the function of resilience as a personal strength is contingent on the support and opportunities available in the context and the program. When the context or program encourages or requires resilience, resilience would become a determinant of positive youth development. The theory also posits the presence of multiple systems, each of which interactively contributes to positive youth development. Therefore, the personal strength of resilience is one factor, playing the role of a contributor, collaborating with other factors in the production of positive youth development.

Resilience as a *concomitant* that follows positive youth development means that positive youth development is a sufficient condition for resilience. That is, positive youth development alone is capable of generating resilience. This is the view of the solution-focused model of resilience, which regards resilience as a success in development, adaptation, or overcoming problems or simply as a solution to problems (Simon et al. 2005). In this view, positive youth development means resilience, as a result of successfully encountering developmental tasks or problems (Benson 2007; Scales et al. 2000; Wagener et al. 2003). In other words, because of difficulties in development, resilience takes shape in the success of positive youth development or in solutions to developmental problems. Resilience is, therefore, not separate from positive youth development. Possibly, positive youth development is a process that results in the development of resilience.

Resilience as an *indicator* of positive youth development means that positive youth development is a necessary condition for resilience, and resilience necessarily reflects positive youth development. This is the view of the adaptation and competence models of positive youth development. The adaptation model holds that adaptation to myriad developmental tasks is imperative for positive youth development and the adaptation generates competence, which upholds resilience (Guerra and Bradshaw 2008). Such competence comprises abilities to maintain a positive self-image, self-control, decision-making, moral reasoning, and social connectedness. Similarly, the competence model includes resilience as one among many forms of competence, including social competence, emotional competence, moral competence, self-determination, spirituality, and belief in the future. Together the developments of these characteristics are indicative of positive youth development (Catalano et al. 2004). In this model, positive youth development is a latent variable, which is identifiable by resilience and other forms of competence.

Resilience as a *derivative* or probabilistic consequence of positive youth development means that human development is likely to engender resilience. This implies that resilience and positive youth development are conceptually separate and related only contingently. This implication inheres in self-regulation theory, which posits that positive youth development generates resilience in the presence of problems and alternative goal evaluations (Scheier and Carver 2001). Self-regulation theory essentially holds that proactive action and expectation play a contributory role in tackling contextual problems. Relevant to positive youth development are selection, optimization, and compensation in the presence of problems (Balsano et al. 2009; Lewin-Bizan et al. 2010). Accordingly, problems limit choices such that the selection of options for their best use and disallowing forbidden options is necessary. Self-regulation demonstrates its usefulness in tackling problems, creating the need for change or self-regulation. Key to the probabilistic influence of positive youth development is confidence, which indicates thriving or flourishing (Balsano et al. 2009; Gestsdóttir and Lerner 2007; Phelps et al. 2009).

Resilience holds a spurious relationship with positive youth development because their *common effect* means that the common effect is responsible for maintaining a relationship that otherwise does not hold. This is possible based on the citizenship model, which posits that both resilience and positive youth development are contributors to citizenship in terms of personal and social responsibility (Balsano et al. 2009; Hines et al. 2005; Lerner 2004; Mullin and Arce 2008). Hence, both resilience and positive youth development serve a similar role in satisfying societal needs (Lerner 2004). This similarity forms a relationship between resilience and positive youth development because of their common role.

Resilience has a spurious relationship with positive youth development due to their *common cause* which means that the common cause implies a relationship that would not otherwise exist. This common causation is proposed in control theory, which posits that control is a common cause of both resilience and positive youth development (Heckhausen 2002). Accordingly, control involves primary and secondary forms of control dealing with selection and compensation of factors and resources used to facilitate resilience and positive youth development. All these factors lead to coping, which is then conducive to resilience and positive youth development (Anthony 2008; Aspinwall and Taylor 1992; Göral et al. 2006; Swanson et al. 2002). Hence, control and coping are common causes of both resilience and positive youth development, thus creating an illusion of relationship.

Discussion

The aforementioned eight possible relationships between resilience and positive youth development are not necessarily mutually exclusive, since they can operate at the same time in an additive way. This is because both resilience and positive youth development can take many forms, as either dynamic processes or static conditions. Nevertheless, the most viable, suitable, reasonable, and popular possibility is that resilience is a contributor to positive youth development, as based on developmental systems theory. This conceptualization has the advantage of treating resilience and positive youth development as separate concepts, which avoids confusion and overlap. The separation is vital for establishing discriminant validity and thereby the unique value of the two concepts. In this conceptualization, positive youth development has its own indicators. Consistent with developmental systems theory, the indicators are the six Cs: confidence, competence, connection, character, caring, and contribution (Balsano et al. 2009; Gestsdóttir and Lerner 2007; Phelps et al. 2009). They make positive youth development conceptually different from resilience. Moreover, the contributory relationship does not require either a sufficient or a necessary condition in the relationship between resilience and positive youth development. This condition is easily and commonly met in empirical research (Gestsdóttir and Lerner 2007; Göral et al. 2006). Most importantly, this formulation has a strong theoretical base in developmental systems theory (Balsano et al. 2009). The theory tends to be realistic in regarding youth development as a product of interactions among multiple systems. Another strong justification is the differentiation of views that resilience deals with the removal of negative development problems and that positive youth development is about the positive side of development beyond problem resolution (Bogenschneider 1996; Lerner et al. 2009; Luthar et al. 2000; Rutter 1999). Accordingly, the removing of problems in resilience is unlikely to represent or create positive youth development immediately. Furthermore, a third forceful justification is that resilience contributes to positive youth development only conditionally, in the presence of adversity or problems (Luthar et al. 2000; Rutter 1999). This view is also consistent with developmental systems theory, which envisions positive youth development as a contingent outcome resulting from interactions among systems.

Evidence supporting the conditional or probabilistic contribution of resilience to positive youth development, including its five major indicators competence, confidence, connectedness, character, and caring, includes the following. First, resilience in terms of controllability over stress appears be more conducive to youth development in relation to stress-related growth when the youth has practiced problem-focused coping strategies. This is evidenced by enhanced competence. Controllability itself has not shown a main effect (Göral et al. 2006). This conditional contribution implies that stress or adversity is needed for coping and that enhanced competence is the successful consequence. When coping and controllability fit the need for coping, youth development emerges. Second, resilience in terms of residential stability in a disadvantaged neighborhood has appeared to be particularly conducive to positive youth development in terms of competence (Elliott et al. 2006). In this case, the disadvantaged neighborhood would be a source of adversity, giving rise to the opportunity for resilience to manifest. Third, resilience in terms of the absence of social anxiety has appeared to be more conducive to positive youth development in terms of the character of moral behavior when the youth has had a chronic illness (McCarroll et al. 2009). In this connection, chronic illness as adversity combined with resilience can reduce social anxiety and improved character, another major indicator of positive youth development. Fourth, resilience in terms of belief in a just world has appeared to be particularly conducive to self-esteem development in terms of anger induction (Dalbert 2002). As such, anger induction is an adversity, and the resilient response leads to enhanced confidence. Fifth, resilience in terms of absence of worry about illness appears conducive to the childhood cancer survivor's confidence (Zebrack and Chesler 2001). Sixth, resilience in terms of morale in the presence of illness has appeared to foster development in terms of social interaction and relationship quality, which are defining characteristics of connectedness (Davies et al. 2000). The latter two findings consistently show that illness can be an adverse condition which, when responded to with resilience, provides an important developmental contribution.

One of the factors that may hinder the development of resilience research is the complexity of adversity. Future theoretical development needs to clearly define adverse events in the external world. Within a life-span developmental perspective, the context of the adversity could be biological, psychological, economic, or social. A major concern is that it will be inappropriate to apply the concept of resilience if a stressor does not require adaptation or does not lead to negative outcomes (Roisman 2005). Not all adversities are equivalent in severity (Vanderbilt-Adriance and Shaw 2008). Therefore, research methodologies should carefully consider the identification of the specific adversity along with its severity and duration when constructing measurement instruments.

References

American Psychological Association. (n.d.). *The road to resilience*. Retrieved from http://www. apa.org/helpcenter/road-resilience.aspx

Anthony, E. K. (2008). Cluster profiles of youths living in urban poverty: Factors affecting risk and resilience. *Social Work Research, 32*(1), 6–17.

Aspinwall, L. G., & Taylor, S. E. (1992). Modeling cognitive adaptation: A longitudinal investigation of the impact of individual differences and coping on college adjustment and performance. *Journal of Personality and Social Psychology, 63*(6), 989–1003.

Balsano, A. B., Phelps, E., Theokas, C., Lerner, J. V., & Lerner, R. M. (2009). Patterns of early adolescents' participation in youth development programs having positive youth development goals. *Journal of Research on Adolescence, 19*(2), 249–259.

Benson, P. L. (1997). *All kids are our kids*. Minneapolis: Search Institute.

Benson, J. E. (2007). Make new friends but keep the old: Peers and the transition to college. *Advances in Life Course Research, 12*, 309–334.

Bogenschneider, K. (1996). Family related prevention programs: An ecological risk/protective theory for building prevention programs, policies, and community capacity to support youth. *Family Relations, 45*(2), 127–138.

Bradshaw, C. P., Brown, J. S., & Hamilton, S. F. (2008). Bridging positive youth development and mental health services for youth with serious behavior problems. *Child & Youth Care Forum, 37*(5-6), 209–226.

Brendtro, L., & Larson, S. (2004). The resilience code: Finding greatness in youth. *Reclaiming Children and Youth, 12*(4), 194–200.

Catalano, R. F., Berglund, M. L., Ryan, J. A., Lonczak, H. S., & Hawkins, J. D. (2004). Positive youth development in the United States: Research findings on evaluations of positive youth development programs. *The Annals of the American Academy of Political and Social Science, 591*, 98–124.

Choi, P. Y. W., Au, C. K., Tang, C. W., Shum, S. M., Tang, S. Y., Choi, F. M., & Lee, T. C. (2003). *Making young tumblers: A manual of promoting resilience in schools and families* (in Chinese). Hong Kong: Breakthrough.

Cicchetti, D. (2010). Resilience under conditions of extreme stress: A multilevel perspective. *World Psychiatry, 9*(3), 145–154.

Cohen, P., Cohen, J., Teresi, J., Marchi, M., & Velez, C. N. (1990). Problems in the measurement of latent variables in structural equations causal models. *Applied Psychological Measurement, 14*(2), 183–196.

Compas, B. E. (2006). Psychobiological processes of stress and coping. *Annals of the New York Academy of Sciences, 1094*(1), 226–234.

Dalbert, C. (2002). Beliefs in a just world as a buffer against anger. *Social Justice Research, 15*(2), 123–145.

Davies, B., Fernandez, J., & Nomer, B. (2000). *Equity and efficiency policy in community care: Needs, service productivities, efficiencies, and their implications*. Ashgate: University of Kent at Canterbury Personal Social Services Research Unit.

Dixon, N. (1980). Humor: A cognitive alternative to stress. In C. D. Spielberger & I. G. Sarason (Eds.), *Anxiety and stress* (pp. 281–289). Washington: Hemisphere.

Elliott, D. S., Menard, S., Elliott, A., Rankin, B., Huizinga, D., & Wilson, W. J. (2006). *Good kids from bad neighborhoods: Successful development in social context.* New York: Cambridge University Press.

Fonagy, P., Steele, M., Steele, H., Higgitt, A., & Target, M. (1994). The Emanuel Miller Memorial lecture 1992: The theory and practice of resilience. *Journal of Child Psychology and Psychiatry, 35*(2), 231–257.

Garmezy, N. (1996). Reflections and commentary on risk, resilience, and development. In R. J. Haggerty, L. R. Sherrod, N. Garmezy, & R. Rutter (Eds.), *Stress, risk, and resilience in children and adolescents* (pp. 1–15). New York: Cambridge University Press.

Genero, N. P. (1995). Culture, resiliency, and mutual psychological development. In H. I. McCubbin, E. A. Thompson, A. I. Thompson, & J. A. Futrell (Eds.), *Resiliency in ethnic minority families: African-American families* (Vol. 2, pp. 31–48). Thousand Oaks: Sage.

Gestsdóttir, S., & Lerner, R. M. (2007). Intentional self-regulation and positive youth development in early adolescence: Findings from the 4-H study of positive youth development. *Developmental Psychology, 43*(2), 508–521.

Gitterman, A. (Ed.). (1991). *Handbook of social work practice with vulnerable populations.* New York: Columbia University Press.

Gomez, B. J., & Ang, P. M. M. (2007). Promoting positive youth development in schools. *Theory Into Practice, 46*(2), 97–104.

Göral, F. S., Kesimci, A., & Gençöz, T. (2006). Roles of the controllability of the event and coping strategies on stress-related growth in a Turkish sample. *Stress and Health, 22*(5), 297–303.

Grotberg, E. H. (1999). *Tapping your inner strength: How to find the resilience to deal with anything.* Oakland: New Harbinger Publications.

Guerra, N. G., & Bradshaw, C. P. (2008). Linking the prevention of problem behaviors and positive youth development: Core competencies for positive youth development and risk prevention. *New Directions for Child and Adolescent Development, 2008*(122), 1–17.

Hage, J., & Meeker, B. F. (1988). *Social causality.* Boston: Unwin Hyman.

Haskett, M. E., Nears, K., Sabourin Ward, C., & McPherson, A. V. (2006). Diversity in adjustment of maltreated children: Factors associated with resilient functioning. *Clinical Psychology Review, 26*(6), 796–812.

Heckhausen, J. (2002). 10 developmental regulation of life-course transitions: A control theory approach. In L. Pulkkinen & A. Caspi (Eds.), *Paths to successful development: Personality in the life course* (pp. 257–280). New York: Cambridge University Press.

Heise, D. R. (1972). Employing nominal variables, induced variables, and block variables in path analyses. *Sociological Methods & Research, 1*(2), 147–173.

Hepworth, D. H., Rooney, R. H., Rooney, G. D., Strom-Gottfried, K., & Larson, J. (2006). *Direct social work practice: Theory and skills* (7th ed.). Belmont: Thomson Brooks/Cole.

Hines, A. M., Merdinger, J., & Wyatt, P. (2005). Former foster youth attending college: Resilience and the transition to young adulthood. *American Journal of Orthopsychiatry, 75*(3), 381–394.

Kaplan, H. B. (1999). Toward an understanding of resilience: A critical review of definitions and models. In M. D. Glantz & J. R. Johnson (Eds.), *Resilience and development: Positive life adaptations* (pp. 17–83). New York: Plenum Press.

Larson, R. (2006). Positive youth development, willful adolescents, and mentoring. *Journal of Community Psychology, 34*(6), 677–689.

Lee, T. Y., Kwong, W. M., Cheung, C. K., Ungar, M., & Cheung, M. Y. (2010). Children's resilience-related beliefs as a predictor of positive child development in the face of adversities: Implications for interventions to enhance children's quality of life. *Social Indicators Research, 95*(3), 437–453.

Lerner, R. M. (2004). *Liberty: Thriving and civic engagement among America's youth.* Thousand Oaks: Sage.

Lerner, J. V., Phelps, E., Forman, Y. E., & Bowers, E. P. (2009). Positive youth development. In R. M. Lerner & L. Steinberg (Eds.), *Handbook of adolescent psychology* (3rd ed., pp. 524–558). Hoboken: Wiley.

Lewin-Bizan, S., Bowers, E. P., & Lerner, R. M. (2010). One good thing leads to another: Cascades of positive youth development among American adolescents. *Development and Psychopathology, 22*(4), 759–770.

Luthar, S. S., & Zigler, E. (1991). Vulnerability and competence: A review of research on resilience in childhood. *American Journal of Orthopsychiatry, 61*(1), 6–22.

Luthar, S. S., Cicchetti, D., & Becker, B. (2000). The construct of resilience: A critical evaluation and guidelines for future work. *Child Development, 71*(3), 543–562.

Masten, A. S. (1986). Humor and competence in school-aged children. *Child Development, 57,* 461–473.

Masten, A. S. (2007). Resilience in developing systems: Progress and promise as the fourth wave rises. *Development and Psychopathology, 19*(3), 921–930.

Masten, A. S., & Obradović, J. (2006). Competence and resilience in development. *Annals of the New York Academy of Sciences, 1094*(1), 13–27.

Masten, A. S., & Reed, M. G. J. (2002). Resilience in development. In C. R. Snyder & S. J. Lopez (Eds.), *Handbook of positive psychology* (pp. 74–88). New York: Oxford University Press.

Masten, A. S., Best, K. M., & Garmezy, N. (1990). Resilience and development: Contributions from the study of children who overcome adversity. *Development and Psychopathology, 2*(4), 425–444.

McCarroll, E. M., Lindsey, E. W., MacKinnon-Lewis, C., Chambers, J. C., & Frabutt, J. M. (2009). Health status and peer relationships in early adolescence: The role of peer contact, self-esteem, and social anxiety. *Journal of Child and Family Studies, 18*(4), 473–485.

Moran, C. C., & Massam, M. M. (1999). Differential influences of coping humor and humor bias on mood. *Behavioral Medicine, 25*(1), 36–42.

Mullin, W. J., & Arce, M. (2008). Resilience of families living in poverty. *Journal of Family Social Work, 11*(4), 424–440.

Noller, P., Feeney, J. A., & Peterson, C. (2001). *Personal relationships across the lifespan.* Sussex: Psychology Press.

Nolte, T., Guiney, J., Fonagy, P., Mayes, L. C., & Luyten, P. (2011). Interpersonal stress regulation and the development of anxiety disorders: An attachment-based developmental framework. *Frontiers in Behavioral Neuroscience, 5,* a55.

Phelps, E., Zimmerman, S., Warren, A. E. A., Jeličić, H., von Eye, A., & Lerner, R. M. (2009). The structure and developmental course of positive youth development (PYD) in early adolescence: Implications for theory and practice. *Journal of Applied Developmental Psychology, 30*(5), 571–584.

Richardson, G. E. (2002). The metatheory of resilience and resiliency. *Journal of Clinical Psychology, 58*(3), 307–321.

Roisman, G. I. (2005). Conceptual clarifications in the study of resilience. *American Psychologist, 60*(3), 264–265.

Roth, J., Brooks-Gunn, J., Murray, L., & Foster, W. (1998). Promoting healthy adolescents: Synthesis of youth development program evaluations. *Journal of Research on Adolescence, 8*(4), 423–459.

Ruch, W., & Köhler, G. (1998). A temperament approach to humor. In W. Ruch (Ed.), *The sense of humor: Explorations of a personality characteristic* (pp. 203–230). New York: Mouton de Gruyter.

Rutter, M. (1987). Psychosocial resilience and protective mechanisms. *American Journal of Orthopsychiatry, 57*(3), 316–331.

Rutter, M. (1999). Resilience concepts and findings: Implications for family therapy. *Journal of Family Therapy, 21*(2), 119–144.

Scales, P. C., Benson, P. L., Leffert, N., & Blyth, D. A. (2000). Contribution of developmental assets to the prediction of thriving among adolescents. *Applied Developmental Science, 4*(1), 27–46.

Scheier, M. F., & Carver, C. S. (2001). Adapting to cancer: The importance of hope and purpose. In A. Baum & B. L. Andersen (Eds.), *Psychosocial interventions for cancer* (pp. 15–36). Washington, DC: American Psychological Association.

Simon, J. B., Murphy, J. J., & Smith, S. M. (2005). Understanding and fostering family resilience. *The Family Journal, 13*(4), 427–436.

Smith, B. W., & Zautra, A. J. (2008). Vulnerability and resilience in women with arthritis: Test of a two-factor model. *Journal of Consulting and Clinical Psychology, 76*(5), 799–810.

Sun, J., & Stewart, D. (2007). Development of population-based resilience measures in the primary school setting. *Health Education, 107*(6), 575–599.

Swanson, D. P., Spencer, M. B., Harpalani, V., & Spencer, T. R. (2002). Identity processes and the positive youth development of African Americans: An explanatory framework. *New Directions for Youth Development, 2002*(95), 73–100.

Vanderbilt-Adriance, E., & Shaw, D. S. (2008). Conceptualizing and re-evaluating resilience across levels of risk, time, and domains of competence. *Clinical Child and Family Psychology Review, 11*(1–2), 30–58.

Wagener, L. M., Furrow, J. L., King, P. F., Leffert, N., & Benson, P. (2003). Religious involvement and developmental resources in youth. *Review of Religious Research, 44*(3), 271–284.

Windle, G. (2011). What is resilience? A review and concept analysis. *Reviews in Clinical Gerontology, 21*(2), 152–169.

Wong, K. Y., & Lee, T. Y. (2005). Professional discourse among social workers working with at-risk adolescents in Hong Kong. In M. Ungar (Ed.), *Pathways to resilience: A handbook of theory, methods, and intervention* (pp. 313–327). Thousand Oaks: Sage.

Zebrack, B. J., & Chesler, M. (2001). Health-related worries, self-image, and life outlooks of long-term survivors of childhood cancer. *Health & Social Work, 26*(4), 245–256.

Part II
Student Well-Being and Developmental Issues in Hong Kong: Primary Prevention

Prevention of Drug Abuse Among Young People in Hong Kong: The P.A.T.H.S. Program

Tak Yan Lee and Diego Busiol

Abstract Adolescents' use of drug is influenced by peer influence and (lack of) school support as well as by students' and students' families' characteristics. P.A.T.H.S. program helps students to develop self-determination in achieving their goals and being less subjected to peer influence and enhances emotional competence to recognize, name, and transform negative feelings into more constructive attitudes. The following chapter attempts to construct a conceptual framework of adolescent drug abuse by integrating existing theories and the positive youth development perspective; further, it reports with illustrations how each of the 20 units on drug prevention introduced in the extension phase of Project P.A.T.H.S. is inspired by the 15 PYD constructs. It is argued that primary intervention developed under this framework will fulfill four functions: (1) prevention of the use of psychotropic drugs, (2) victimization protection, (3) strengthening support system, and (4) promotion of biopsychosocial aspects of health.

Introduction

Project P.A.T.H.S. is a school-based program designed to prevent, among others, drug use in youth and combines features of ecological and social cognitive theories. The ecological perspective leads to a consideration of the complexity of the personal, sociocultural, policy, and physical-environmental factors within and beyond youth that contribute to drug use. Students' use of drug is influenced by peer influence and

The preparation for this work and the Project P.A.T.H.S. were financially supported by The Hong Kong Jockey Club Charities Trust.

This paper is partially based on an article originally published by *The Scientific World Journal*: Lee, T. Y. (2011). Construction of an integrated positive youth development conceptual framework for the prevention of the use of psychotropic drugs among adolescents. *The Scientific World Journal, 11*, 2403–2417.

T.Y. Lee (✉) • D. Busiol
Department of Applied Social Sciences, City University of Hong Kong,
Kowloon, Hong Kong, China
e-mail: ty.lee@cityu.edu.hk

(lack of) school support as well as by students' and students' families' characteristics. Social cognitive theory indicates that teachers' delivery of the P.A.T.H.S. program helps students to develop self-determination in achieving their goals and being less subjected to peer influence and enhances emotional competence to recognize, name, and transform negative feelings into more constructive attitudes. P.A.T.H.S. is inspired by the concept of *positive youth development* (Table 1). It is based on a comprehensive framework and adopts a "strengths" perspective, that is, it aims at enhancing youth's attributes and resources. It focuses on prevention rather than on responding to needs or problem solving (Lam et al. 2011). Indeed, it is grounded on the principle that if psychosocial competencies in adolescents can be promoted, adolescent risky behavior such as drug taking will be greatly reduced.

Research on the development of adolescents' risky behavior over a period of 5 years demonstrated that students receiving the program had significantly slower increases in substance use as compared to the control participants (Shek and Yu 2012). Shek (2006) described objective outcome evaluation findings based on the first six waves of data (i.e., Secondary 1 to Secondary 3 data) of Project P.A.T.H.S. and revealed that students in the experimental schools displayed a lower level of risky behavior (including substance abuse behavior) than did students in the control group in terms of abuse of ketamine, cannabis, pills, and heroin (i.e., illegal psychotropic substances) as well as delinquent behavior. Obviously, the positive evaluation findings in Project P.A.T.H.S. suggest that it is a promising program which can be used as an effective antidrug education program in Hong Kong. Different evaluation studies consistently show that Project P.A.T.H.S. can promote psychosocial competencies and reduce risky behavior (including substance abuse) in early adolescents in Hong Kong (Shek 2006, 2008, 2009a, b; Shek and Ma 2010; Shek and Ng 2009; Shek and Sun 2008, 2010; Shek et al. 2007, 2008).

An Integrated Positive Youth Development Conceptual Framework for Primary Prevention of Adolescent Drug Use

By further linking the 15 positive youth development constructs, an integrated positive youth development conceptual framework for primary prevention of adolescent drug abuse has been developed (Fig. 1). It hypothesizes that drug use in adolescence is a result of the interaction between genetic and biological vulnerabilities with contextual, lifestyle, and sociological factors which will also further condition drug dependency.

According to this framework, an adolescent who is biologically and psychologically vulnerable (factors (A)–(D), (F), and (M), Fig. 1) living in deprived social circumstances (factors (G)–(L), Fig. 3) who is exposed to certain psychoactive chemicals (structural barriers, factor (N)) will promote adolescent drug use, continuous use, and subsequent abuse (relapse, factor (E)).

Theoretically, personal cognitions and perceptions are influenced by several factors (factors (E), (F), (K), (L), and (M), Fig. 1). According to social learning theory (Blumer 1969), drug abuse is a behavior that an adolescent is taught by his/

Table 1 Dealing with the causes of adolescents' use of psychotropic drugs through the promotion of 15 positive youth development constructs

Code	Positive youth development constructs	Content	Responding to relevant causes
BO	Bonding	Promotion of relationships with healthy adults and positive peers	Alienated family relationship; delinquent peers
RE	Cultivation of resilience	Enhancing the capacity to adapt to change and stressful events in healthy and adaptive ways	Weak resilience
SC	Social competence	Promotion of interpersonal skills and providing opportunities to practice such skills	Difficult interpersonal relationships
EC	Emotional competence	Promotion of emotional maturity and management	Boredom; complex situations; weak emotional control and expression
CC	Cognitive competence	Promotion of development of cognitive skills and thinking	Weak analytical ability
BC	Behavioral competence	Cultivation of verbal and nonverbal communication skills and initiatives in taking action	Weak will power; weak problem-solving ability
MC	Moral competence	Development of a sense of right and wrong	Peer pressure; weak problem-solving ability; weak moral competence
SD	Self-determination	Promoting a sense of autonomy	Peer pressure
SE	Development of self-efficacy	Promotion of coping and mastery skills	Peer pressure; low self-esteem
SP	Spirituality	Development of purpose and meaning in life, hope or belief in a higher power	Curiosity and ostentation; complex situations; weak future direction
BF	Belief in the future	Development of future potential goals, choices, or options	Low self-esteem; curiosity and ostentation
ID	Development of clear and positive identity	Promotion of healthy identity	Delinquent peers; low self-esteem
PI	Providing opportunities for prosocial involvement	Designing activities and events for program participants to make positive contributions to groups	Low self-esteem; boredom
PN	Fostering prosocial norms	Encouraging program participants to develop clear and explicit standards for prosocial engagement	Alienated family relationships; quick money; social exclusion
	Recognition for positive behavior	Developing systems for rewarding positive behavior	Since the last construct, recognition for positive behavior is relevant to all other constructs, it is excluded

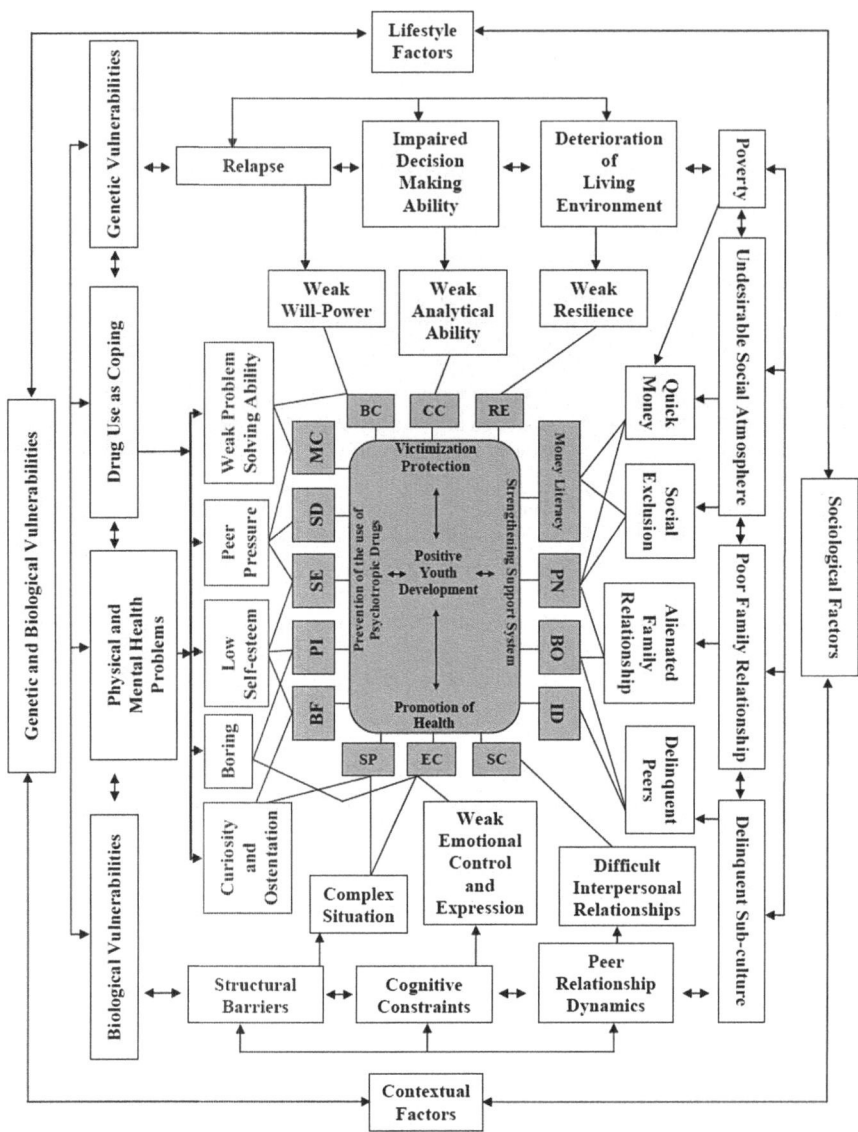

Fig. 1 Integrated positive youth development conceptual framework for primary prevention of adolescent drug use

her surroundings to adopt. This means that drug abuse is partly due to direct (e.g., friends' influence, ineffective parental control, parental attitudes and availability) and indirect stimuli (e.g., delinquent peer models). Moreover, symbolic interaction (Skinner 1953) postulates that an adolescent's action is based on his/her interpretation of settings, symbols, and meanings. Factors (B), (C), and (F)–(M) also find their grounds from the perspective of symbolic interaction. Furthermore, the operant conditioning theory explains why an adolescent tends to repeat drug-taking behavior that is rewarded. These rewards can be of both a social and a biological nature, for example, the social acceptance gained when taking drugs or the sensation of well-being when under a drug's influence (Becker and Murphy 1988). The value of taking drugs, and the rationality in achieving this, is discussed in the theory of rational choice theory (Polansky 1986).

The links between the 15 positive youth development constructs and causes of the use of psychotropic drugs indicate how the constructs are used to tackle such causes as prevention measures. The lines denote linkages but by no means are the only connections. Significant linkages are shown diagrammatically in the elaborated conceptual framework presented in Fig. 1.

Project P.A.T.H.S.

The following table (Table 2) describes how each of the 20 units on drug prevention is inspired by the 15 PYD constructs. Each unit has a specific goal and is based on one principal PYD construct and one or more secondary constructs (in brackets). Each unit aims at responding to different risk factors, among those described by the literature. To do this, a number of activities are suggested, as reported in the table.

Year 1 to Year 3 students are expected to shift their attention from their inner state and emotions to the outside values and needs of society.

In the first year (Fig. 2), students are helped to know more about themselves and their personality and how this may affect their relationships. They are initially guided to identify different emotional states and coping methods (Units 1–3: Choosing a Better Way; Emotion, Your Name Is…; Emotional Survival Guide) and encouraged to think of the consequences of disruptive emotions (i.e., substance abuse). Then, they are encouraged to think critically about drugs (Unit 4: Facts Are Facts), their peers (Unit 5: At Sixes and Sevens), and the influence that the two can have on them. Finally, they are helped to distinguish between desirable and undesirable friends, prefer healthy relations to drug temptation (Units 6–7: Find a Good Friend; Say No to Undesirable Friends), and reflect on consequences of making a choice (Unit 8: What Should I Do?).

In year two (Fig. 3), students are helped to shift their focus from themselves to others, from the individual level to the community in which they live. Students are invited to observe and understand the standards in the community as well as recognize expectations from society (Unit 1: Is It Okay?). Then they are helped to recognize conforming behavior and ethical standards of the community (Unit 2: Is It Right or Wrong to Follow the Trend?). Then they are helped to find productive ways for facing frustrations and resist temptations when they are facing difficulties (Unit 3: What Are frustrations?). To enhance their own sense of responsibility, students are invited to think about their own strengths and they are helped to enhance their critical-thinking and

Table 2 Structure of the program across the 3 years

Unit	Goal of the unit	PYD constructs	Risk factors	Questions/activities
Secondary one curriculum				
Choosing a Better Way (AD 1.1)	To enable students to understand that emotions may affect our ability to solve problems and thus lead to different consequences	EC (MC, RE)	Emotional detachment Unengaged youths Exclusion Isolation, depression, anxiety, stress Low self-control Peer influence Susceptibility to peer pressure	A group discussion to understand the relationship between coping methods and consequences A group game to understand the possible consequences of emotions
Emotion, Your Name Is… (AD 1.2)	To help students understand their emotions, identify different emotional states caused by different conditions, and realize that individuals in certain emotional states are easily influenced by drugs	EC (RE, ID)	Emotional detachment Unengaged youths Exclusion Isolation, depression, anxiety, stress Low self-control Peer influence Susceptibility to peer pressure	A group game and a class sharing to improve the ability to describe and identify emotions Class discussion and games to identify various emotional states and their causes
Emotional Survival Guide (AD 1.3)	To understand that choosing a smarter coping method can make life better	RE (BC, BF)	Emotional detachment Unengaged youths Exclusion Isolation, depression, anxiety, stress Low self-control Peer influence Susceptibility to peer pressure	Group creative activity and sharing to explore different ways of solving problems and coping with emotions creatively Class discussion to identify the benefits and drawbacks of "forgetting/detaching" as a coping method Group work to analyze the use of drugs as a coping method

Facts Are Facts (AD 1.4)	To understand that clarifying facts is the first step of critical thinking	CC (BO, SD)	Unawareness of the consequences of drug use	Class discussion to identify the facts and myths about drugs Group discussion and self-reflection to improve the use of critical thinking in daily life
At Sixes and Sevens (AD 1.5)	To encourage students when they face peer pressure	CC (RE, SD)	Peer influence Susceptibility to peer pressure	Role play and class discussion to familiarize students with persuasion strategies and evaluate their judgment standards A game to improve students' critical thinking when facing peer pressure
Find a Good Friend (AD 1.6)	To enhance students' understanding of their own personality and to investigate the effect of personality on interpersonal relationships	BO	Exclusion Isolation, depression, anxiety, stress Emotional detachment	Group discussion and role play to learn about the four major types of personality Role play to understand the effects of personality on interpersonal relationships and review their own personality and individual behavior (including illegal behavior)
Say No to Undesirable Friends (AD 1.7)	To show students how to recognize desirable friends from undesirable ones and encourage them to choose the right friends and establish a healthy relationship To show students the required skills to resist temptation	BO (BC)	Peer influence Susceptibility to peer pressure Isolation, depression, anxiety, stress Exclusion from school and from nondrug-using peer groups Underachievement	Class game to identify desirable and undesirable friends Group discussion and role play to learn how to practice refusal principles and skills
What Should I Do? (AD 1.8)	To explore vital areas in decision-making in order to be able to make positive decisions in daily life	SD (CC)	Peer influence Peer drug use Low self-control Low self-esteem Perceived control to gain access to drugs	Group discussion to learn and to consider and analyze others' opinions and the consequences of making a choice

(continued)

Table 2 (continued)

Unit	Goal of the unit	PYD constructs	Risk factors	Questions/activities
Secondary two curriculum				
Is It Okay? (AD 2.1)	To let students understand and encourage students to observe the clear, positive, healthy, and ethical standards in the community	PN	Peer influence Family drug use Perceived control to gain access to drugs Susceptibility to peer pressure Intention to try other substances Unawareness of the consequences of drug use	Group discussion to learn that society holds different standards toward different people/issues Role play to understand that people of different age groups/backgrounds have different social responsibilities Case study and group discussion to understand that the court imposes heavy penalties on drug traffickers and the reasons for this
Is It Right or Wrong to Follow the Trend? (AD 2.2)	To distinguish the expectations of society toward conforming behavior	PN	Peer influence Family drug use Perceived control to gain access to drugs Susceptibility to peer pressure Intention to try other substances Unawareness of the consequences of drug use	Group discussion to understand that conforming behavior can be good or bad and to understand the importance of not following trends blindly but making rational choices
What Are Frustrations? (AD 2.3)	To reconstruct students' awareness of what frustrations are and to let them understand how to learn from the experience of frustrations	RE	Low self-esteem Low self-control Underachievement Study stress Negative labeling from teachers Suspension from school Isolation, depression, anxiety, and stress Physical maltreatment	Class game and group discussion to understand how to face failures and to find out the learning points from the experience of frustrations

General's Choice (AD 2.4)	To learn that we should not accept any temptations when we are facing difficulties just to obtain excitement as we are creating greater problems for the future	RE	Low self-esteem Low self-control Underachievement Study stress Negative labeling from teachers Suspension from school Isolation, depression, anxiety, and stress Physical maltreatment	Class game and personal reflection to understand the luring effects of temptations and how to reject them and to stay away from short-term happiness that comes from avoidance of adversity
Think Twice! (AD 2.5)	To enhance students' competence in self-determination by sharpening their decision-making skills	SD	Peer influence Low self-esteem Low self-control Isolation, depression, anxiety, and stress	Group discussion to sharpen decision-making skills Class discussion to handle peer pressure by making use of decision-making skills and to understand that each person should be responsible for his/her decisions and accept the consequences
I Am Precious! (AD 2.6)	To rediscover self-worth, as a means of resisting the temptation to take drugs	ID	Peer influence Low self-esteem Low self-control Isolation, depression, anxiety, and stress	Personal reflection to understand that each person can overcome the past and rediscover their self-worth and direction in life; to discover one's strengths; and to understand that everyone is unique
Secondary three curriculum				
Opium Trade War (AD 3.1)	To reflect on how we can contribute to a society that is being harmed	SC (MC)	Lack of values Lack of responsibility Peer influence Exclusion from schools and from nondrug-using peer groups Low self-esteem Low self-control Unawareness of the consequences of drug use Isolation	Group discussion to know the stories of some "nobodies" in Chinese history and cultivate our sense of responsibility when facing social problems To think about our own roles when the community is being harmed

(continued)

Table 2 (continued)

Unit	Goal of the unit	PYD constructs	Risk factors	Questions/activities
Encountering a Friend (AD 3.2)	To facilitate students' empathetic understanding of others and to encourage them to help themselves and others when there are problems caused by emotions	EC (SE)	Emotional detachment Unengaged youths Peer drug use Isolation, depression Low self-esteem Psychosomatic symptoms	Role play and class discussion to develop empathy by illustrating and explaining the mind-set of the youngsters who use drugs and to realize that these emotions may be ways of adapting to life Personal reflections to take action to support friends facing emotional problems in order to reduce their need for drugs
Believe It or Not (AD 3.3)	To facilitate students' use of critical thinking, realize there are various causes of deviant behavior, and help students enhance their empathy for parents	CC (EC)	Single-parent family Family drug use Physical maltreatment Low self-esteem Emotional detachment	Group discussion to apply critical-thinking skills and analyze the responsibility of parents for a young person's drug use Class discussion to understand the aim of developing critical-thinking abilities and to understand the real world and take responsibility for our actions
This Is My Badge (AD 3.4)	To assist students to establish positive and feasible objectives of life in order for them to understand that they have the ability to face challenges and enrich their life	BF (SE)	Unengaged youths Underachievement Exclusion Isolation, depression Low self-esteem	Group sharing to consider which characteristics can let them better face challenges in life and not to solve problems by abusing drugs and to enhance students' confidence and expectation in nurturing their good quality through creative activities

The New Biography of Sisyphus (AD 3.5)	To cultivate the ability to face and handle misery and adversity	RE	Low self-esteem Unengaged youths Underachievement Isolation, depression, anxiety, and stress	Group discussion to understand that our mind affects our behavior Class sharing to understand how to face misery and adversity
A U-Turn in Life (AD 3.6)	To understand that there is always a way out of adversity. Do not use negative ways to "solve" problems in times of difficulty	SD (SE)	Low self-esteem Childhood experience of school suspension Corporal punishment Negative labeling from teachers Perceived control to gain access to drugs Intention to try other substances Unawareness of the consequences of drug use	Group discussion to understand that every person has choices and is able to find positive solutions in times of difficulty

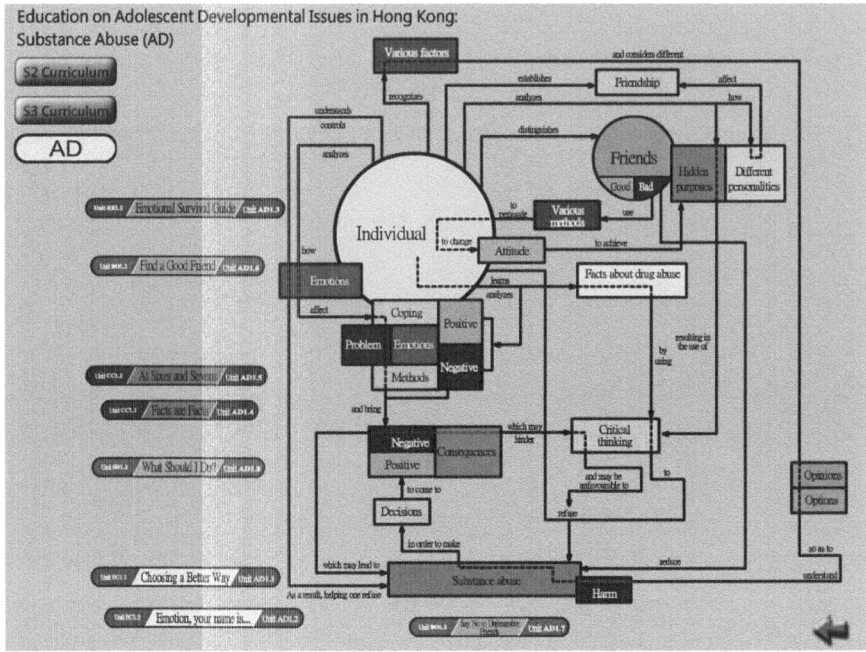

Fig. 2 S1 curriculum design

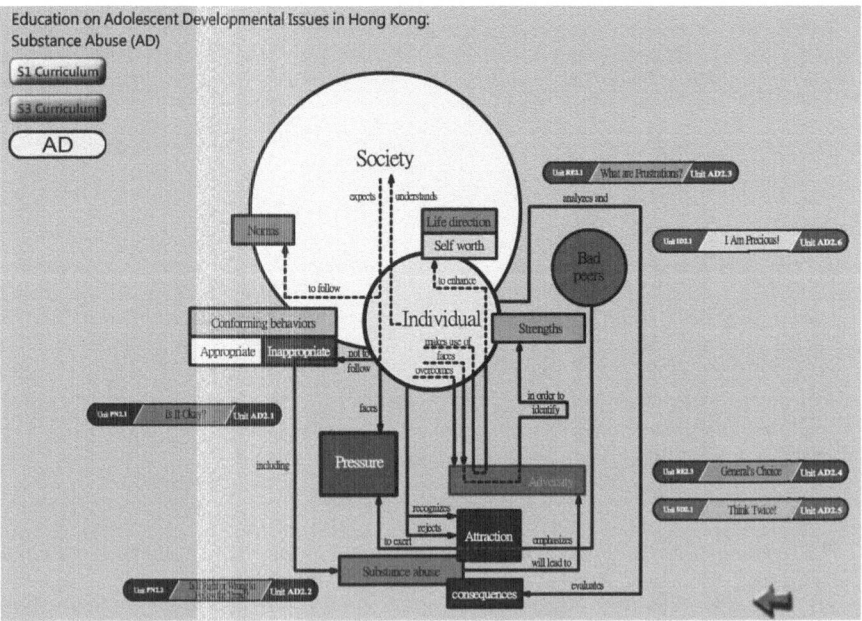

Fig. 3 S2 curriculum design

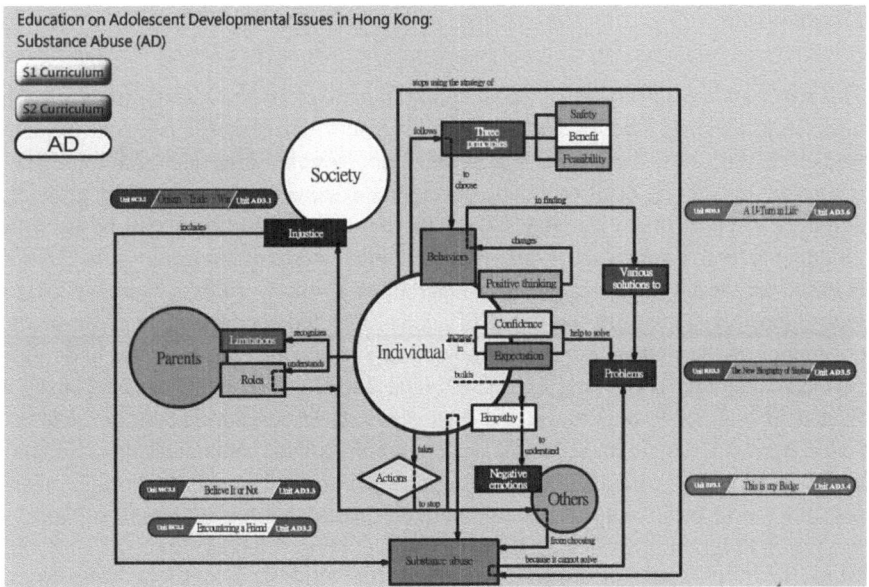

Fig. 4 S3 curriculum design

decision-making skills (Unit 4: General's Choice). This should help them to better recognize bad influences and distance themselves from them, enhancing instead their self-worth (Unit 5: Think Twice!). Finally, they are supported to find their own values and strengthen self-determination (Unit 6: I Am Precious!).

In the third and last year (Fig. 4), students are expected to be no longer spectators of what happens to them or to people around them, but to become the protagonist of their life and active participants in their community. They are invited to critically think how they could contribute to their society and their peers: what can they give? Thus, they are expected to develop different perspectives and a sense of empathy, so to understand others' problems and behavior and help them when needed. They are encouraged to think how our actions can contribute to a society that is being harmed (Unit 1: Opium Trade War); one of the goals is to enhance students' empathy toward friends who may face emotional problems (Unit 2: Encountering a Friend) as well as toward parents (Unit 3: Believe It or Not). Students are then supported to think about the feasible objectives of life (Unit 4: This Is My Badge), so to enhance their confidence and their ability to face challenges (Unit 5: The New Biography of Sisyphus). Students are encouraged to think that there is always a way out of adversities and that they can find it improving their social and cognitive skills (Unit 6: A U-Turn in Life).

Discussion

This paper attempts to construct a conceptual framework of adolescent drug abuse by integrating existing theories and the positive youth development perspective. The framework specifies the plausible causes of adolescents' drug use and abuse. By incorporating the 15 positive youth development constructs, which find growing empirical support in Project P.A.T.H.S., the integrated framework can be used in guiding preventive work. There are several unique features of the framework. First, it is based on the model developed by Logan et al. (Volkow 2006; Abadinsky 2011) with minor revisions to fit the target of adolescents and accommodate adolescents' conception of the causes of drug use and abuse. Second, the revised model finds support from major psychological and sociological theories. Third, it echoes Abadinsky's (Bukstein et al. 1989) hypothesis that drug use in adolescence is a result of the interaction between genetic and biological vulnerabilities with contextual, lifestyle, and sociological factors which will also further condition drug dependency. Fourth, incorporating the 15 positive youth development constructs that find empirical support in the Tier 1 Program of Project P.A.T.H.S. into the revised model (Shek 2006, 2008, 2009a, b, 2010; Shek and Ma 2010; Shek and Ng 2009; Shek and Sun 2008, 2010; Shek et al. 2007, 2008), the integrated conceptual framework is a comprehensive and coherent one in responding to the different causes of adolescents' drug use and abuse.

The construction of the framework has two implications. First, it delineates mezzo- and microlevels of factors and causes of adolescent drug abuse while accepting multiple causation and interactions among factors and causes. The second implication is on a practical level. It provides a solid foundation for guiding the development, implementation, and evaluation of program-level primary intervention. While we have little control over the external environment (i.e., macro-level implication and dosage) in primary prevention, sound theoretical support is sought in developing the program (Vaughan and Buss 1998). The integrated conceptual framework adopting a positive youth development perspective can be applied in other social work or health science contexts, especially in educational and developmental issues of adolescence. It is particularly critical for classroom-based psychosocial primary intervention programs.

There are several controversies with regard to the integrated conceptual framework. The first, an insignificant one, is that there are very often different opinions regarding how the factors and causes are categorized. Second, although the links between 15 positive youth development constructs and causes of the use of psychotropic drugs have been identified, they are only indicative and they are by no means absolute connections. While this ambiguity may be a weakness to a comprehensive primary prevention program, the advantage of having such an all-round development is that it increases the amount of relevant intervention to the target system (e.g., knowledge, values, beliefs, emotions, and behavior) or the abilities of the adolescent. It should be noted that even though 20 new curriculum units of 35 min each will be designed with a view to strengthen the effect of drug prevention, all other units of the curriculum in the Tier 1 Program of Project P.A.T.H.S. were designed to strengthen the relevant abilities of the adolescent which would help participants resist drug use. All of the 120 curriculum units of the Tier 1 Program will contribute to dealing with different causes of psychotropic drug use in Hong Kong. Third, with regard to the all-inclusive manner in incorporating different theories, the integrated framework is considered not parsimonious. However, any perspective on adolescent drug abuse is bound to have limitations because it is just one way of examining reality. Theoretically, the ability of psychological theories to explain is inhibited by environmental influences. The parable of the blind men and the elephant illustrates the importance of generating understanding and creating knowledge about reality through interdisciplinary dialogue and debate. Although different theories of drug abuse may find limited support from their practical application and empirical testing, they are falsifiable in different psychological, social, cultural, legal, and economic contexts. Intervention programs based only on single theories usually fail to handle properly the multiple, qualitatively different layers of context. By incorporating sociological, contextual, and lifestyle factors, elements of preventive intervention programs can target all alleged and real causes for drug abuse. From the developmental and preventive perspective, the 15 positive youth development constructs may act like a master key to fit all locks. Capacity building including enhancement in values, knowledge, and skills in one developmental issue may facilitate learning in another issue. Fourth, one of the major difficulties for the evaluation of a comprehensive program is that it is difficult to delineate which elements of the primary prevention program designed according to the framework would produce a more significant intervention effect. Systematically planned empirical studies are needed to resolve the issue. Finally, this framework does not particularly address the issue of gender. A theory that accounts for an isolated clinical phenomenon, that is, drug-taking behavior of male or female adolescents, does not have as wide reaching an impact as one that considers the drug use of all adolescents. However, at the intervention level, gender-sensitive program designs are necessary. This helps the program designers and implementers avoid the risk of overgeneralization and gender bias.

There are several limitations of this integrated conceptual framework. First, there may be initial bias in its construction because it relies only on limited empirical evidence from Project P.A.T.H.S. in preventing the problem of adolescents' drug use. Further effort in refining the framework is deemed necessary to avoid ongoing bias. The framework has to be rigorously tested before it can be improved or falsified. Moreover, qualitative studies on how participants learn and apply what they have learned in the real-life context are essential for refining the framework. Second, although the genetic factor is important, its interactive effects with biological, psychological, and social factors, that is, living in deprived social circumstances and exposure to certain psychoactive chemicals, are yet to be established. At this stage, it is premature to establish a conclusive presumption of genetic control. The development of neuropsychological research has a long past but a short history, and many questions are not yet adequately answered. Therefore, Abadinsky's hypothesis (Bukstein et al. 1989) that a biologically and psychologically vulnerable adolescent living in deprived social circumstances who is exposed to certain psychoactive chemicals will promote drug use and abuse is valid and thus adopted. Finally, the two-dimensional figure cannot adequately handle some extra connections between a particular positive youth development construct and a certain cause. For example, the construct "development of clear and positive identity" (ID) can also tackle other relevant causes including "low self-esteem" and "boring" as positive identity is associated with personal goals and achievement. Since the framework is used for guiding the development of preventive programs, the link between the literature, the constructs, and the intended outcomes should be carefully delineated before program development. Further research on how each of the 15 positive youth development constructs and the construct of money literacy should be used to tackle different causes of drug use is recommended. Such studies will shed light on previously unexplored issues.

To conclude, the integrated framework can be used as the guiding theoretical framework to develop primary intervention at program level for Project P.A.T.H.S. In the context of antidrug education, the framework provides justifications that primary intervention developed under this framework will fulfill four functions: (1) prevention of the use of psychotropic drugs, (2) victimization protection, (3) strengthening support system, and (4) promotion of biopsychosocial aspects of health. It delineates the influences of psychosocial factors of adolescents' drug use and its risks. It also provides practical guidance for developing primary prevention practice of adolescents' use and abuse of psychotropic drugs.

References

Abadinsky, H. (2011). *Drug use and abuse: A comprehensive introduction* (7th ed.). Belmont: Wadsworth.

Becker, G. S., & Murphy, K. M. (1988). A theory of rational addiction. *Journal of Political Economy, 96*, 675–700.

Blumer, H. (1969). *Symbolic interactionism: Perspective and method*. Englewood Cliffs: Prentice Hall.

Bukstein, O. G., Brent, D. A., & Kaminer, Y. (1989). Comorbidity of substance abuse and other psychiatric disorders in adolescents. *American Journal of Psychiatry, 146*(9), 1131–1141.

Lam, C. M., Lau, P. S., Law, B. M., & Poon, Y. H. (2011). Using positive youth development constructs to design a drug education curriculum for junior secondary students in Hong Kong. *The Scientific World Journal, 11*, 2339–2347.

Polansky, N. A. (1986). There is nothing so practical as a good theory. *Child Welfare, 65*(1), 3–15.

Shek, D. T. L. (2006). Effectiveness of the Tier 1 program of the project P.A.T.H.S.: Preliminary objective and subjective outcome evaluation findings. *The Scientific World Journal, 6*, 1466–1474.

Shek, D. T. L. (2008). Special issue: Evaluation of project P.A.T.H.S. in Hong Kong. *The Scientific World Journal, 8*, 1–94.

Shek, D. T. L. (2009a). Effectiveness of the tier 1 program of project P.A.T.H.S.: Findings based on the first 2 years of program implementation. *The Scientific World Journal, 9*, 539–547.

Shek, D. T. L. (2009b). Using students' weekly diaries to evaluate positive youth development programs: The case of project P.A.T.H.S. in Hong Kong. *Adolescence, 44*(173), 69–85.

Shek, D. T. L. (2010). Objective outcome evaluation of the project P.A.T.H.S. in Hong Kong: Findings based on individual growth curve models. *The Scientific World Journal, 10*, 182–191.

Shek, D. T. L., & Ma, H. K. (2010). Editorial: Evaluation of the project P.A.T.H.S. in Hong Kong: Are the findings replicable across different populations? *The Scientific World Journal, 10*, 178–181.

Shek, D. T. L., & Ng, C. S. M. (2009). Secondary 1 program of project P.A.T.H.S.: Process evaluation based on the co-walker scheme. *The Scientific World Journal, 9*, 704–714.

Shek, D. T. L., & Sun, R. C. F. (2008). Evaluation of project P.A.T.H.S. (Secondary 1 program) by the program participants: Findings based on the full implementation phase. *Adolescence, 43*(172), 807–822.

Shek, D. T. L., & Sun, R. C. F. (2010). Effectiveness of the tier 1 program of project P.A.T.H.S.: Findings based on three years of program implementation. *The Scientific World Journal, 10*, 1509–1519.

Shek, D. T. L., & Yu, L. (2012). Longitudinal impact of the project P.A.T.H.S. on adolescent risk behavior: What happened after five years? *The Scientific World Journal, 2012*, 1–13.

Shek, D. T. L., Siu, A. M. H., & Lee, T. Y. (2007). The Chinese positive youth development scale: A validation study. *Research on Social Work Practice, 17*(3), 380–391.

Shek, D. T. L., Siu, A. M. H., Tak, Y. L., Chau, K. C., & Chung, R. (2008). Effectiveness of the Tier 1 program of project P.A.T.H.S.: Objective outcome evaluation based on a randomized group trial. *The Scientific World Journal, 8*, 4–12.

Skinner, B. F. (1953). *Science and human behavior*. New York: Free Press.

Vaughan, R. J., & Buss, T. F. (1998). *Communicating social science research to policymakers*. Thousand Oaks: Sage.

Volkow, N. D. (2006). NIDA Director's report to CPDD meeting: Progress, priorities, and plans for the future. In W. L. Dewey (Ed.), *Problems of drug dependence. Proceedings of the 67th annual scientific meeting, the college on problems of drug dependence* (pp. 70–79). Bethesda: U.S. Department of Health and Human Services, National Institutes of Health, National Institute on Drug Abuse.

Promotion of Sex Education: The P.A.T.H.S. Program

Diego Busiol and Tak Yan Lee

Abstract In Hong Kong the majority of youth have not many opportunities to receive appropriate support about sexuality. To fill this gap a total of 15 units (five for each year) on sex education are included in the extension phase of Project P.A.T.H.S. Sex education is intended as a moment of personal growth in which pupils have the chance to reflect on gender differences, love, relationships, dating, diversity, and all areas related to sexuality (rather than just sexual intercourse or the biology of the body). This chapter illustrates the guiding principles for the construction of the conceptual framework, structure of the course, operationalization of the 11 PYD constructs in the sex education curriculum, and implementation of the protective factors in the teaching units. Concept maps of the curriculum for each school year are also presented.

P.A.T.H.S. to Sex Education

As reported by the literature, in Hong Kong the majority of youth have not many opportunities to receive appropriate support about sexuality and relationships from parents, and they may find it hard to openly discuss them even with peers (Lau and Lee 1993; Fok 2005). Some people have a negative perspective toward sex education and claim that it urges pupils to anticipate with eagerness to have sexual intercourse. As a consequence, issues related to sex and sexuality often remain a taboo, both at home and at school (Ip et al. 2001; Ng 1998; Wong 2000; Ying Ho and Tsang 2002). How can pupils be released from such stigma, and how can they be given the opportunity to be informed about sex and to discuss issues concerning love, gender, friendships, and loving relationships? Everyone would benefit from

The preparation for this work and the Project P.A.T.H.S. were financially supported by The Hong Kong Jockey Club Charities Trust.

D. Busiol • T.Y. Lee (✉)
Department of Applied Social Sciences, City University of Hong Kong,
Kowloon, Hong Kong, China
e-mail: ty.lee@cityu.edu.hk

© Springer Science+Business Media Singapore 2015   147
T.Y. Lee et al. (eds.), *Student Well-Being in Chinese Adolescents in Hong Kong*,
Quality of Life in Asia 7, DOI 10.1007/978-981-287-582-2_12

positive and appropriate sex attitude and behavior, and there is no evidence to show that an informed sexual life may in any way disrupt the ethical value system of society or marriage or the traditional family system.

To fill this gap a total of 15 units (five for each year) on sex education are included in the extension phase of Project P.A.T.H.S. which is designed to promote holistic development among Grade 7–9 students. These special units were created to help students strengthen their sex education and relational skills using a progressive approach. The goal of P.A.T.H.S. is to explore sexuality in its complexity, anticipating the situation that young students may face. The course is oriented to set a boundary in a clear and firm manner. Indeed, it is rather directive in giving youth "positive values" which help them to grow. Indeed, although students have room for developing their own ideas, the moral values sustaining the course are clear. Out of the original 15 constructs encompassed by the project, 11 are directly related to these units: behavioral competence, prosocial norms, self-determination, clear and positive identity, social competence, emotional competence, cognitive competence, moral competence, spirituality, bonding, and resilience. Each unit encompasses different constructs.

Unlike other contexts, sex education in Hong Kong cannot merely be limited to giving information on contraception and prevention of STDs. Sex, love, and relationships are at best regarded as a continuum. There is no point below which we could say that someone has no literacy, and there is no point at the high end where we can claim that we are fully literate.

Conceptual Framework

These special teaching units developed within the broader framework of the Project P.A.T.H.S. are based on focus on positive development, ecological emphasis, developmental assets, psychosocial competence, character strengths, thriving and spirituality, and engagement and connectedness.

The 15 units are designed for students, focusing on different aspects of human sexuality; it is not simply a matter of head knowledge. Instead, sex education is intended as a moment of personal growth in which pupils have the chance to reflect on gender differences, love, relationships, dating, diversity, and all areas related to sexuality (rather than just sexual intercourse or the biology of the body). At the same time, the course aims at training the teachers and suggesting to them a number of activities to approach sexuality issues with students. Indeed, the course is not addressed solely to youth, but was developed bearing in mind also the needs of the teachers, the institutions, and all the actors involved. The greatest challenge was to develop a specific framework for the sex education curriculum that would be in consonance with Hong Kong's Chinese cultural setting as well as in tune with the school education system (including the institutions and the teachers/ principals).

Guiding Principles for the Construction of the Conceptual Framework

The framework evolved within an ecological perspective and a positive youth developmental approach. Thus, it was developed in consideration of:

- A literature review of sexual education in Chinese societies
- The literature about risk factors and protective factors in relation to sexual behavior
- The most recent literature on youth sexuality, with particular attention to emerging phenomena like compensated dating, pornography, premarital sex, etc.
- The previous conceptual frameworks and the current guidelines from the Education Bureau
- The necessity to train the trainers and to overcome resistances from institutions
- The 14 constructs inspired by positive psychology and founding the entire P.A.T.H.S. program
- The need to develop an interactive and age-appropriate course free of gender bias

Religious beliefs and moral values play important roles in the debate on sex education in Hong Kong. However, the pragmatic nature of Hong Kong helps to maintain a balance between the needs of the individual (exploring and discovering one's own sexuality and the relations with others) and the needs of society (developing positive values shared by society, religion and Chinese culture, and respect for others), so that sex education can find its place within a comprehensive approach. P.A.T.H.S. does not encourage pupils to engage in more or less relationships and does not promote a more libertine or conservative view on sexuality. Instead, the program aims at enhancing a more informed and responsible attitude from youths toward friendship, loving relationships, and sexuality-related issues (Shek et al. 2013). Youths are given the opportunity to share and discuss their beliefs and opinions with their peers, under the supervision of teachers, so that they can find out more about their own feelings and values. Guidance is provided with respect to the different individuals' values. P.A.T.H.S. is not in opposition to different cultures or religions. P.A.T.H.S. aims at promoting positive development among secondary school students, just like religious education aims at enhancing adolescents' spiritual, moral, emotional, and cultural development (Shek et al. 2011). It is then not surprising that some of the 15 constructs of P.A.T.H.S. are intimately related to the principles of religious education. The first is *spirituality*, which is strongly related to what is the core of any religion, the quest for meaning in life, and the development of faith (students are invited to learn about all of the main religions practiced in Hong Kong, not any specific one); another construct is *belief in the future*, which is also very much related to a long-term perspective normally held by religions. Both constructs emphasize the sense of moral development and the rightness of certain behavior (although these might be codified by religions more than P.A.T.H.S. does so); furthermore, both give importance to cultivation of the person as well as cultivation of relational skills and a sense of understanding, compassion, forgiveness, and piety. It has also to be noted that *religiosity* has been largely described by the literature as a protective factor for STDs, undesirable pregnancy, multiple sex partners, and other risky sex behavior; then, it would be incorrect to say that cultivation of values (like in religious education) and psychosocial competencies (as the PYD) is incompatible (Shek et al. 2011). Sex education is sometimes even requested by institutions with religious backgrounds, so as to complete their educational program. This is part of the experience in Hong Kong, where P.A.T.H.S. has also been implemented in a high-band Christian school for girls; however, at that time education on human sexuality was not included in the program, and teachers expressly suggested that the program content and teaching materials should be updated and revised, incorporating sex education into the curriculum (Shek et al. 2011).

Structure of the Course

The course is structured over 3 years (Fig. 1). Adolescence is a process of growth and opening to the world, from the "I" to the others. Thus, educational processes should support this process of opening up to the world, building values, knowledge, attitudes, and skills that can help to move from "me" to "we." Coherently with this perspective, teachers too should give youth their own space for experiment and act as their support system and not as authority. Acceptance and inclusion are the basis of this course, and these principles should inspire both young students and teachers.

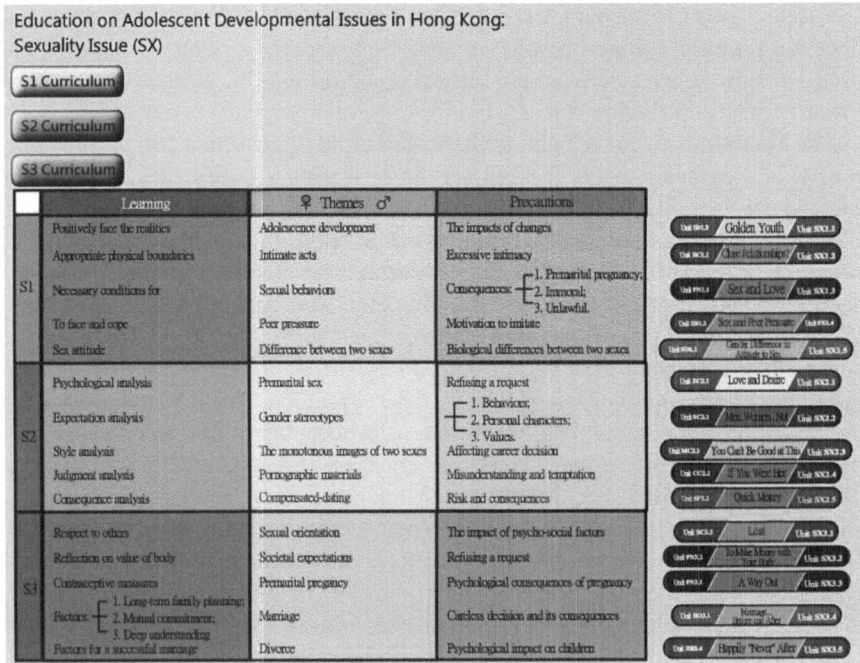

Fig. 1 Sex education curriculum design

Table 1 Constructs guiding the curriculum units in years 1, 2, and 3

S1	S2	S3
Behavioral competence	Social competence	Bonding
Prosocial norms	Emotional competence	Behavioral competence
Self-determination	Cognitive competence	Prosocial norms
Clear and positive identity	Moral competence	Resilience
	Spirituality	

The structure of the course reflects this direction from the "me" to the "we," as reflected by the constructs undergoing the different teaching units (Table 1). Gradually, students are introduced to consider the relationships with their peers and friends of both genders.

Year 1

In the first year (Fig. 2), emphasis is given to build a clear and positive identity and to self-determination. At this stage youth are mainly learning about their self and their bodies.

Learning targets include:

- To understand that adolescent development varies from person to person and that we should not make comparisons or ridicule others for how they are changing and to understand what leads to these changes and learn to face them positively (SX 1.1)
- To understand that excessive intimacy with the opposite sex may lead to misunderstanding and to learn about appropriate physical boundaries for getting along with the opposite sex (SX 1.2)
- To understand the definition of sex and how it is related to everyday living, to learn to respect and consider other people's feelings before deciding sexual behavior, and to understand the consequences and responsibilities after sexual behavior (SX 1.3)
- To know how peer pressure affects our decisions and behavior and to think about the motives and attitudes before we face sexual behavior (SX 1.4)
- To understand the differences between how men and women choose their partners and to understand the biological differences between the genders and how they affect their attitudes toward sex (SX 1.5)

Year 2

In the second year (Fig. 3), the individual is confronted with the world around him/her, and emphasis is placed on the social, emotional, and moral competence. Furthermore, youth are expected to develop appropriate reasoning and critical thinking (cognitive competence) and may develop a more profound sense of spirituality.

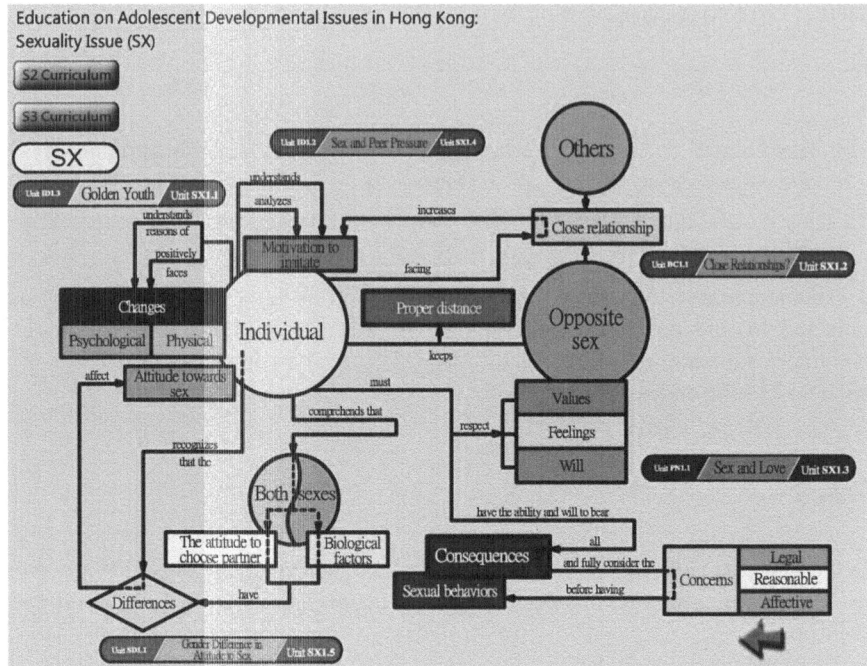

Fig. 2 S1 curriculum design

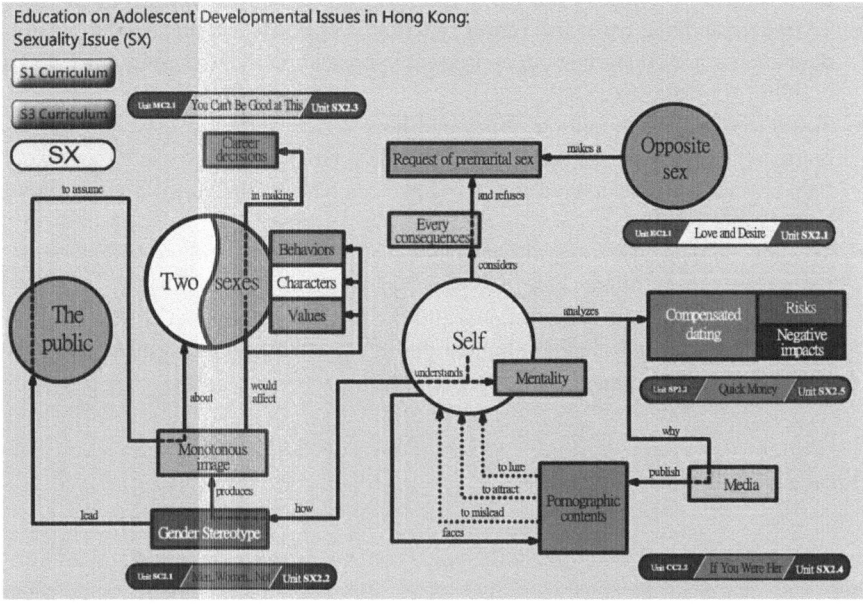

Fig. 3 S2 curriculum design

Learning targets include:

- To understand intimate relationships between the genders (SX 2.1)
- To understand gender stereotypes and to understand views and values on gender roles (SX 2.2)
- To understand how stereotyping affects career decisions and to learn the importance of gender equality (SX 2.3)
- To understand the purpose why media publish pornographic information and to cultivate criticizing attitudes toward pornographic information (SX 2.4)
- To understand the motives why teenagers engage in compensated dating and to analyze the dangers and impacts that compensated dating may cause (SX 2.5)

Year 3

Finally, in the third year (Fig. 4), pupils are expected to improve their bonding skills and relate to others. At the same time they are expected to be more mature and more capable to face frustrations and develop resilience skills.

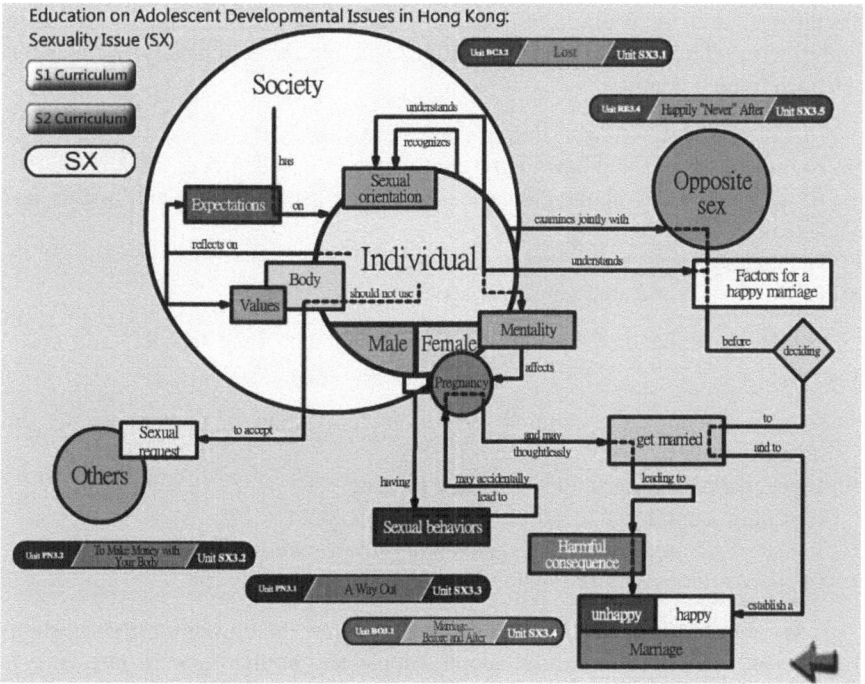

Fig. 4 S3 curriculum design

Learning targets include:

- To understand different sexual tendencies and to reflect on the attitudes toward homosexuality (SX 3.1)
- To learn appropriate attitudes toward the values of one's own body and to learn how to make choices appropriately and not to exchange one's own body for any benefits (SX 3.2)
- To examine one's views on and feelings about premarital pregnancy and to analyze the psychological and developmental impact of premarital pregnancy on young people (SX 3.3)
- To understand the similarities and differences between dating relationships and marriage and to clarify one's values on sexual relationships in dating or before marriage (SX 3.4)
- To learn the factors contributing to happy marriages and those to divorces and to find out how one could be affected by the marriage of parents or close family members (SX 3.5)

Operationalization of the Constructs

On the one hand, the course aims at guiding students to reflect on themselves, their body, their feelings, as well as their relations with others. Specifically, the course is intended to help youths:

- To understand the changes they are undergoing
- To recognize risks and how to prevent them
- To feel confident about themselves and not ashamed of their bodies and sexuality
- To make decisions and negotiate with others
- To have a safe and nonjudgmental space for discussion

On the other hand, the course is also intended to help teachers and social workers:

- To gain a better understanding of what students know or think about sex and sexuality issues
- To receive professional and structured training
- To acquire confidence to handle such sensitive topic
- To learn teaching strategies and techniques of providing sex education
- To choose the most appropriate teaching methods

Every unit presents a topic to be discussed in class and poses several questions for students. The course, which adopts simple and straightforward language, is intended to be interactive. Furthermore, it refers to the present language and current phenomena in society, for example, compensated dating. As the new generations face challenges that are new to society, teachers are not expected to be experts. This course was not intended simply as a transfer of information or standard teaching. Thus, teachers should suggest a number of scenarios in which students may try to articulate their ideas and opinions, sharing and debating with others, under the guidance and supervision of one or more adults. Teaching methods include: group discussion, role play, class discussion, class sharing, and class games. Teaching materials include: PowerPoint slides, video clips, and group worksheets.

Operationalization of the PYD Constructs in the Sex Education Curriculum

The following table (Table 2) describes how each PYD construct finds its place in the 15 units on sex education of the P.A.T.H.S. program, from theory to practice. First, each construct is presented in terms of what it can help to achieve, and how it can be implemented in the teaching curriculum. Then it is reported what unit is inspired by such construct, what risk factors it is intended to address, and what goals/aims it is to serve. Finally, a list of specific activities to operationalize the construct is presented.

Implementation of the Protective Factors in the Teaching Units

The 15 PYD constructs represent a comprehensive approach in that they reflect a plurality, if not a totality, of protective factors. For what concerns sex education specifically, 11 PYD constructs are essential for operationalizing the majority of the protective factors highlighted by literature in the teaching units, as shown by Fig. 5.

Protective Factors and PYD Constructs: Evidence from the Literature

The following table (Table 3) sums up and shows: (1) the protective factors for healthy sexual development of youth (left column), as they emerge from the literature review both from Hong Kong and abroad; (2) the related PYD constructs (middle column); and (3) their link and evidence from the literature. Each construct includes two or more protective factors. Finally, the construct "recognition for positive behavior" is directly related to all of the protective factors that emerge. Indeed, this last construct is not specific to one single unit of the program only but inspires the whole program.

Table 2 Operationalization of the PYD constructs in the sex education curriculum

PYD	Guidelines to operationalization	Unit	Risk factor	Goal of the unit	Questions/activities
EC	Provide a platform for discussing emotions Promote skills to listen, to feel committed and responsible for work, to rein in impulses, and to cope with upsetting events	2.1	Confusion between love and sex	To help students distinguish between love and sex and to communicate effectively their emotions with others	Group discussion on the differences between love and sex Analysis of typical mentalities; what boys and girls normally think about love and sex Case analysis: a young couple talking about intimacy
SD	Include activities to develop skills in goal setting, planning, evaluating and monitoring, and choice making	1.5	Gender differences Sex	To understand that the two genders have different attitudes to sex	Group discussion to understand the inclinations of the two genders in mate selection Group activity and following class discussion about differences in sexual development between the two genders
ID	Promoting self-esteem Fostering exploration and commitment Reducing self-discrepancies (between ideal self, self-perceived self, etc.)	1.1	Physical changes Sense of inferiority and low self-esteem	Unit aim: to understand and to learn how to go through the physical and psychological changes of adolescence	Group discussion to understand what leads to changes in adolescence, to encourage students to share worries and concerns, and to face these changes positively Presentation of typical changes and problems that adolescents encounter: case studies Ask students to suggest solutions to their classmates to overcome problems in their puberty
		1.4	Sex Peers sexually active	To understand how friends affect our decision-making and behavior	Group discussion to understand how friends affect our decisions and behavior in love Individual home activity; the questionnaire is intended to allow students to experience self-reflection when facing peer pressure Video "stuck with virginity" and following individual questions

PN		No.	Topic	Objective	Activities
Impart clear-cut boundaries against problem behavior Promote young people's commitment to valued relationships Help students to: Apply moral reasoning skills in the face of peer pressure Evaluate incentives and sanctions when following group norms How to make choices when personal values conflict with group norms		1.3	Sex Love	To understand the meaning of sex and love	Group discussion to introduce what sex and intimate behavior are Definitions of some common terms related to sex and intimacy Some possible consequences of sexual behavior: legal consequences, illnesses, pregnancy
		3.2	Being attracted by money and gifts Easily available pornography Physical changes	To understand the attitude of today's teenagers toward their own bodies To learn the appropriate attitudes toward the values of one's own body and to learn how to make choices appropriately and not to exchange one's own body for any benefits	Group discussion to understand that one's body cannot be used in exchange for any benefits Case study: a young girl starts working as a model. Will you be a young model? What requests will you accept? Analysis of some recent news about teen models
		3.3	Youth's conception of procreation and contraception Youth's conception of marriage Sex	To understand how premarital pregnancy may affect one's well-being and evaluate the options available	Group discussion to understand the psychological and physical consequences of abortion Further reflections about the meaning and implications of a relationship What is life? And what are the consequences of early pregnancies? The case of adoption News from the media concerning some consequences of teen pregnancy

(continued)

Table 2 (continued)

PYD	Guidelines to operationalization	Unit	Risk factor	Goal of the unit	Questions/activities
RE	Promote positive social connections between teachers and students and among students. Nurture positive qualities, such as forgiveness. Teach by example which is an effective approach. Notice and reinforce qualities that are keys to resilience. Avoid focusing on failure or negative behavior. Foster feelings of competence and self-efficacy	3.5	Youth's conception of love. Youth's conception of marriage	To know the factors contributing to happy marriages and those to divorces; to find out how one could be affected by the marriage of one's parents or close family members	Group discussion to find out how one's conception of marriage is affected by the marriages of one's parents or close family members. Group discussion to understand roles in a marriage and learn how to resolve disputes. Self-reflection: what are the benefits of marriage? Case studies for students: to love or not to love?
BO	Cultivation of supportive relationships. Creating opportunities to belong. Promoting positive social norms. Support for efficacy	3.4	Youth's conception of dating. Youth's conception of marriage. Desire and intimacy. Sex	To understand the similarities and differences between dating relationships and marriage. To examine the relationships among family, marriage, and sex	Group discussion to understand the impacts of sexual relationships on marriage. Self-reflection: what are the changes, if any, required for a person to get married? Case study: two young lovers decide to get married. How will their life change?
MC	Presents students real-life cases to let students consider multiple perspectives and different points of views	2.3	Youth's conception of gender differences and stereotypes	To understand sex equality and discrimination. To understand how stereotyping affects career decisions	Group discussion on sex discrimination. Group work on men's careers and women's careers. Reflections on gender equality

CC	Provide social opportunities for adolescents to master these skills. Thinking skills can be taught by: Direct teaching (bolt-on approach) Embedded approach (practiced within a subject in the school curriculum) Infusion approach (within subjects across the curriculum)	2.4	Easily available pornography	To cultivate a criticizing attitude toward pornographic information and learn to distinguish the right information from bad	Group discussion to increase students' awareness of the use of pornography by media and society Give students information related to the impacts of pornographic information and examples
BC	Develop a curriculum which encompasses: Knowledge course Project-based learning Practicum	1.2	Desire and intimacy Youth's conception of friendship Gender differences	To understand that opposite-sex and same-sex friendships require different attitudes and behavior	Group discussion on the possible consequences of excessive intimacy with the opposite sex and the necessity to set appropriate boundaries Group discussion to understand that opposite-sex and same-sex friendships require different attitudes and behavior
		3.1	Youth's conception of heterosexuality and homosexuality Gender differences and stereotypes	To understand different sexual tendencies; to reflect on the attitudes toward homosexuality	Group discussion to understand different definitions of sexual orientation Self-reflection: what if your friend has a homosexual orientation, what will you do? How is your attitude? Case study: being uncertain of one's own sexual orientation Discussion about common stereotypes on homosexuality Case study: what will you do if…?

(continued)

Table 2 (continued)

PYD	Guidelines to operationalization	Unit	Risk factor	Goal of the unit	Questions/activities
SP	Promote active reflection and experience to promote spiritual growth: why do we exist; where are we going; what is really important in life?	2.5	Being attracted by money and gifts Dating	To understand the motives why teenagers engage in compensated dating; to analyze the dangers and impacts that compensated dating may cause	A group discussion to understand the motives why teenagers engage in compensated dating Case study: a young girl has decided to start compensated dating
SC	Promote a positive attitude toward what is "different"; analyze how people live in different contexts, cultures, and societies Let students express their stereotypes and see how they limit their social life	2.2	Gender differences and stereotypes Dating	To understand gender stereotypes; to understand views and values on gender roles	A group discussion to understand views and values on gender roles, particularly on "family roles" and "roles in dating"

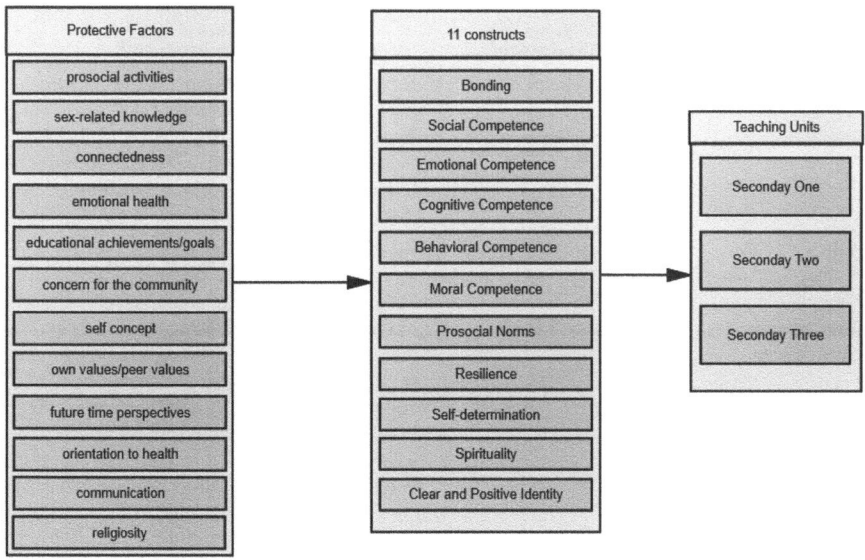

Fig. 5 Protective factors and PYD constructs implemented in the teaching units

Table 3 Relation between protective factors and PYD constructs

Protective factors	PYD construct	Evidence from the literature
Emotional health Communication	*Emotional competence*	Ineffective orientation to emotional-related problems is related to the difficulty in identifying, recognizing, and naming the emotions (Lau and Wu 2013). Ineffective orientation may lead an individual to avoid thoughts and feelings related to the problem (Frauenknecht and Black 1995). People with effective problem orientation are less likely to experience stress, depression, and anxiety (Ciarrochi and Scott 2006)
Self-concept Academic achievements and goals	*Self-determination*	A better knowledge of oneself facilitates goal-directed behavior. Self-determination is associated with academic performance and success, independence, quality of life, choice making, and self-awareness (for a review, see Hui and Tsang 2013)
Self-concept Connectedness Own values/peer values	*Clear and positive identity*	Positive indicators for identity are self-esteem, life satisfaction, positive affect, quality of life, and positive relations with parents and others (Tsang et al. 2013). Self-esteem can influence identity formation and the emotions and performances related to it (Harter 1999)

(continued)

Table 3 (continued)

Protective factors	PYD construct	Evidence from the literature
Prosocial activities Own values/peer values	*Prosocial norms*	Empathy, perspective taking, and sympathy are often related to development of prosocial dispositions (for a review, see Siu et al. 2013). Peer relationships are also shown to be largely influential toward prosocial dispositions (Ma 2003)
Connectedness Future-time perspectives Orientation to health Emotional health Self-concept	*Resilience*	Research has shown that better health is correlated to optimism, perception of control, self-efficacy, and active coping (Smith 2002). Major components of resilience have been identified in bonding or emotional attachment to caregivers, emotional/moral/cognitive competence, spirituality and sense of meaning in life, and environmental variables related to socioeconomic and health conditions (Masten and Reed 2002). In addition, resilience has been described as being related to psychological support and self-concept (Ruch and Köhler 1998)
Prosocial activities Connectedness Future-time perspectives Concern for the community Communication	*Bonding*	Several factors promote bonding: open and frequent communication, connectedness, availability of guidance, creating opportunities to belong, promotion of positive social norms, and self-efficacy (Lee and Lok 2013) as well as active listening, mutual affection, and emotional support (Choi et al. 2003; Cheng et al. 1995)
Self-concept Own values/peer values Connectedness Prosocial activities	*Moral competence*	Studies show that moral competence is related to acceptance of paternal authority and adult guidance (Eisenberg et al. 2006) and to prosocial behavior (Ma et al. 2000). Furthermore, it can be enhanced by peer interaction (Ma et al. 1996). Moral competence encompasses several relational dimensions, like empathy and sense of the other (Hoffman 2000); then it is included in school-based programs so as to promote prosocial attitudes (Ma 2005)
Sex-related knowledge Academic achievements and goals Self-concept	*Cognitive competence*	Cognitive competence encompasses critical thinking and creative thinking, which are reputed to facilitate knowledge construction, task completion, problem-solving, and decision-making (Sun and Hui 2013). Cognitive competence is related to academic achievement, self-esteem, emotion management, cognitive development, and identity development (Zhang and Sternberg 1998)

(continued)

Table 3 (continued)

Protective factors	PYD construct	Evidence from the literature
Sex-related knowledge Own values/peer values Concern for the community	*Behavioral competence*	Behavioral competence is related to moral competence, emotional competence, and social competence. Skills and knowledge are necessary for taking an appropriate decision; however, behavioral competence means that one is able to act accordingly. Indeed, behavioral competence encompasses four dimensions: knowledge, social skills, positive attributes, and action taking (for a review, see Ma 2013). Peer influences on behavioral competence are significant (Ma et al. 1996, 2000)
Own values/peer values Religiosity Future-time perspectives Orientation to health Connectedness	*Spirituality*	Three factors strongly related to spirituality are connectedness, peer values, and beliefs or religiosity (Scott 1997). Furthermore, an orientation to health is also related to spirituality (Shek et al. 2013). Spirituality emphasizes a feeling of connectedness to the sacred, to the mankind, to nature, or to the whole of creation (Worthington Jr and Sandage 2001). A belief in the future and a meaning and purpose in life are also important dimensions of spirituality (Lewis 2001)
Self-concept Concern for the community Connectedness Prosocial activities Communication Academic achievements and goals	*Social competence*	Social competence refers to a clear self-identity or group identity, the ability to solve conflicts, positive interpersonal relationships, and the orientation to be a responsible citizen (Ma 2006). Prosocial activities are often used as a measure of social competence (Eisenberg et al. 2006). Some suggest that a strategy to promote the sense of self of students, and thus their social competence, is to promote success on academic, social, and physical tasks (McDevitt and Ormrod 2009)
Prosocial activities Sex-related knowledge Connectedness Emotional health Educational achievements and goals Concern for the community Self-concept Future-time perspectives Orientation to health Communication Own values/peer values	*Recognition of positive behavior*	Recognition of positive behavior promotes identity formation, moral reasoning, and social perspective thinking. As such, it encompasses several socio-cognitive and interpersonal skills and behavior that aim at enhancing an individual's quality of life: physical health, academic pursuit, following cultural norms, contemplating transcendental values, and getting along with family members (Law et al. 2013)

References

Cheng, C., Bond, M. H., & Chan, S. C. (1995). The perception of ideal best friends by Chinese adolescents. *International Journal of Psychology, 30*(1), 91–108.

Choi, P. Y. W., Au, C. K., Tang, C. W., Shum, S. M., Tang, S. Y., Choi, F. M., & Lee, T. C. (2003). *Making young tumblers: A manual of promoting resilience in schools and families.* Hong Kong: Breakthrough.

Ciarrochi, J., & Scott, G. (2006). The link between emotional competence and well-being: A longitudinal study. *British Journal of Guidance and Counselling, 34*(2), 231–243.

Eisenberg, N., Fabes, R. A., & Spinrad, T. L. (2006). Prosocial development. In N. Eisenberg (Ed.), *Handbook of child psychology vol. 3: Social, emotional, and personality development* (6th ed., pp. 646–718). New York: Wiley.

Fok, C. S. (2005). A study of the implementation of sex education in Hong Kong secondary schools. *Sex Education, 5*(3), 281–294.

Frauenknecht, M., & Black, D. R. (1995). Social Problem-Solving Inventory for Adolescents (SPSI-A): Development and preliminary psychometric evaluation. *Journal of Personality Assessment, 64*(3), 522–539.

Harter, S. (1999). *The construction of the self: A developmental perspective.* New York: Guilford Press.

Hoffman, M. L. (2000). *Empathy and moral development: Implications for caring and justice.* New York: Cambridge University Press.

Hui, E. K., & Tsang, S. K. (2013). Self-determination as a psychological and positive youth development construct. In D. T. L. Shek, R. T. F. Sun, & J. Merrick (Eds.), *Positive youth development. Theory, research and application* (pp. 65–77). New York: Nova Publishers.

Ip, W. Y., Chau, J. P., Chang, A. M., & Lui, M. H. (2001). Knowledge of and attitudes toward sex among Chinese adolescents. *Western Journal of Nursing Research, 23*(2), 211–222.

Lau, J., & Lee, S. S. (1993). *Evaluation of AIDS educational programs for secondary schools in Hong Kong.* Paper presented at Yokohama conference on AIDS, Japan.

Lau, P. S., & Wu, F. K. (2013). Emotional competence as a positive youth development construct: A conceptual review. In D. T. L. Shek, R. T. F. Sun, & J. Merrick (Eds.), *Positive youth development. Theory, research and application* (pp. 39–51). New York: Nova Publishers.

Law, B. M., Siu, A. M., & Shek, D. T. (2013). Recognition for positive behavior as a critical youth development construct: Conceptual bases and implications on youth service development. In D. T. L. Shek, R. T. F. Sun, & J. Merrick (Eds.), *Positive youth development. Theory, research and application* (pp. 117–127). New York: Nova Publishers.

Lee, T. Y., & Lok, D. P. (2013). Bonding as a positive youth development construct: A conceptual review. In D. T. L. Shek, R. T. F. Sun, & J. Merrick (Eds.), *Positive youth development. Theory, research and application* (pp. 145–162). New York: Nova Publishers.

Lewis, M. M. (2001). Spirituality, counseling, and elderly: An introduction to the spiritual life review. *Journal of Adult Development, 8*(4), 231–240.

Ma, H. K. (2003). The relation of moral orientation and moral judgment to prosocial and antisocial behaviour of Chinese adolescents. *International Journal of Psychology, 38*(2), 101–111.

Ma, H. K. (2005). Moral competence as a positive youth development construct: Conceptual bases and implications for curriculum development. *International Journal of Adolescent Medicine and Health, 18*(3), 371–378.

Ma, H. K. (2006). Social competence as a positive youth development construct: Conceptual bases and implications for curriculum development. *International Journal of Adolescent Medicine and Health, 18*(3), 379–386.

Ma, H. K. (2013). Behavioral competence as a positive youth development construct: A conceptual review. In D. T. L. Shek, R. T. F. Sun, & J. Merrick (Eds.), *Positive youth development. Theory, research and application* (pp. 189–200). New York: Nova Publishers.

Ma, H. K., Shek, D. T., Cheung, P. C., & Lee, R. Y. (1996). The relation of prosocial and antisocial behavior to personality and peer relationships of Hong Kong Chinese adolescents. *The Journal of Genetic Psychology, 157*(3), 255–266.

Ma, H. K., Shek, D. T., Cheung, P. C., & Lam, C. O. B. (2000). Parental, peer, and teacher influences on the social behavior of Hong Kong Chinese adolescents. *The Journal of Genetic Psychology, 161*(1), 65–78.

Masten, A. S., & Reed, M. G. J. (2002). Resilience in development. In C. R. Snyder & S. J. Lopez (Eds.), *Handbook of positive psychology* (pp. 74–88). New York: Oxford University Press.

McDevitt, T. M., & Ormrod, J. E. (2009). *Child development and education*. Upper Saddle River: Pearson.

Ng, M. L. (1998). School and public sexuality education in Hong Kong. *Journal of Asian Sexology, 1*, 32–35.

Ruch, W., & Köhler, G. (1998). A temperament approach to humor. In W. Ruch (Ed.), *The sense of humor: Explorations of a personality characteristic* (pp. 203–230). New York: Mouton de Gruyter.

Scott, A. B. (1997). *Categorizing definitions of religion and spirituality in the psychological literature: A content analytic approach*. Unpublished manuscript.

Shek, D. T. L., Ng, C. S., & Chak, Y. L. (2011). Implementation of the Project PATHS in a school with a religious background: A case study. *International Journal of Adolescent Medicine and Health, 23*(4), 341–349.

Shek, D. T. L., Sun, R. T. F., & Merrick, J. (2013). Introduction: Positive youth development constructs: Conceptual review and application. In D. T. L. Shek, R. T. F. Sun, & J. Merrick (Eds.), *Positive youth development. Theory, research and application* (pp. 1–12). New York: Nova Publishers.

Siu, A. M. H., Shek, D. T. L., & Law, B. (2013). Prosocial involvement as a positive youth development construct: A conceptual review. In D. T. L. Shek, R. T. F. Sun, & J. Merrick (Eds.), *Positive youth development. Theory, research and application* (pp. 105–115). New York: Nova Publishers.

Smith, B. W. (2002). Vulnerability and resilience as predictors of pain and affect in women with arthriti. *Dissertation Abstracts International Part B, 63*(3), article 1575.

Sun, R. C., & Hui, E. K. (2013). Cognitive competence as a positive youth development construct: A conceptual review. In D. T. L. Shek, R. T. F. Sun, & J. Merrick (Eds.), *Positive youth development. Theory, research and application* (pp. 27–38). New York: Nova Publishers.

Tsang, S. K., Hui, E. K., & Law, B. (2013). Positive identity as a positive youth development construct: A conceptual review. In D. T. L. Shek, R. T. F. Sun, & J. Merrick (Eds.), *Positive youth development. Theory, research and application* (pp. 79–92). New York: Nova Publishers.

Wong, V. (2000). A never-ending obsession with breasts. In V. Wong, W. Shiu, & H. Har (Eds.), *From lives to critique*. Hong Kong: Hong Kong Policy Viewers (In Chinese).

Worthington, E. L., Jr., & Sandage, S. J. (2001). Religion and spirituality. *Psychotherapy: Theory, Research, Practice, Training, 38*(4), 473.

Ying Ho, P. S., & Tsang, A. K. T. (2002). The things girls shouldn't see: Relocating the penis in sex education in Hong Kong. *Sex Education: Sexuality, Society and Learning, 2*(1), 61–73.

Zhang, L. F., & Sternberg, R. J. (1998). Thinking styles, abilities, and academic achievement among Hong Kong university students. *Educational Research Journal, 13*(1), 41–62.

Contrasting School Bullying: The P.A.T.H.S. Program

Sandra K.M. Tsang and Eadaoin K. Hui

Abstract The P.A.T.H.S. project aims at enhancing students' understanding and awareness of the nature of bullying and cyberbullying, the needs of the bullies and the victims, the role of the bystanders in bullying, the moral responsibility to stop bullying, the respect for others, and cyber ethics. It is a preventive program using positive youth development (PYD) approach because it suggests solutions for reducing bullying (remedial level), suggests activities for weakening risk factors (preventive level), is based on PYD constructs, and gives tools for strengthening protective factors (developmental level). This chapter illustrates strategies for enhancing positive identity, self-efficacy, and self-determination in bystanders' position taking. Further, the importance of the teacher and peers support in anti-bullying intervention is stressed. Besides the focus on bullying and cyberbullying, the P.A.T.H.S. project aims at enhancing essential competencies in social bonding, emotional competence, and moral judgments that both victims and bullies lack. To illustrate this, the concept map of the curriculum for each school year is presented.

The preparation for this work and the Project P.A.T.H.S. were financially supported by The Hong Kong Jockey Club Charities Trust. This paper is based on two articles originally published by the Scientific World Journal: Hui, E. K., Tsang, S. K., & Law, B. (2011). Combating school bullying through developmental guidance for positive youth development and promoting harmonious school culture. *The Scientific World Journal*, *11*, 2266–2277. Tsang, S. K., Hui, E. K., & Law, B. (2011). Bystander position taking in school bullying: the role of positive identity, self-efficacy, and self-determination. *The Scientific World Journal*, *11*, 2278–2286.

S.K.M. Tsang (✉)
Department of Social Work and Social Administration,
The University of Hong Kong, Pok Fu Lam, Hong Kong, China
e-mail: sandratsang@hku.hk

E.K. Hui
Faculty of Education, The University of Hong Kong, Pok Fu Lam, Hong Kong, China

© Springer Science+Business Media Singapore 2015
T.Y. Lee et al. (eds.), *Student Well-Being in Chinese Adolescents in Hong Kong*,
Quality of Life in Asia 7, DOI 10.1007/978-981-287-582-2_13

Introduction

In addressing the problem of bullying, the newly devised P.A.T.H.S. units share functions similar to classroom-based intervention. As shown in Table 1, these units aim to enhance students' understanding and awareness of the nature of bullying and cyberbullying, the needs of the bullies and the victims, the role of the bystanders in bullying, the moral responsibility to stop bullying, the respect for others, and cyber ethics (Hui et al. 2011). As a PYD program, these units foster the psychological constructs of bonding, resilience, social competence, emotional competence, behavioral competence, moral competence, and prosocial norms.

In addition, the P.A.T.H.S. curriculum aims at facilitating students to become helpful prosocial bystanders (Tsang et al. 2011). The curriculum, as a psychoeducational program, aims to enhance students' positive identity, self-efficacy, and self-determination. With reference to Salmivalli's recommendations (1999) in the case of school bullying, the P.A.T.H.S. curriculum helps to: (1) raise students' general awareness of bullying, (2) offer them chances for self-reflection, and (3) provide possibilities to rehearse new behavior (Table 1).

In this newly revised curriculum, Secondary 1 students are introduced to basic knowledge on bullying, including what it is and what its effects are as well as the dos and don'ts when facing bullying. Through understanding the effects of bullying, students can understand how bullying harms themselves and others, which help to deter them from turning into or taking side with the bullies. Teaching students dos and don'ts may also help them protect themselves when being bullied. The focus shifts to bystanders in Secondary 2 and Secondary 3, with four goals: (1) to understand that peer bystanders play an important role in bullying and can alter the outcome of bullying, (2) to learn to be a wise and sensible bystander in school bullying, (3) to be a responsible bystander in cyberbullying, and (4) to learn to understand and accept the differences and constraints of others. Since these units are taught as a classroom curriculum for all students in their respective class levels, the students will acquire competence, positive skills, and strategies to face bullying and school violence. Hence, these PYD units also tackle bullying from a developmental guidance perspective through a systematic curriculum targeting all students.

There are several merits in adopting the positive approach to tackling bullying (Hui et al. 2011). First, it addresses bullying from a positive youth development paradigm, stressing the importance of competency building. Issues relating to bullying are used as a context through which students learn appropriate social skills, emotional management skills, and the ability to understand others' emotions as well as to appreciate and forgive others. In addition, units target at helping students to explore proper attitudes and skills when facing unjust and violent situations, to learn to see things from other people's perspectives, and to consider appropriate ways of responding. Through enhancing students' moral, social, and behavioral competence, the incidences of bullying can be prevented. Second, this is a deliberate attempt to incorporate anti-bullying elements in the schools' regular curriculum in the form of a classroom curriculum. Indeed, enhancing students' knowledge about

Table 1 Anti-bullying (AB) units overview

	Unit code/unit name	Construct	Unit aim	Learning targets
Secondary 1	1.1 Incidents of bullying	Behavioral competence, emotional competence, resilience	To understand what is meant by bullying and its consequences, to avoid being a bully or a victim	1. To understand the definition of bullying 2. To investigate the behavioral and emotional reactions of the bully, the victim, and bystanders in bullying incidents and the consequences of bullying
	1.2 Behind the mask of bullying	Emotional competence Behavioral competence	To understand the true needs of the bullies and identify proper approaches to minimize bullying	1. To understand the reasons for bullying and the mentality of the bullies 2. To identify suitable approaches to fulfill the underlying needs of the bullies in order to reduce bullying
	1.3 A secret book of bullying prevention	Social competence Behavioral competence	To learn what should be done in the face of bullying	To learn dos and don'ts in the face of bullying
Secondary 2	2.1 I can make a difference	Moral competence, prosocial norm	To understand that bystanders play an important role in bullying	1. To understand that the "bystander effect" has a significant impact on a person's decisions and behavior 2. To understand that the consequences of a bullying incident vary with the attitudes and responses of the bystanders
	2.2 Make a smart move	Moral competence Behavioral competence	To learn to be a wise and responsible bystander	1. To understand the factors affecting the attitudes and responses of bystanders to bullying incidents 2. To investigate how to stop school bullying wisely
Secondary 3	3.1 Online buddies	Moral competence	To learn to be a responsible bystander in cyberbullying	1. To know the tremendous harm that cyberbullying can cause 2. To investigate the proper attitude for bystanders in cyberbullying incidents
	3.2 Alien	Social competence	To learn and practice the motto "seek common ground and respect differences; seek harmony but not uniformity"	1. To understand that everyone has his/her own limitations and is different from others 2. To learn to understand, tolerate, and accept those who are different from us

bullying and positive ways of handling it through classroom discussion and activities has been found to be more effective as an intervention strategy (Mishna 2008). Students can be equipped with knowledge and skills to foster a positive and culturally appropriate learning environment. Cooperative group work and activities which enhance students' intrapersonal and interpersonal skills can reduce the extent of victimization of vulnerable students and promote a peaceful, loving, and respectful classroom environment (Wong et al. 2008). Third, building students' assets and strengths in interpersonal relationships, bonding, and competence will help build a caring school ethos, leading to a more harmonious school culture.

Project P.A.T.H.S. is a comprehensive program because it suggests solutions for reducing bullying (remedial level), suggests activities for weakening risk factors (preventive level), is based on PYD constructs, and gives tools for strengthening protective factors (developmental level). Project P.A.T.H.S. adopts an ecological perspective and is addressed to all the actors involved in the context: bullies, victims, and bystanders. In broader terms, in addition to fellow students, teachers and staff at school as well as parents who interact in their children's lives at school can be considered "bystanders." Yet, this group has often been excluded from intervention programs.

Roles of Bystanders in the Course of Bullying

Peer bystanders in schools can decisively influence the intensity and outcome of bullying by assuming different roles or positions in the bullying process (Davis and Davis 2007; Stueve et al. 2006; Twemlow et al. 2004). Twemlow et al. (2004) have identified several roles which different bystanders can assume. Bully (aggressive) bystanders may sustain bullying by offering positive feedback, such as joining in or actively reinforcing the act through laughs or encouraging gestures. Victim (passive) bystanders may simply stand aside and keep silent while observing, which actually renders silent consent (Salmivalli et al. 1996, 1999; Schwartz et al. 1993) and making them part of the victimizing process. Avoidant bystanders may facilitate victimizing by denying personal responsibility. Abdicating bystanders may use scapegoating to shed responsibility. In contrast to these first four types, altruistic bystanders may mobilize personal or social resources to help reduce or even stop bullying, for example, defending victims, taking sides with victims, informing and seeking help from adults, comforting victims, or trying to make bullies stop (Salmivalli 1999). In many incidents, when peer bystanders intervene against bullying, it tends to stop quickly (Hawkins et al. 2001).

After acknowledging the pivotal function of peer bystanders in influencing the course of school bullying and identifying the different positions of such bystanders, it is logical to ask whether bystanders can be helped to take up the altruistic position to reduce school bullying, and how this can be achieved. According to Twemlow et al. (2004), bystanders are actually uncomfortable in non-altruistic roles or are at least caught in the dilemma of choosing among the different roles.

Therefore, they are motivated to seek effective ways out. This search (i.e., a bystander taking a position) is affected by various external or environmental factors. Physical environmental factors include classroom spaciousness and even home proximity to bullies and victims. Social factors include the availability of parents, teachers, other adults, or peers for protection or role modeling of different attitudes and skills of coping.

In addition, personal factors of the bystanders, such as physical characteristics, social and academic status (Davis and Davis 2007), and even social skills (Stueve et al. 2006), are variables that influence bystanders' position taking. Further, the personal qualities of the individual bystander (e.g., positive self-identity, self-efficacy, and self-determination) are even more pertinent, according to psychoeducational and clinical literature on bystanders (Gini et al. 2008; Hawkins et al. 2001; Kohut 2007; Lodge and Frydenberg 2005; Nickerson et al. 2008). In a bystander's spontaneous position taking, the possession of these personal qualities would affect the way they act when facing bullying. And these factors are most amenable to the control of the bystander.

Enhancing Positive Identity, Self-efficacy, and Self-determination in Bystanders' Position Taking

Positive Identity

Identity is a constellation of personality characteristics and social styles through which one defines oneself and is recognized by others. The development of a clear and positive self-identity rests on the building of self-esteem, facilitation of the exploration of and commitment to self-definition, and reduction of inconsistencies in the self to enhance role formation and achievement (Tsang and Yip 2006; Tsang et al. 2012). This definition of positive identity gives three clues to how bystanders can be constructive helpers in school bullying. The first strategy is to enhance the bystander's positive self-esteem, which is highly correlated with prosocial behavior and positive well-being (Lodge and Frydenberg 2005; Salmivalli et al. 1999). The second strategy is to engage the bystander in thinking through and working out responses to situations like bullying and upholding such options. Finally, the bystander needs to see the gaps between their ideal, real, and perceived selves, seeking to sort out such gaps in order to achieve peace of mind (Tsang et al. 2011). To activate such strategies, it has been effective to present the potential bystanders with case scenarios for guided discussion and self-reflection on the choice of response. The evaluation findings of Project P.A.T.H.S. reveal that students participating in the program performed better than their counterparts in different areas of psychosocial competencies and strengths, including positive identity, self-efficacy, and self-determination (Shek 2009; Shek and Ma 2011; Shek and Sun 2010). They also had lower intention to engage in problem behavior and higher life satisfaction (Shek and Sun 2010).

Self-efficacy

Bandura (1997) defined self-efficacy as "beliefs in one's capabilities to organize and execute the courses of action required to produce given attainments." Self-efficacy plays a central role in the "exercise of personal agency" and revolves around the idea that "unless people believe that they can produce desired effects by their actions, they have little incentive to act" (Bandura et al. 1996, p. 1206). It functions as a multilevel and multifaceted set of beliefs that can include a global self-efficacy and self-efficacy regarding different domains of the self (Tsang and Hui 2006). Self-efficacy has been shown in both Hong Kong (Wong 2004) and overseas (Gini et al. 2008) studies to positively affect prosocial behavior, including bullying defending behavior. Students high in social self-efficacy are likely to try to help victims in bullying situations, whereas students with low levels of self-efficacy are more reluctant to intervene and help, regardless of their level of empathic responsiveness (Schwarzer et al. 1992). Even if peer bystanders know how to intervene effectively, if they believe that they will be ineffective or that other bystanders are more competent, they will be less likely to take action against bullying (Stueve et al. 2006).

Self-determination

Self-determination is defined by Catalano and his colleagues (2002) as "the ability to think for oneself, and to take action consistent with that thought" (p. 19). It refers to the competence in thinking for oneself and autonomy in choice making. People who are self-determined are able to make choices according to their own thinking and are less likely to submit to outside pressure. Group norms and school culture often create pressure for certain behavior. Bystanders' position taking in bullying is very much the result of peer pressure and the desire to be accepted by peers (Nickerson et al. 2008). Besides group norms, school culture also contributes to the social pressure on bystanders. In school environments where speaking up against injustice is clearly accepted and valued, the risk of social rejection for active bystanders is reduced. However, in environments which allow bullies to hold the power of determining acceptance or rejection, the risks of speaking up for bystanders are greater (Davis and Davis 2007). Hence, it is pertinent for schools to cultivate students with self-determination and values for justice so that they are less likely to acquiesce to negative peer pressure and are more able to take the positive side when they witness bullying.

Social Support of Teachers

Social support has been found to be an important contextual factor in countering bullying, yet there is a lack of explicit application of social support in anti-bullying programs and interventions (Demaray and Malecki 2006). Research studies have demonstrated that students' perceived school satisfaction is related to supportive teacher-student relationships (Baker 1999), teacher support (Danielsen et al. 2009), and a caring and supportive school climate (Baker 1998). Teacher support has been found to be a protective factor against students' suicidal ideation (Sun and Hui 2007), has acted as a significant predictor of students' perceived school satisfaction (Hui and Sun 2010), and played a mediating role in the relationship between victimization and school maladjustment (Demaray and Malecki 2006). However, not all teachers perceive bullying as serious, know how to intervene and prevent bullying, or have the confidence to manage disruptive behavior (Atlas and Peper 1998). This goes to show the importance of educating teachers about bullying and strengthening teachers as support in the school setting.

A whole-school intervention program by Olweus (1993) incorporated teachers to provide support at the whole-school level by, for example, identifying bullying incidents, providing increased supervision in secluded areas, and coordinating with parents, school staff, and students. At the classroom level, teacher support includes establishing class rules against bullying and setting consequences for violating the rules. However, simply setting rules or holding a one-off discussion in the classroom or at the whole-school level is not sufficient. Involving teachers in delivering guidance programs that address bullying has further benefits. Teachers may integrate anti-bullying themes within the school developmental guidance programs and values education programs so that nonviolence and tolerance can be presented as a consistent message to all students and highlighted as the ethos of the school. Supportive teacher-student relationships will encourage students, whether victims or bystanders, to seek help. Teachers may foster attitudes such as acceptance, respect, tolerance, and forgiveness and relate their importance to interpersonal relationships and social harmony (Hui et al. 2011). At the individual student level, teachers may offer support to bullies, victims, and the peers of bullies and victims, in dealing with bullying and conflicts. Involving teachers systematically on all three levels is a more comprehensive strategy to prevent bullying. As peer victimization is an important determinant leading to school dissatisfaction (Verkuyten and Thijs 2002) and peer conflicts lower students' liking of their schools (Ladd et al. 1996), ongoing efforts and social support from teachers are pertinent to building a positive and caring classroom and school climate.

Involving Peers as Support

Students value having a peer to listen to their experience of being bullied (Cowie and Olafsson 2000). Peer-led anti-bullying interventions, such as peer counseling and peer mediation, have been found to have positive outcomes, which also lead to an improvement of school climate (Mishna 2008). Peer counseling is increasingly being used in schools in Hong Kong and elsewhere as a form of peer support to facilitate junior students' adjustment and learning. Such support can be extended to include anti-bullying. In recruitment of peer counselors, attention needs to be paid to identifying students who are trustworthy. The training of counselors needs to

address issues including maintenance of confidentiality, skills such as active listening and empathy, as well as the provision of advice on solving bullying-related
problems (Boulton et al. 2007). Further, the units which address school bullying in
Project P.A.T.H.S. can be incorporated into the training program to enhance peer
counselors' knowledge and understanding of the nature of bullying, the feelings and
emotions of the victims, the needs and mentalities of the bullies, and proper
approaches to minimize bullying. Nonetheless, the provision of support from adults
such as teachers and social workers to these peer counselors is essential.

Furthermore, support needs to go beyond the peer counselors recruited for anti-
bullying intervention to other peers in the school community, as not all students use
peer counseling due to the fear of being stigmatized (Boulton et al. 2007). Project
P.A.T.H.S. includes units addressed specifically to the role of bystanders in bullying
and the factors affecting the attitudes and responses of bystanders to bullying
incidents. All students, whether victims, bullies, or bystanders, will be taught explicitly in classroom guidance programs about bullying as a form of violence and its
effects on the school community. Such an approach targeting all students will further enhance peers as a support system in the school community. Further, school-
wide developmental guidance programs educating students about respect for
individual differences and the value of harmony, justice, and responsibility will help
to build a more tolerant and caring school climate.

Promoting Nonviolence and Harmony as a Whole-School Approach to Counter Bullying

Research and practices in school guidance and pastoral care have affirmed the
importance of having a whole-school approach to facilitate students' whole-person
development (Hui 2000, 2002, 2010). Under the framework of a whole-school
approach, guidance and support are provided to all students, not merely students
who are at risk, and are the responsibility of all teachers, not only the guidance personnel and professionals. Guidance can be delivered at individual student level and
classroom and whole-school levels. Developing a systematic and planned guidance
curriculum and integrating guidance themes into the school's formal and informal
curriculum are essential elements under this framework. Such an approach also
requires schools to have a whole-school policy which details the goals, system of
management, coordination, and communication among teachers, parents, and professionals. Promoting a whole-school approach to guidance is a way to cultivate a
positive school ethos (Hui 2010). Hence, this approach is very much in line with
promoting nonviolence and harmony as a positive way to combat school bullying.

Cultivating a harmonious school culture needs to be done as a whole-school
approach, ranging from the individual student and class levels to the school-wide
program level as discussed above. Such an endeavor needs to be further supported
at the whole-school system level. First, a whole-school policy which stresses nonviolence and tolerance needs to be integrated into the school's guidance policy so

that there will be consensus and consistency among all staff in their responses to the problems of bullying and peer victimization and the promotion of nonviolence. Such a policy needs to be communicated to the students and parents. Second, in addition to cultivating the values of harmony and nonviolence through schools' values and moral education curricula, the implementation of the PYD anti-bullying program at classroom level which fosters students' bonding, competencies, and self-determination will contribute to a more positive and caring class ethos. Further, the integration of themes such as respect, tolerance, forgiveness, and justice with academic subject teaching will help enhance effectiveness, as the teaching of values must be ongoing and integrated into the school curriculum so that the values can be kept front and center (Mishna 2008). Third, at the management level, another essential element that needs to be dealt with from a whole-school system perspective is collaboration with professionals, such as school psychologists, school counselors, and social workers, in identifying students at risk of bullying and victimization and offering timely intervention. The implementation of the Tier II program of Project P.A.T.H.S., for example, will require teachers and professionals to work in collaboration. Fourth, as mentioned above, teachers play a very important role in fostering values through classroom teaching and delivering classroom guidance programs such as the PYD anti-bullying programs and forgiveness education. This will require the school to plan and organize professional development programs to enhance teachers' knowledge and skills and to offer individual support. Involving peers as support and working with parents are other essential elements under the framework of a whole-school approach, which have been adopted in whole-school anti-bullying intervention. Lastly, the involvement of the entire school community, students, parents, teachers, administrators, professionals, and adjunct school staff in the practice and support of such a school policy is crucial in building a safer, more caring, responsive, and harmonious school culture (Elinoff et al. 2004; Mishna 2008). Combating bullying as a whole-school approach to guidance is therefore a matter of cultivating a guidance-oriented ethos, in which concern, love, and compassion are advocated as values for students' whole-person development.

Cyberbullying

As highlighted by the literature, a school-based comprehensive prevention program is potentially the most effective option to tackle cyberbullying. Schools are in the position to educate, prevent, and when necessary take action against bullying and cyberbullying. However, it should be clear that cyberbullying does not simply concern the use of digital media, like the Internet and smartphones. Although some unique features of the new technologies need to be investigated in more depth, bullying and cyberbullying largely overlap; thus, when thinking of cyberbullying, the stress should be on contrasting *bullying* more than *cyber*. Literature shows a correlation between time spent on devices and risks of being harassed, threatened, or bullied. However, trying to simply limit youth's access to the Internet or use of technology is anachronistic, ineffective, and probably unfair. Furthermore, Slonje and Smith (2008) identified three significant challenges faced by schools to address cyberbullying: (1) social network and digital devices are extremely popular so that the victim of cyberbullying finds it hard to escape from digital messages; (2) because of the nature of electronic devices, it is impossible to determine who has received the messages aside from the intended recipient; and (3) the anonymity among cyberbullies adds to the complexity of defining and implementing a successful prevention plan.

Instead, Couvillion and Ilieva (2011) suggest that for a quality and successful cyberbullying prevention program, it is critical to focus on developing, maintaining, practicing, and promoting appropriate behavior. Specifically, they suggest: (1) do not ban the use of electronic devices, because this will not solve the problem; (2) teach and model practices of digital citizenship and appropriate social behavior and emphasize that they are even more important when one acts/participates in electronic communication with anonymity; (3) communicate clearly the consequences and effects of cyberbullying as no one is immune to becoming a target; (4) teach that cyberbullying is hurtful and unethical in multiple ways; (5) teach what messages are attempts at cyberbullying and that not taking part in spreading these messages further is an appropriate step; and (6) stay informed about new social environments and understand the constantly growing features of formerly basic digital tools; do not make the prevention a one-time event with limited scope; do it 24 h a day, 7 days a week, and 365 days of the year.

Conceptual Map for Cyberbullying

Technically, only one of the seven units on bullying is dedicated to cyberbullying (AB3.1), which reflects the overlap between the two forms of harassment. Specifically, the different forms of cyberbullying (texts, images, videos, spamming, human flesh search, hacking, and Internet trial) are discussed with students in year 3 (Fig. 4). Students are invited to consider the differences between face-to-face bullying and cyberbullying and the consequences that the latter can cause. Students are invited to discuss and share in groups about recent incidents of local people who have been involved in harassment on the Internet. The goal is to let students empathize with the misery of the victims of cyberbullying and to avoid being involved in or encouraging cyberbullying in the future. Then students are taught some of the main causes for being targeted by cyberbullies and how to avoid such unpleasant situations. Because one may happen to become a victim (or be a friend of a victim or a bystander) of cyberbullying, students are also told about some practical ways to handle it. Altogether, students are expected to have a better understanding of the needs of the bullies and the victims, the role of the bystanders in bullying (so as to become a responsible bystander themselves), the moral responsibility to stop bullying, the respect for others, cyber ethics, and the laws of Hong Kong.

Besides the focus on bullying and cyberbullying, the P.A.T.H.S. project aims at enhancing essential competencies in social bonding, emotional competence, and moral judgments that both victims and bullies lack, as highlighted by the literature. In many cases cyberbullying is retaliatory behavior that follows students' inabilities to handle social tensions and relationship issues. It might be either a way to vent frustration and take revenge on others, the product of low self-esteem, or a way of letting another person experience the feelings that the perpetrator feels. Thus, while technology training is necessary, it is not enough to make a real change. What is central is to address and tackle the causes of bullying behavior. The 15 PYD constructs of the P.A.T.H.S. project can effectively address such critical areas so that it can be said that not only the special units on bullying are effective against a bullying attitude in students, but the entire course is relevant for weakening the risk factors as well as for strengthening the protective factors of bullying.

Concluding Remarks

The literature has shown that adolescents involved in bullying, whether as bullies, victims, or bystanders, are all at risk of psychiatric disorders and might even show antisocial behavior. As most of such peer bullying occurs in schools, the way in which schools respond to school bullying is pertinent. A whole-school approach to guidance takes into account the fact that school bullying is a highly social process. It stresses the involvement of fellow students, teachers, and staff at school as well as parents who interact in their children's lives at school in prevention. Project P.A.T.H.S. is a proactive approach that fosters positive youth development, and its units can be implemented as a comprehensive school guidance program to combat school bullying. It is based on psychoeducational principles with demonstrated effectiveness and presents a positive paradigm shift to prevent peer bullying, in both physical and cyber space.

Concept Map of the Curriculum

Figure 1 presents the complexity of the bullying situations and thus the complexity of an anti-bullying prevention program like P.A.T.H.S. Students are expected to be familiar with this complexity and make informed choices. Bullying involves several more actors than just bullies and victims. In fact, bullying is largely possible because there is an audience for the bully; while the bully seems to address his/her actions toward a victim, it might be that actually his/her attention is oriented toward a third party. The role of the bystanders has been largely ignored by the literature on bullying. However, the bystanders can decide to either become part of the problem (by doing nothing or just being spectators) or by referring to external parties, like teachers, parents, social workers, good friends, or the police.

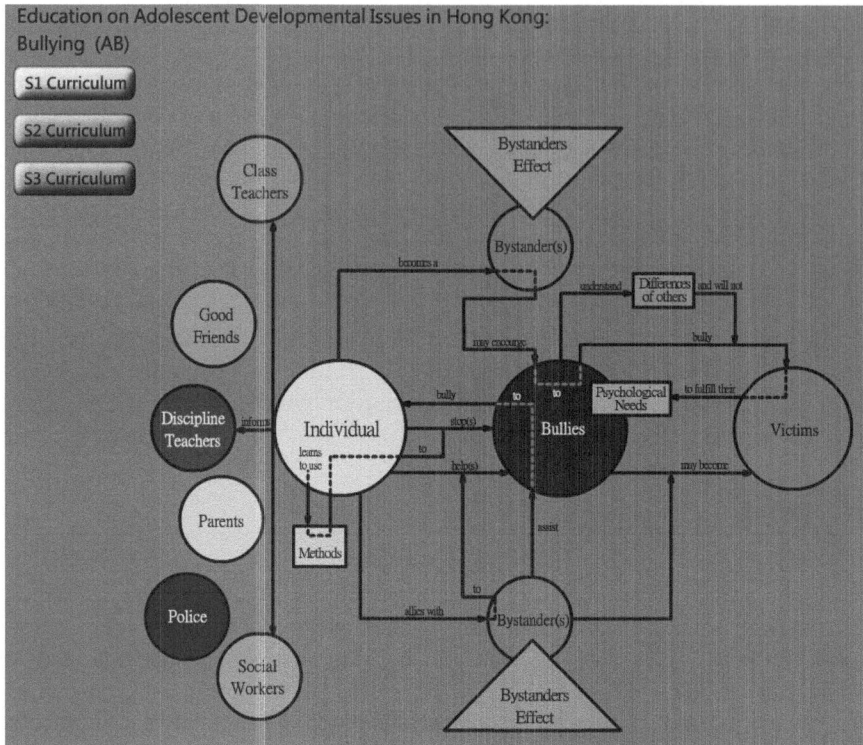

Fig. 1 Concept map of anti-bullying education

Students as bystanders need to learn methods to effectively stop bullying. On the other hand, bullies cannot be simply seen as the origin of the problem or the deviants. It is pertinent to attend to the psychological needs of the bullies (Elinoff et al. 2004) and to help them express their needs differently. Similarly, victims of bullying can sometime retaliate, and the spiral of bullying behavior may never come to an end. Project P.A.T.H.S. as a comprehensive program has the advantage of tackling bullying from a developmental and preventive perspective in addition to being a remedial intervention, thus contributing to breaking this spiral.

Year 1

During the first year (Fig. 2), students are helped to understand and make sense of bullying behavior. Because bullying is aggressive and violent behavior, it may provoke fear and anxiety in victims and bystanders, and it may cause feelings of punishment and repression in adults. However, the reasons that lead the youth to become bullies, victims, or bystanders remain unexplored. Although the roles seem to be well defined, bullies, not any less than victims and bystanders, also have their

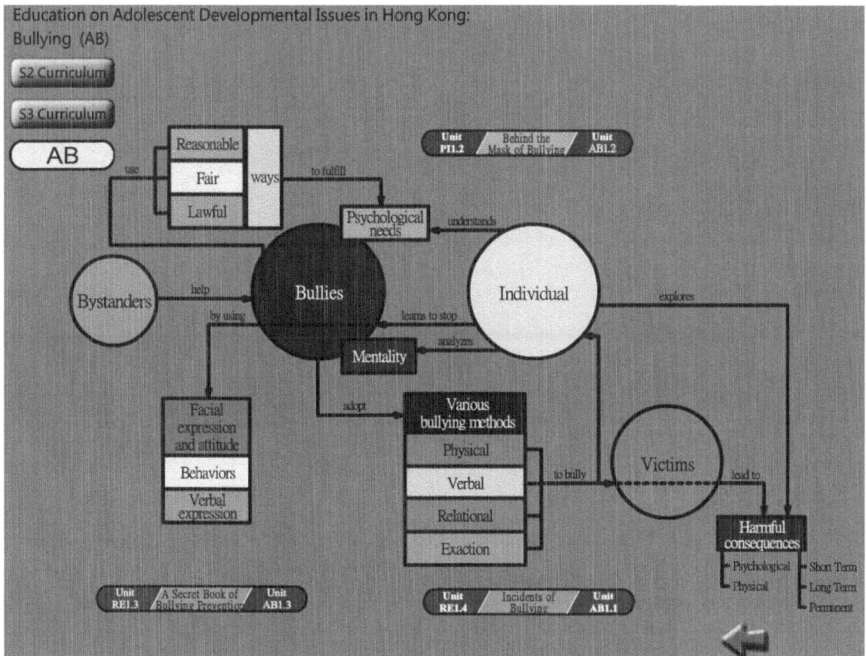

Fig. 2 S1 curriculum design

weaknesses and strengths as well as risk and protective factors, and all of them will experience the consequences of bullying. Therefore, students are invited to consider what bullying is; what are the most common bullying methods; what they think causes such behavior; what separates jokes, conflicts, and bullying; what are the underlying intentions; what are the possible consequences, physically and psychologically as well as in the short/long term and permanently; what are the dos and don'ts in the face of bullying; and how should one defend against bullying. They are guided to think not in terms of chastising the bullies, but instead what possibly lies behind that mask, what other problems exist, and how can such situations be prevented. Furthermore, they are encouraged to express care and concern for other classmates, so to strengthen bonding with peers and lower the risk of bullying.

Year 2

In the second year (Fig. 3), students are invited to consider the role of the bystanders, which is often underestimated, although it may largely affect the outcomes and the consequences of the bullying behavior. Students are informed that a person's intention to offer help is reduced when other people are present, and they are invited to consider some common group dynamics. Then they are asked to think about what personal factors (responsibility, benefits, safety, authority, friendship)

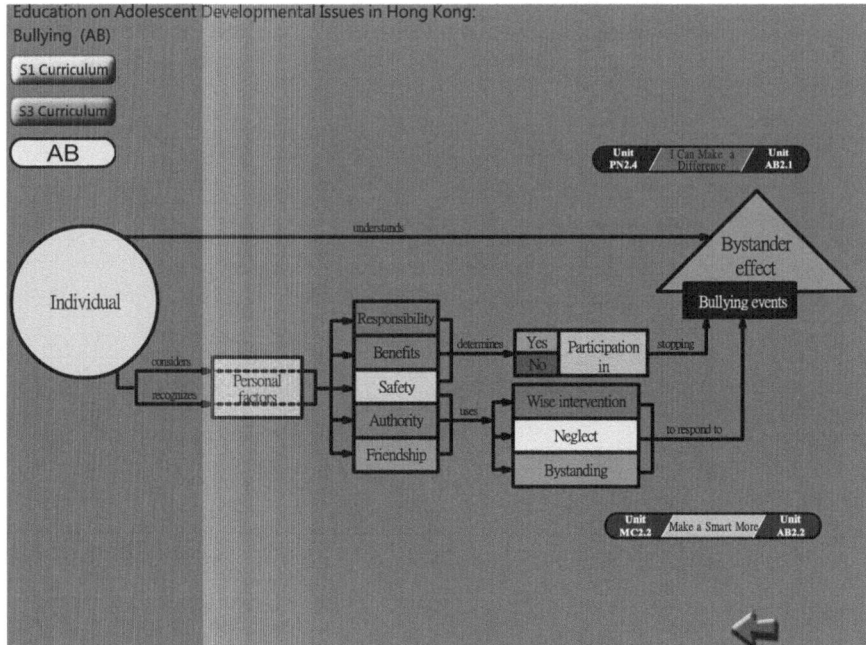

Fig. 3 S2 curriculum design

may influence a bystander as to whether they participate in bullying, how they might participate, and how they might perceive their own responses. Students are invited to give examples of such processes and decide whether it is really possible to avoid taking part in bullying or whether turning a blind eye is likely to encourage bullying and escalate the problem. Finally, they are asked to suggest strategies to stop bullying.

Year 3

In the final year (Fig. 4), students are introduced to a different form of bullying that is perpetrated through electronic devices (computers and mobile phones) and is normally played out on the Internet: cyberbullying. Again, particular emphasis will be given to the role of the bystanders; in year 3 students are asked what the proper attitude for bystanders in cyberbullying is, and how they can actively reduce such bullying behavior by refusing to participate and informing teachers or social workers to take action. It has been argued that bullying behavior is generally addressed toward those who are "different" (because of their religion, sexual orientation, or any other discrepancy from the "standards"). Thus, an important step in bullying prevention is the acceptance of differences and to emphasize that everyone has his/her own idiosyncrasies.

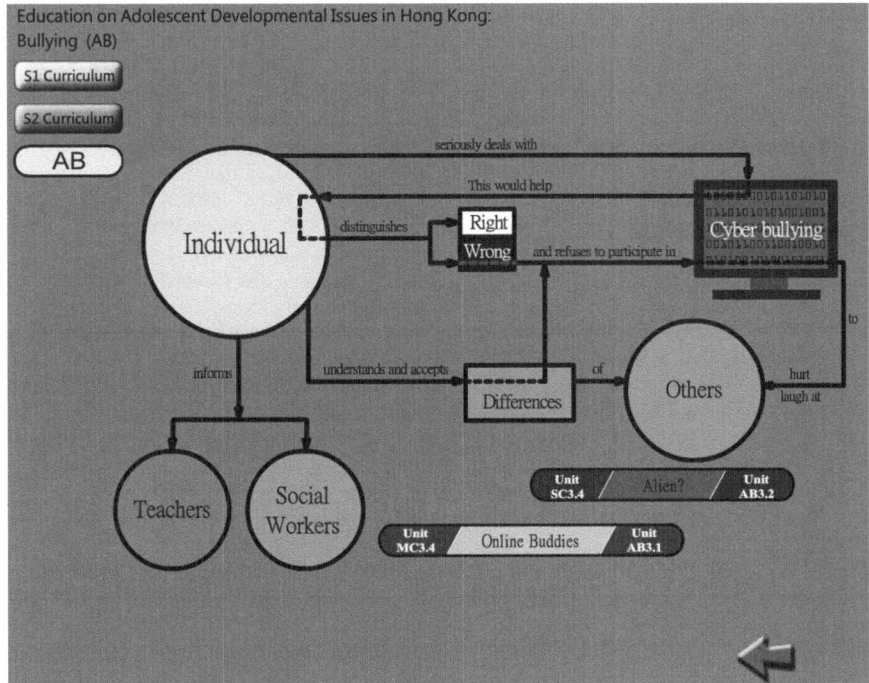

Fig. 4 S3 curriculum design

References

Atlas, R. S., & Pepler, D. J. (1998). Observations of bullying in the classroom. *The Journal of Educational Research, 92*(2), 86–99.

Baker, J. A. (1998). The social context of school satisfaction among urban, low-income, African-American students. *School Psychology Quarterly, 13*(1), 25.

Baker, J. A. (1999). Teacher-student interaction in urban at-risk classrooms: Differential behavior, relationship quality, and student satisfaction with school. *The Elementary School Journal, 100*(1), 57–70.

Bandura, A. (1997). *Self-efficacy: The exercise of control.* New York: WH Freeman.

Bandura, A., Barbaranelli, C., Caprara, G. V., & Pastorelli, C. (1996). Multifaceted impact of self-efficacy beliefs on academic functioning. *Child Development, 67*(3), 1206–1222.

Boulton, M. J., Trueman, M., Bishop, S., Baxandall, E., Holme, A., Smith, S. L., Vohringer, F., & Boulton, L. (2007). Secondary school pupils' views of their school peer counselling for bullying service. *Counselling and Psychotherapy Research, 7*(3), 188–195.

Catalano, R. F., Berglund, M. L., Ryan, J. A., Lonczak, H. S., & Hawkins, J. D. (2002). Positive youth development in the United States: Research findings on evaluations of positive youth development programs. *Prevention and Treatment, 5*(1), 15a.

Couvillon, M. A., & Ilieva, V. (2011). Recommended practices: A review of schoolwide preventative programs and strategies on cyberbullying. *Preventing School Failure: Alternative Education for Children and Youth, 55*(2), 96–101.

Cowie, H., & Olafsson, R. (2000). The role of peer support in helping the victims of bullying in a school with high levels of aggression. *School Psychology International, 21*(1), 79–95.

Danielsen, A. G., Samdal, O., Hetland, J., & Wold, B. (2009). School-related social support and students' perceived life satisfaction. *The Journal of Educational Research, 102*(4), 303–320.

Davis, S., & Davis, J. (2007). *Schools where everyone belongs: Practical strategies for reducing bullying.* Campaign: Research Press.

Demaray, M. K., & Malecki, C. K. (2006). A review of the use of social support in anti-bullying programs. *Journal of School Violence, 5*(3), 51–70.

Elinoff, M. J., Chafouleas, S. M., & Sassu, K. A. (2004). Bullying: Considerations for defining and intervening in school settings. *Psychology in the Schools, 41*(8), 887–897.

Gini, G., Albiero, P., Benelli, B., & Altoe, G. (2008). Determinants of adolescents' active defending and passive bystanding behavior in bullying. *Journal of Adolescence, 31*(1), 93–105.

Hawkins, D. L., Pepler, D. J., & Craig, W. M. (2001). Naturalistic observations of peer interventions in bullying. *Social Development, 10*(4), 512–527.

Hui, E. K. (2000). Guidance as a whole school approach in Hong Kong: From remediation to student development. *International Journal for the Advancement of Counselling, 22*(1), 69–82.

Hui, E. K. (2002). A whole-school approach to guidance: Hong Kong teachers' perceptions. *British Journal of Guidance and Counselling, 30*(1), 63–80.

Hui, E. K. (2010). Guiding students for positive development. In L. F. Zhang, J. Biggs, & D. Watkins (Eds.), *Learning and development of Asian students: What the 21st century teachers need to think about* (pp. 221–244). Singapore: Pearson Education South Asia.

Hui, E. K., & Sun, R. C. (2010). Chinese children's perceived school satisfaction: The role of contextual and intrapersonal factors. *Educational Psychology, 30*(2), 155–172.

Hui, E. K., Tsang, S. K., & Law, B. C. (2011). Combating school bullying through development guidance for positive youth development and promoting harmonious school culture. *The Scientific World Journal, 11*, 2266–2277.

Kohut, M. R. (2007). *The complete guide to understanding, controlling, and stopping bullies & bullying: A complete guide for teachers & parents.* Ocala: Atlantic Publishing Company.

Ladd, G. W., Kochenderfer, B. J., & Coleman, C. C. (1996). Friendship quality as a predictor of young children's early school adjustment. *Child Development, 67*(3), 1103–1118.

Lodge, J., & Frydenberg, E. (2005). The role of peer bystanders in school bullying: Positive steps toward promoting peaceful schools. *Theory Into Practice, 44*(4), 329–336.

Mishna, F. (2008). An overview of the evidence on bullying prevention and intervention programs. *Brief Treatment and Crisis Intervention, 8*(4), 327.

Nickerson, A. B., Mele, D., & Princiotta, D. (2008). Attachment and empathy as predictors of roles as defenders or outsiders in bullying interactions. *Journal of School Psychology, 46*(6), 687–703.

Olweus, D. (1993). *Bullying at school: What we know and what we can do.* Cambridge, MA: Blackwell.

Salmivalli, C. (1999). Participant role approach to school bullying: Implications for interventions. *Journal of Adolescence, 22*(4), 453–459.

Salmivalli, C., Lagerspetz, K., Björkqvist, K., Österman, K., & Kaukiainen, A. (1996). Bullying as a group process: Participant roles and their relations to social status within the group. *Aggressive Behavior, 22*(1), 1–15.

Salmivalli, C., Kaukiainen, A., Kaistaniemi, L., & Lagerspetz, K. M. (1999). Self-evaluated self-esteem, peer-evaluated self-esteem, and defensive egotism as predictors of adolescents' participation in bullying situations. *Personality and Social Psychology Bulletin, 25*(10), 1268–1278.

Schwartz, D., Dodge, K. A., & Coie, J. D. (1993). The emergence of chronic peer victimization in boys' play groups. *Child Development, 64*(6), 1755–1772.

Schwarzer, R., Dunkel-Schetter, C., Weiner, B., & Woo, G. (1992). Expectancies as mediators between recipient characteristics and social support intentions. In R. Schwarzer (Ed.), *Self-efficacy: Thought control of action* (pp. 65–87). Washington, DC: Hemisphere Publishing.

Shek, D. T. L. (2009). Effectiveness of the tier 1 program of project P.A.T.H.S.: Findings based on the first 2 years of program implementation. *The Scientific World Journal, 9*, 539–547.

Shek, D. T. L., & Ma, C. M. S. (2011). Impact of the project P.A.T.H.S. in the junior secondary school years: Individual growth curve analyses. *The Scientific World Journal, 11*, 253–266.

Shek, D. T. L., & Sun, R. C. F. (2010). Effectiveness of the tier 1 program of project P.A.T.H.S.: Findings based on three years of program implementation. *The Scientific World Journal, 10*, 1509–1519.

Slonje, R., & Smith, P. K. (2008). Cyberbullying: Another main type of bullying? *Scandinavian Journal of Psychology, 49*, 147–154.

Stueve, A., Dash, K., O'Donnell, L., Tehranifar, P., Wilson-Simmons, R., Slaby, R. G., & Link, B. G. (2006). Rethinking the bystander role in school violence prevention. *Health Promotion Practice, 7*(1), 117–124.

Sun, R. C., & Hui, E. K. (2007). Building social support for adolescents with suicidal ideation: Implications for school guidance and counselling. *British Journal of Guidance and Counselling, 35*(3), 299–316.

Tsang, S. K., & Hui, E. K. (2006). Self-efficacy as a positive youth development construct: Conceptual bases and implications for curriculum development. *International Journal of Adolescent Medicine and Health, 18*(3), 441–450.

Tsang, S. K., & Yip, F. Y. (2006). Positive identity as a positive youth development construct: Conceptual bases and implications for curriculum development. *International Journal of Adolescent Medicine and Health, 18*(3), 459–466.

Tsang, S. K., Hui, E. K., & Law, B. C. (2011). Bystander position taking in school bullying: The role of positive identity, self-efficacy, and self-determination. *The Scientific World Journal, 11*, 2278–2286.

Tsang, S. K. M., Hui, E. K. P., & Law, B. C. M. (2012). Positive identity as a positive youth development construct: A conceptual review. *The Scientific World Journal*, doi:10.1100/2012/529691

Twemlow, S. W., Fonagy, P., & Sacco, F. C. (2004). The role of the bystander in the social architecture of bullying and violence in schools and communities. *Annals of the New York Academy of Sciences, 1036*(1), 215–232.

Verkuyten, M., & Thijs, J. (2002). School satisfaction of elementary school children: The role of performance, peer relations, ethnicity and gender. *Social Indicators Research, 59*(2), 203–228.

Wong, D. S. W. (2004). School bullying and tackling strategies in Hong Kong. *International Journal of Offender Therapy and Comparative Criminology, 48*(5), 537–553.

Wong, D. S. W., Lok, D. P., Lo, T. W., & Ma, S. K. (2008). School bullying among Hong Kong Chinese primary school children. *Youth and Society, 40*(1), 35–54.

Prevention of Internet Addiction: The P.A.T.H.S. Program

Diego Busiol and Tak Yan Lee

Abstract The effects and consequences of Internet addiction might seem less showy and dramatic than, for example, the effects of substance abuse or bullying. Internet addiction is a much more silent problem, and as such, it might be more easily ignored or even not recognized as a problem. In this chapter, it is argued that an effective prevention program against Internet addiction should first of all promote positive youth development among adolescents. Results from previous research showed that students participating in Project P.A.T.H.S. showed higher levels of psychosocial competencies and less problem behavior than students in a control group. Project P.A.T.H.S. aims at reducing adolescents' antisocial behavior, substance use, and Internet addiction primarily by improving their psychosocial competencies. This chapter will illustrate how these developmental issues are explored within the special teaching units included in the extension phase of Project P.A.T.H.S. on Internet addiction.

Necessity of Educational Programs and Current Programs

The problem of the misuse, or even abuse, of the Internet has been largely underestimated. A digital divide between people exists (Christakis 2010), and it is what separates in most cases parents from their children as well as educators, teachers, and policymakers from younger generations. This could explain the delay in research on Internet addiction and why the field is in its infancy. So, it is not surprising that Internet abuse prevention programs are almost completely lacking in the literature.

Although the large majority of the population may not be said to be addicted to it, still, in recent years, the pervasive use of technology has profoundly shaped the way people interact and relate; this is particularly true for the new generations, as

Author contributed equally with all other contributors.

The preparation for this work and the Project P.A.T.H.S. were financially supported by The Hong Kong Jockey Club Charities Trust.

D. Busiol • T.Y. Lee (✉)
Department of Applied Social Sciences, City University of Hong Kong,
Kowloon, Hong Kong, China
e-mail: ty.lee@cityu.edu.hk

© Springer Science+Business Media Singapore 2015   185
T.Y. Lee et al. (eds.), *Student Well-Being in Chinese Adolescents in Hong Kong*,
Quality of Life in Asia 7, DOI 10.1007/978-981-287-582-2_14

they were born after the beginning of the digital era and have no memory of life without the Internet and mobile phones.

The effects and consequences of Internet abuse might seem less showy and dramatic than, for example, the effects of substance abuse or bullying. Drug abuse usually has a remarkable physical impact and normally is related to several other types of crimes and offenses. Bullying too is a rather striking phenomenon that involves violence and might have serious consequences for victims and society. Both drug abuse and bullying have clear manifestations that cannot be ignored. Instead, Internet abuse might be more easily underestimated because it might lead to retiring or even disappearing from social life (e.g., this is the case of the so-called hikikomori). Indeed, Internet abuse is a much more *silent* problem, and as such, it might be more easily ignored or even not recognized as a problem.

Internet addiction has oftentimes been considered a pathology with mechanisms similar to other compulsive behavior, like eating disorders, substance abuse, and pathological gambling. Researchers have proposed different intervention strategies to treat Internet addiction, such as cognitive behavior therapy and motivational enhancement therapy (Orzack and Orzack 1999; Young 2007). For example, in cognitive behavior therapy, addicts are taught to identify the distorted thoughts that trigger Internet addictive behavior and are provided with training in coping strategies to help them effectively deal with real or perceived problems. Motivational enhancement therapy allows Internet abusers and therapists to collaborate on treatment plans and set achievable goals (Orzack and Orzack 1999). Young (2007) also suggested several specific treatment techniques, like constructing new schedules for using the Internet, setting clear and achievable goals to give the addict a sense of control, and providing social support to decrease addicts' dependence on the Internet as well as family therapy. There are reports of treatments of Internet addiction with CBT (Pujol et al. 2009) and even pharmacotherapy (Han et al. 2009); however, as noted by some (Weiss et al. 2011; Fu et al. 2010), there is a general lack of prevention programs or even guidelines. Only a few school-based programs have been developed in Korea, where Internet addiction is considered one of the most serious public health issues (Ahn 2007; Joo and Park 2010).

Although these techniques have been demonstrated to be effective in treating Internet addicts, it is more important to prevent adolescents who have not yet fulfilled the criteria to be considered an Internet addict from developing such behavioral pattern. Based on the "problem behavior theory" that Internet addiction is an intersection of multiple physical, psychological, and technological phenomena instead of a single problem, it has been suggested that prevention programs directed at the organization of different problem behaviors (e.g., substance use, delinquency) may be more appropriate than those which target specific behavior alone (Yen et al. 2007).

As has emerged from the literature, students who are addicted to the Internet normally show weaknesses in school performances, poor family relationships, and mood problems. Thus, prevention of Internet addiction should address these underlying issues, rather than be focused on the use of technological devices. Yu and Shek (2013) suggest that improving the parent–child relation, communication, and understanding among family members can be the right direction for preventing youth Internet addiction. Iskender and Akin (2010) suggest that prevention for students should aim at improving communication with family members and should develop social skills and self-efficacy.

A Comprehensive Approach to Adolescents' Internet Addiction

Nowadays, particularly in places like Hong Kong, almost the entirety of the youth population make use of the Internet and technology devices, and although only a relatively small percent may be described as addicts, education in technology and healthy relationships is the cornerstone for living in society (Shek et al. 2008). Thus, a prevention program may not just be beneficial, but highly recommended.

It is argued that an effective prevention program against Internet addiction should first of all promote positive youth development among adolescents. Project P.A.T.H.S. (Fig. 1) aims at reducing adolescents' antisocial behavior, substance use, and Internet addiction primarily by improving their psychosocial competencies. As has emerged from the literature, Internet addiction shares several similarities with adolescents' other forms of addictions; this suggests that particular attention should be paid to the "addiction" issue, rather than focusing on the substance abused. However, different forms of addiction are not completely overlapping; for instance, they may affect very different user populations, they may be rooted in different causes, and they may also be perceived differently by society.

Project P.A.T.H.S. aims at helping students to recognize and distinguish the practical benefits of being connected to the Internet (and what a proper use of it could be) from being dependent on it (what leads to an improper or even a pathological use). A proper use of the Internet is understood as when it remains a tool for expanding social relations, communicating with distant friends, acquiring knowledge, and

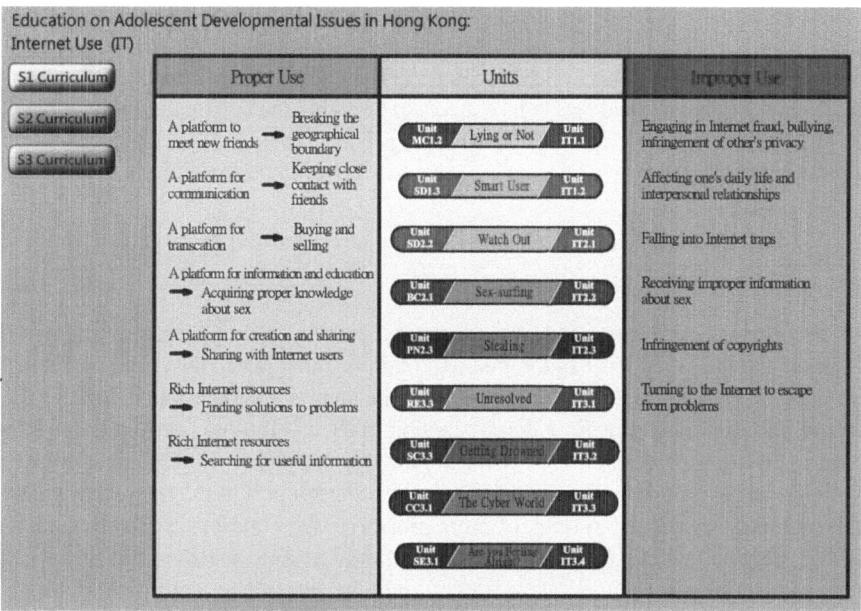

Fig. 1 Internet use curriculum design

trading or sharing ideas. Instead, an improper use is when the Internet becomes a defense from "real" life, a way of escaping problems and difficulties, a place for infringing laws and bullying others, and finally a tool for avoiding any kind of sharing or communication with others.

The following table (Table 1) shows how these developmental issues are explored within the special teaching units on Internet addiction.

Year 1

In Secondary 1 (Fig. 2), students are introduced to basic knowledge about the Internet and are taught to become responsible users, to reflect and understand the impact of improper use of the Internet in their own as well as others' daily life (Unit 1: Lying or Not). Students are led to consider how to allocate their time to the Internet and other daily activities and how their behavior and attitude should or should not change in relation to the Internet and everyday life (Unit 2: Smart User).

Year 2

In Secondary 2 (Fig. 3), students should develop more critical thinking and self-determination to recognize the potential threats of the Internet (pseudo-identity and cyberbullying) and be self-protective (Unit 1: Watch Out). This implies acquiring self-reflection, becoming more able to enquire and understand more and, most importantly, to distinguish whether the information obtained from websites is suitable and appropriate (Unit 2: Sex Surfing). Finally, students are encouraged to consider carefully any ethical and legal aspects of breaking the law on the Internet, such as infringement of copyright or cyberbullying (Unit 3: Stealing?).

Year 3

In Secondary 3 (Fig. 4), students are invited to think more critically about the Internet and not consider it as the first and main resource when they face problems. To many students, the Internet can represent the answer to boredom or the solution to overcoming unhappiness or dissatisfaction in their life. As a consequence, they might acquire a passive attitude toward their life and develop a low resilience to stress, becoming more and more addicted to finding support in the Internet. Against this, students are invited to think of more proactive ways (various methods, such as doing exercise or taking a rest) to face their weaknesses, and they are invited to reconsider critically those who instead indulge in online activities (Unit 1: Unresolved). For example, a number of characteristics (symptoms) of teenagers

Table 1 Internet use (IT): unit overview

	Unit code/unit name	Construct	Unit aim	Learning targets
Secondary 1	1.1 Lying or Not	Moral competence (Behavioral competence) (Social competence)	To learn to be respectful and responsible when using the Internet	1. To understand that lying online is irresponsible and disrespectful 2. To learn to respect privacy
	1.2 Smart User	Self-determination (Social competence) (Belief in the future)	To learn how to use the Internet with self-control and to prevent it from interrupting our daily life	1. To understand how excessive Internet activities affect daily life and interpersonal relationships 2. To understand that we have other activities apart from surfing the Internet, and we should know how to make choices
Secondary 2	2.1 Watch Out	Self-determination	To learn about the potential traps on the Internet so students should know how to protect themselves and handle the issue carefully	1. To learn how one should surf websites and handle the information carefully 2. To be self-protective against loss from all online trading
	2.2 Sex Surfing	Behavioral competence (Moral competence)	To cultivate the right attitude toward searching for sex-related information on the Internet	1. To learn not to totally trust the sex-related information offered on the Internet as well as to learn how to distinguish between the right information and wrong
	2.3 Stealing?	Prosocial norms	To enhance students' knowledge of proper Internet use	1. To understand that infringement of copyright is unethical 2. To understand the consequences of illegal Internet use
Secondary 3	3.1 Unresolved	Resilience	To enhance the self-reflection on using the Internet as the only way to solve daily problems	1. To understand how to solve problems 2. To discuss whether to enhance self-reflection on using the Internet is a good way or not to solve personal problems in daily life
	3.2 Getting Drowned	Social competence	To look into the impacts of devoting oneself to the Internet world and reflect on one's habit of surfing the Internet	1. To understand the features of overusing the Internet and do self-evaluation 2. To understand the impacts of devoting oneself to the Internet world and think of some ways to improve
	3.3 The Cyber World	Cognitive competence	To reflect on the impact of violent and virtual reality games on mental and physical health	1. To learn not to indulge in violent and virtual reality computer games 2. To know how to distinguish the virtual world and reality
	3.4 Are You Feeling Alright?	Self-efficacy	To become a healthy high-tech user	1. To understand the potential impact of prolonged use of computers and digital and gaming devices on our health 2. To learn how to use computers and digital and gaming devices properly in order to avoid adverse effects on health

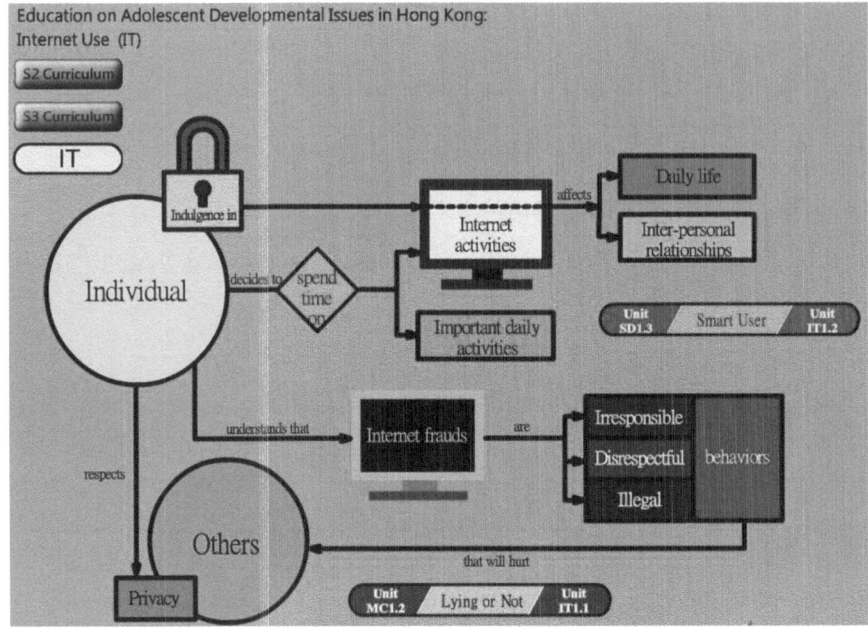

Fig. 2 S1 curriculum design

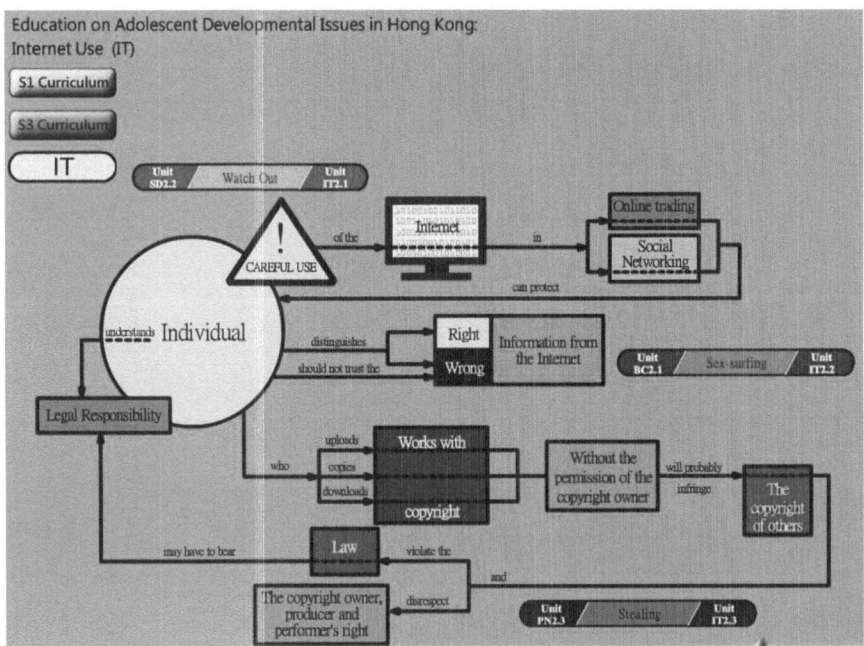

Fig. 3 S2 curriculum design

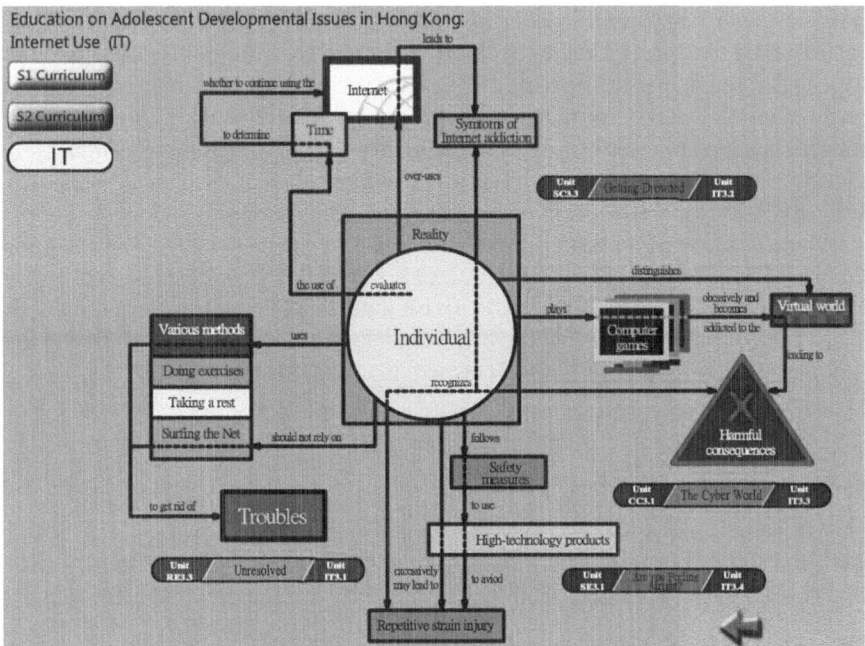

Fig. 4 S3 curriculum design

indulging in the Internet are presented, like lack of sleep, lack of concentration, no time for other activities, fluctuating moods, anger or aggressiveness when prohibited from using the Internet, and going online being the sole objective of the day. The aim is to describe some common experiences shared by peers of the same age, so that students can better identify the risks of abuse of the Internet by identifying some distinctive signs (Unit 2: Getting Drowned). Consequently, they are invited to reflect on the different spheres that can be affected (harmful consequences) by Internet abuse, like their academic performance, family, personal relationships, mood and emotions, health, and legal offenses (Unit 3: The Cyber World). Not only students are led to consider the negative effects of prolonged use of their computer and gaming devices, but more specifically, they are invited to think of all the other aspects of their lives that in doing so are being neglected and how the virtual life little by little tends to substitute their life (Unit 4: Are You Feeling Alright?).

Efficacy of Project P.A.T.H.S.

Based on a longitudinal randomized controlled group trial, researchers have reported that participants of Project P.A.T.H.S. displayed stronger ability to control their Internet use than did the comparison group (Shek and Yu 2011). It seems that positive youth development programs represent a promising direction for youth Internet addiction prevention in the future (Shek and Ng 2010; Shek et al. 2010). In a recent longitudinal study including eight waves of data collected in Project PATHS, results showed that relative to the control group participants, students in the experimental schools (i.e., students participating in Project P.A.T.H.S.) showed higher levels of psychosocial competencies and less problem behavior (Shek and Yu 2012b). It is argued that the promotion of psychosocial competencies may help to protect young people from risky behavior by enhancing their inner strengths (Sun and Shek 2010; Shek and Merrick 2010; Shek 2010; Yu and Shek 2013). Besides, as different types of youth risky behavior tend to coexist, reduction of other problem behaviors, such as intention to engage in risky behavior, may also lower the risk of developing Internet addiction in the long run (Shek and Ma 2012; Shek and Yu 2012a).

References

Ahn, D. H. (2007). Korean policy on treatment and rehabilitation for adolescents' internet addiction. In *2007 International Symposium on the Counseling and Treatment of Youth Internet Addiction* (p. 49). Seoul, Korea: National Youth Commission.

Christakis, D. A. (2010). Internet addiction: A 21st century epidemic? *BMC Medicine, 8*(1), 61–68.

Fu, K. W., Chan, W. S., Wong, P. W., & Yip, P. S. (2010). Internet addiction: prevalence, discriminant validity and correlates among adolescents in Hong Kong. *The British Journal of Psychiatry, 196*(6), 486–492.

Han, D. H., Lee, Y. S., Na, C., Ahn, J. Y., Chung, U. S., Daniels, M. A., Haws, C. H., & Renshaw, P. F. (2009). The effect of methylphenidate on internet video game play in children with attention-deficit/hyperactivity disorder. *Comprehensive Psychiatry, 50*(3), 251–256.

İskender, M., & Akin, A. (2010). Social self-efficacy, academic locus of control, and internet addiction. *Computers & Education, 54*(4), 1101–1106.

Joo, A., & Park, I. (2010). Effects of an empowerment education program in the prevention of internet games addiction in middle school students. *Journal of Korean Academy of Nursing, 40*(2), 255–263.

Orzack, M. H., & Orzack, D. S. (1999). Treatment of computer addicts with complex co-morbid psychiatric disorders. *Cyberpsychology & Behavior, 2*(5), 465–473.

Pujol, C. D. C., Alexandre, S., Sokolovsky, A., Karam, R. G., & Spritzer, D. T. (2009). Internet addiction: Perspectives on cognitive-behavioral therapy. *Revista Brasileira de Psiquiatria, 31*(2), 185–186.

Shek, D. T. L. (2010). Subjective outcome and objective outcome evaluation findings: Insights from a Chinese context. *Research on Social Work Practice, 20*(3), 293–301.

Shek, D. T. L., & Ma, C. M. S. (2012). Impact of the project PATHS in the junior secondary school years: Objective outcome evaluation based on eight waves of longitudinal data. *The Scientific World Journal, 2012, 12 pages.* doi:10.1100/2012/170345.

Shek, D. T. L., & Merrick, J. (2010). Special issue: Positive youth development and training. *International Journal of Adolescent Medicine and Health, 21*, 341–447.

Shek, D. T. L., & Ng, C. S. (2010). Early identification of adolescents with greater psychosocial needs: An evaluation of the project PATHS in Hong Kong. *International Journal on Disability and Human Development, 9*(4), 291–299.

Shek, D. T. L., & Yu, L. (2011). Prevention of adolescent problem behavior: Longitudinal impact of the project PATHS in Hong Kong. *The Scientific World Journal, 11*, 546–567.

Shek, D. T. L., & Yu, L. (2012a). Internet addiction in Hong Kong adolescents: Profiles and psychosocial correlates. *International Journal on Disability and Human Development, 11*(2), 133–142.

Shek, D. T. L., & Yu, L. (2012b). Longitudinal impact of the project PATHS on adolescent risk behavior: What happened after five years? *The Scientific World Journal, 2012, 13 pages.* doi:10.1100/2012/316029.

Shek, D. T. L., Tang, V. M., & Lo, C. Y. (2008). Internet addiction in Chinese adolescents in Hong Kong: Assessment, profiles, and psychosocial correlates. *The Scientific World Journal, 8*, 776–787.

Shek, D. T. L., Ng, C. S., & Tsui, P. F. (2010). Qualitative evaluation of the project PATHS: Findings based on focus groups. *International Journal on Disability and Human Development, 9*(4), 307–313.

Sun, R. C., & Shek, D. T. L. (2010). Life satisfaction, positive youth development, and problem behaviour among Chinese adolescents in Hong Kong. *Social Indicators Research, 95*(3), 455–474.

Weiss, M. D., Baer, S., Allan, B. A., Saran, K., & Schibuk, H. (2011). The screens culture: Impact on ADHD. *Attention Deficit and Hyperactivity Disorders, 3*(4), 327–334.

Yen, J. Y., Ko, C. H., Yen, C. F., Wu, H. Y., & Yang, M. J. (2007). The comorbid psychiatric symptoms of Internet addiction: Attention deficit and hyperactivity disorder (ADHD), depression, social phobia, and hostility. *Journal of Adolescent Health, 41*(1), 93–98.

Young, K. S. (2007). Cognitive-behavioral therapy with internet addicts: Treatment outcomes and implications. *Cyberpsychology & Behavior, 10*, 671–679.

Yu, L., & Shek, D. T. L. (2013). Internet addiction in Hong Kong adolescents: A three-year longitudinal study. *Journal of Pediatric and Adolescent Gynecology, 26*(3), S10–S17.

Promotion of Money Literacy: The P.A.T.H.S. Program

Tak Yan Lee and Diego Busiol

Abstract Nine units on "Money and Success" are included in the extension phase of P.A.T.H.S. to help students strengthen their money literacy using a progressive approach. Each unit emphasizes one construct more than others, including: self-efficacy, spirituality, belief in the future, cognitive competence, and moral competence. Taken together, all emphasize the self-competence of young people. This chapter briefly introduces the curriculum units on promoting money literacy from year 1 to year 3. The curriculum is based on research findings and is inspired by the 15 PYD constructs; furthermore, its development is informed by psychosocial, developmental, and cultural perspectives. Then, since the Project P.A.T.H.S. is carried out in the Chinese cultural context, examples demonstrating traditional Chinese values are illustrated in the curriculum materials to help students clarify values about money, success, wealth, beauty, power, sex, self-worth, and self-esteem.

Introduction

This framework (Fig. 1) is used for constructing curriculum units on money literacy in the extension phase of Project P.A.T.H.S. in Hong Kong which is designed to promote holistic development among grade 7–9 Chinese students (Shek and Sun 2010; Shek and Ma 2011; Shek and Yu 2011). A total of nine 35-min curriculum units (relatively little when compared to a total of 120 units in the whole curriculum) are included to help students strengthen their money literacy using a progressive approach. The framework is based on research findings and is inspired by the 15 PYD constructs; furthermore, its development is informed by psychosocial,

The preparation for this work and the Project P.A.T.H.S. were financially supported by The Hong Kong Jockey Club Charities Trust.

This paper is based on an article originally published by *The Scientific World Journal*: Lee, T. Y., & Law, M. F. (2011). Teaching Money Literacy in a Positive Youth Development Program: The Project P.A.T.H.S. in Hong Kong. *The Scientific World Journal*, *11*, 2287–2298.

T.Y. Lee (✉) • D. Busiol
Department of Applied Social Sciences, City University of Hong Kong,
Kowloon, Hong Kong, China
e-mail: ty.lee@cityu.edu.hk

© Springer Science+Business Media Singapore 2015
T.Y. Lee et al. (eds.), *Student Well-Being in Chinese Adolescents in Hong Kong*,
Quality of Life in Asia 7, DOI 10.1007/978-981-287-582-2_15

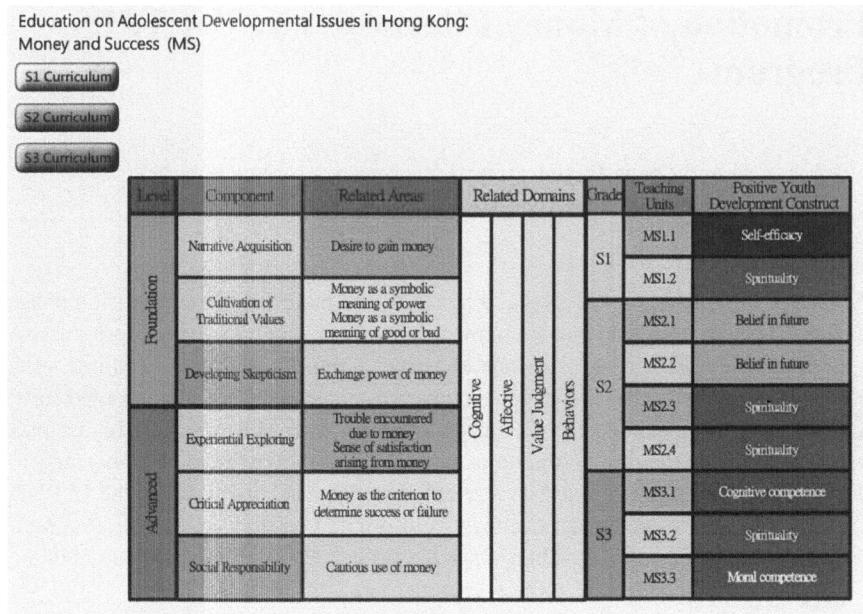

Fig. 1 Conceptual framework on money literacy

developmental, and cultural perspectives. Finally, it provides concrete guides for helping professionals to develop preventive measures for children and adolescents (Shek and Sun 2010; Shek and Ma 2011; Shek and Yu 2011).

Units for grade 7 students are designed using components in the foundation level. For grade 8–9 students, emphasis is put on the advanced level. Each unit emphasizes one construct more than others, including: self-efficacy, spirituality, belief in the future, cognitive competence, and moral competence.

Teenagers' moral values are influenced by their social environment, for example, by financial issues and globalization. Adolescents should have the opportunity to discuss changes resulting from these events in either formal or informal curricula. According to Piaget (1965), mutual discussion and reflection are highly emphasized in the moral development of youth. Similarly, in Chinese moral education, Confucius emphasized the elicitation and thought-provoking methods of teaching; he also stressed teaching students according to their aptitude and setting a good example with one's own conduct (Yin 1998). The curriculum design is inspired by these principles. Teenagers are encouraged to develop their autonomous thoughts and form their value constructs through social interaction with their classmates and teachers. Unwanted value impositions are not recommended.

Hong Kong is an international city which still upholds a predominantly Chinese culture. The traditional Chinese philosophy and values are selectively introduced to children and youth with regard to money and success, such as developing a moral self, promoting counter-materialism, leading a simple life, and encouraging the proper use of money. Some Chinese noble characters' beliefs are embedded in the activities and teaching materials.

The aims and learning targets of the nine curriculum units as well as their linkage to the framework are described in Table 1. A description of how these constructs are used is provided below.

Curriculum Units on Promoting Money Literacy

Year One

Self-efficacy denotes people's beliefs about their capacities to perform in different situations (Tsang and Hui 2006). One unit (I Believe I Can) involving two components, namely, narrative acquisition and cultivation of traditional values, is constructed. The objectives for this unit are (i) to recognize one's efficacy in social and living habits, academic study, appearance, and financial management and (ii) to understand that many essential abilities are not developed with money. It helps students develop an understanding of the differences of needs and wants and clarifies their values about money and success.

A second unit (The Value of Life) focuses on *developing skepticism* and aims to facilitate students' thinking about their life priorities with two objectives: (i) to reflect on materialistic values and their limitations and (ii) to help students explore the value of life (Fig. 2).

Year Two

Belief in the future comprises valued and attainable goals, the ability to plan goal-directed pathways and alternative ones in times of difficulty, positive appraisal of one's capabilities and efforts, and positive and realistic experiences of the future (Sun and Lau 2006). The components of experiential exploring and social responsibility are used to design two units, respectively. The first unit (My Persistence) has two objectives: (i) to understand the two keys to success, persistence and resistance to temptations, and (ii) to understand that money is just a necessary but not a sufficient condition for success in life. The second unit (Drawing the Line at Certain Kinds of Action) aims to help students learn how to make choices and refuse to gain money by illegal means. Three objectives are set for this unit: (i) to let students understand that they should not participate in illegal acts for money, (ii) to teach students to deal with peer pressure by using decision-making skills, and (iii) to understand that everyone should be responsible for his or her own acts for gaining money.

Two more units are based on *spirituality*. Spirituality aims to facilitate students to connect with other people and a higher being and establish personal beliefs and values as well as search for the meaning of life (Lau 2006). These units will help students dispute their beliefs about hedonism and materialism and search for the meaning of life. Unit 2.3 (A Meaningful Life) aims at enhancing critical appreciation and gives students the opportunity to experience managing one's finances through a specially designed board game with two objectives: (i) to understand

Table 1 Aims and learning targets of curriculum units for money literacy

Units	Aim	Learning targets	Positive youth development construct	Elements of money literacy
Secondary One				
I Believe I Can (MS 1.1)	To learn to identify self-efficacy in different domains and the limitations of money	1. To recognize one's self-efficacy in social and living habits, academic study, appearance, and financial management	Self-efficacy	Narrative acquisition and cultivation of traditional values
		2. To understand that many essential abilities are not developed with money		
The Value of Life (MS 1.2)	To facilitate students' thinking about their life priorities	1. To reflect on materialistic values and their limitations	Spirituality	Developing skepticism
		2. To help students to explore the value of life		
Secondary Two				
My Persistence (MS 2.1)	To understand that achieving targets requires persistent hard work	1. To understand two keys to success – persistence and resistance to temptation	Belief in the future	Experiential exploring
		2. To understand money is just a necessary but not a sufficient condition for success in life		
Drawing the Line at Certain Kinds of Action (MS 2.2)	To learn how to make choices and refuse to gain money by illegal means	1. To let students understand that they should not participate in illegal acts to gain money	Belief in the future	Social responsibility
		2. To teach students to deal with peer pressure by using decision-making skills		
		3. To understand that everyone should be responsible for his or her own acts for gaining money		
A Meaningful Life (MS 2.3)	To experience managing one's own finances	1. To understand that good moral character is essential to leading a meaningful life	Spirituality	Critical appreciation
		2. To understand the importance of prudent financial management		
The Story of a Cycling Boy (MS 2.4)	To encourage students to reflect on the meaning of money in their lives	1. To understand the importance of spiritual satisfaction	Spirituality	Experiential exploring
		2. To reflect on the value and meaning of money in life		

Secondary Three

			Cognitive competence	Social responsibility
Know More About Credit Cards (MS 3.1)	To understand consumer loans (e.g., using credit cards) rationally	1. To understand the financial burdens and risks caused by consumer loans 2. To reflect on alternatives to consumer loans	Cognitive competence	Social responsibility
The Kindest Cut (MS 3.2)	To deepen students' understanding toward the meaning of life through a discussion of vocations	1. To introduce Doctor Sidney Chung's work and worldview and probe into conditions of ideal work 2. To deepen students' understanding about the relationship between money and success and reflect on the meaning of life	Spirituality	Critical appreciation
Welcome Everybody to the Party! (MS 3.3)	To understand the styles of consumption that can let everyone contribute to making changes that lead to a better world	1. To nurture the ability of goal achievement and attitudes and skills of good financial management 2. To enhance students' knowledge of responsible consumption with local examples and establish students' belief in civil responsibility with practice in consumption 3. To use the knowledge, skills, and attitude taught in this chapter in real school life	Moral competence	Social responsibility

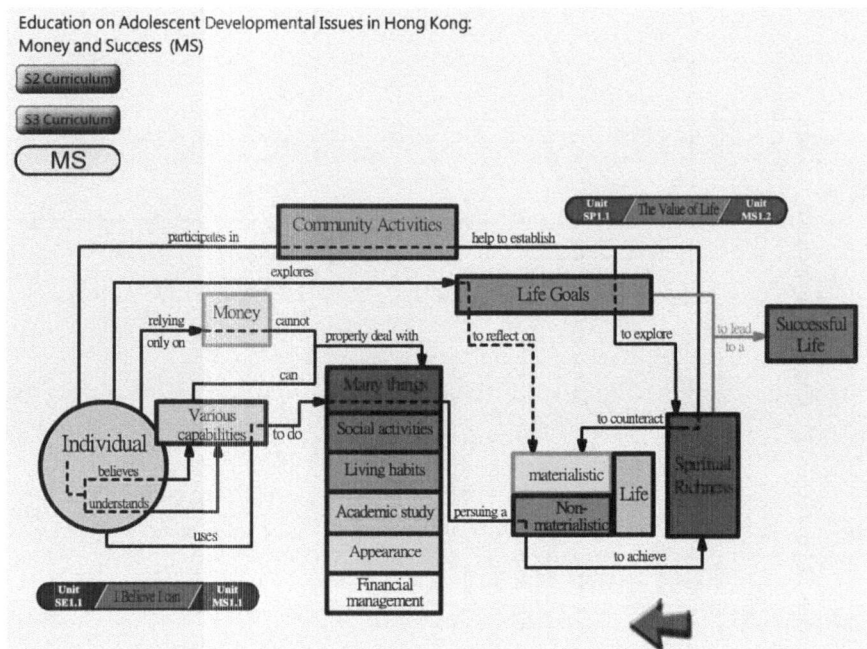

Fig. 2 S1 curriculum design

that good moral character is essential to leading a meaningful life and (ii) to understand the importance of prudent financial management. Unit 2.4 (The Story of a Cycling Boy) adopts experiential exploring and aims to encourage students to reflect on the meaning of money in their lives with two objectives: (i) to understand the importance of spiritual satisfaction and (ii) to reflect on the value and meaning of money in life (Fig. 3).

Year Three

Cognitive competence refers to the cognitive processes that comprise creative thinking and critical thinking (Sun and Hui 2006). Unit one for grade 9 students (Know More about Credit Cards) is designed to help them understand consumer loans rationally with two objectives: (i) to understand the financial burden and risks caused by consumer loans and (ii) to think critically and creatively as to whether there are alternatives to consumer loans through examples of using credit cards. This unit helps students recognize that their own decisions affect peers, family, and society.

Unit 3.2 (The Kindest Cut) is designed with the aim to deepen students' understanding of the meaning of life through a discussion on vocation. It adopts the

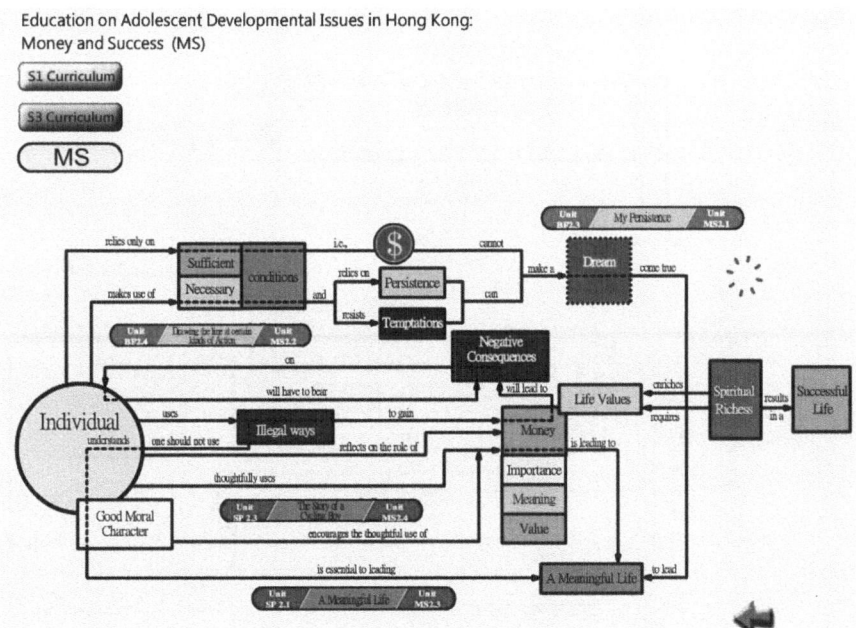

Fig. 3 S2 curriculum design

component of critical appreciation with two objectives: (i) introduce a famous doctor's work and worldview and probe into conditions of ideal work and (ii) deepen students' understanding of the relationship between money and success and reflect on the meaning of life.

Moral competence refers to the orientation to be altruistic and the ability to judge moral issues logically, consistently, and at an advanced level of development (Ma 2006). The last unit (Welcome Everybody to The Party!) also uses the component of social responsibility. The unit objectives are (i) to nurture the ability of goal achievement as well as attitude and skills of good financial management; (ii) to enhance students' knowledge of responsible consumption with local examples and establish students' belief in civil responsibility with practice in consumption; and (iii) to use the knowledge, skills, and attitudes taught in this unit in real school life. This unit helps students recognize that their actions and beliefs may have a constructive or destructive impact on society (Fig. 4).

Cultural Relevance

Since the project is carried out in the Chinese cultural context, examples demonstrating traditional Chinese values are illustrated in the curriculum materials to help students clarify values about money, success, wealth, beauty, power, sex, self-worth, and

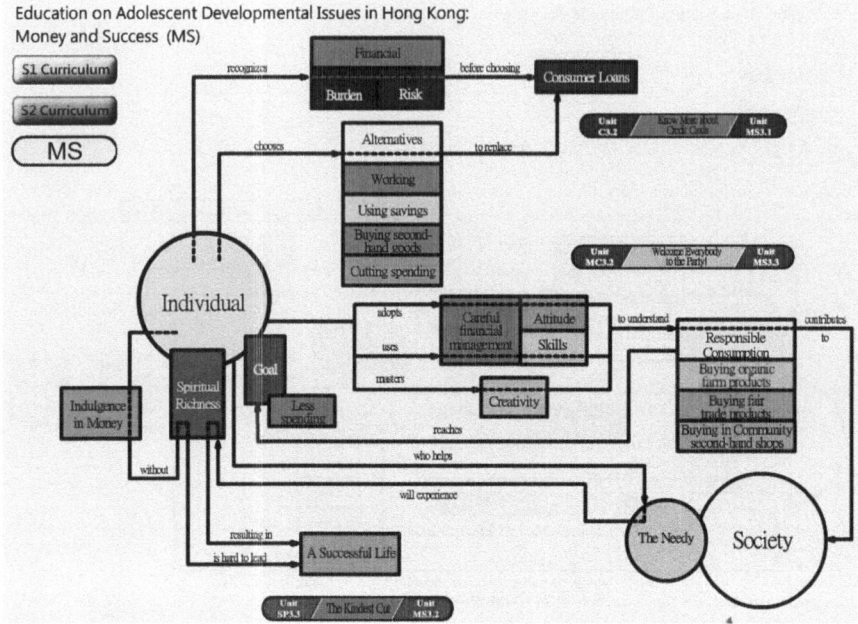

Fig. 4 S3 curriculum design

self-esteem. Since the moral self is highly emphasized in the Chinese culture, materials from Confucianism are used. For example, Confucius said, "The gentleman devotes his mind to attaining the Way and not to securing food. Go and till the land and you will end up by being hungry, as a matter of course; study and you will end up with the salary of an official, as a matter of course. The gentleman worries about the Way, not about poverty" (p. 113) (Lau 2008). Further, he also stated that "There is no point in seeking the views of a gentleman who, though he sets his heart on the Way, is ashamed of poor food and poor clothes (p. 113)" (Lau 2008). Apart from discussing the external social factors, enhancing the internal assets of youth is also one of the major concerns. Nine units on "Money and Success" are designed to promote the moral competence, spirituality, cognitive competence, belief in the future, and self-efficacy of teenagers. All emphasize the self-competence of young people.

In addition, because gender differences regarding money-related issues exist, prominent figures from both genders are used for illustration. Thus, teachers have a choice to select casts from both genders from the audiovisual teaching materials.

References

Lau, P. S. (2006). Spirituality as a positive youth development construct: Conceptual bases and implications for curriculum development. *International Journal of Adolescent Medicine and Health, 18*(3), 363–370.

Lau, D. C. (2008). *Confucius: The analects*. Beijing: Zhonghua Book Company.

Ma, H. K. (2006). Moral competence as a positive youth development construct: Conceptual bases and implications for curriculum development. *International Journal of Adolescent Medicine and Health, 18*(3), 371–378.

Piaget, J. (1965). *The moral judgment of the child*. London: Routledge & K. Paul.

Shek, D. T., & Ma, C. (2011). Impact of the project P.A.T.H.S. in the junior secondary school years: Individual growth curve analyses. *The Scientific World Journal, 11*, 253–266.

Shek, D. T., & Sun, R. C. (2010). Effectiveness of the tier 1 program of project P.A.T.H.S.: Findings based on three years of program implementation. *The Scientific World Journal, 10*, 1509–1519.

Shek, D. T., & Yu, L. (2011). Prevention of adolescent problem behavior: Longitudinal impact of the project P.A.T.H.S. in Hong Kong. *The Scientific World Journal, 11*, 546–567.

Sun, R. C., & Hui, E. K. P. (2006). Cognitive competence as a positive youth development construct: Conceptual bases and implications for curriculum development. *International Journal of Adolescent Medicine and Health, 18*(3), 401–408.

Sun, R. C., & Lau, P. S. Y. (2006). Beliefs in the future as a positive youth development construct: Conceptual bases and implications for curriculum development. *International Journal of Adolescent Medicine and Health, 18*(3), 409–416.

Tsang, S. K., & Hui, E. K. (2006). Self-efficacy as a positive youth development construct: Conceptual bases and implications for curriculum development. *International Journal of Adolescent Medicine and Health, 18*(3), 441–450.

Yin, G. C. (1998). *History of Chinese psychology*. Hangzhou: Zhejiang Education Press.

Promotion of Bonding Among Peers: The P.A.T.H.S. Program

Diego Busiol and Tak Yan Lee

Abstract Project P.A.T.H.S. goes beyond the view of bonding as being solely a stress-reducing system and aims at enabling adolescents to optimize bonding with peers in terms of emotional attachment and commitment during ordinary everyday circumstances. Project P.A.T.H.S. aims at enhancing the process of this developmentally significant network of relationships through various steps: (1) creating opportunities to belong, (2) cultivation of supportive and intimate relationships, (3) promotion of positive social norms, (4) support for efficacy, and (5) promoting skills for involvement and interaction. Ten units are particularly significant for positive development of bonding with peers; however, some other units are informed by the construct of bonding, and they may largely contribute to enhance a positive sense of bonding among students. The rationale behind these units is presented. Concept maps of the curriculum for each school year are also presented.

Ecological Perspectives on Bonding

The ecological perspective emphasizes complex interactions between persons and their environments (Bronfenbrenner 1979, 1986; Collins and Steinberg 2006; Wilks 1986; Sebald 1986). At least two child and adolescent development theories provide a central role for bonding under the ecological perspective: the social control theory and the social development model.

The preparation for this work and the Project P.A.T.H.S. were financially supported by The Hong Kong Jockey Club Charities Trust. The authorship is equally shared between the first author and second author.

D. Busiol • T.Y. Lee (✉)
Department of Applied Social Sciences, City University of Hong Kong,
Kowloon, Hong Kong, China
e-mail: ty.lee@cityu.edu.hk

© Springer Science+Business Media Singapore 2015
T.Y. Lee et al. (eds.), *Student Well-Being in Chinese Adolescents in Hong Kong*,
Quality of Life in Asia 7, DOI 10.1007/978-981-287-582-2_16

Social Control Theory

Hirschi asserted that social bonds explain why adolescents often do not seek immediate gratification in the easiest way possible (Hirschi 1969). As conceived by Hirschi, social bonds promoting socialization and conformity include: involvement, attachment, commitment, and belief. He claimed that the stronger these four bonds, the less likely an adolescent is to become delinquent. The first bond is involvement in the socialization agent. This addresses a preoccupation with activities which stress the conventional interests of society. The second bond is attachment or affective relationships, which refers to one's interest in others, including attachment to parents, to school, and to peers. Acceptance of social norms and the development of a social conscience depend on attachment. The third bond is investment or commitment to the socialization agent which involves time, energy, and effort placed on conventional lines of action. In other words, the support of and participation in social activities ties an individual to the moral and ethical code of society. The final bond is belief in the values of the socialization agent. It deals with the adolescent's assent to society's value system – which entails respect for laws and the people and institutions which enforce such laws. These social bonds, once strongly established, exert an informal control on adolescents' behavior, thereby inhibiting deviant behavior. Implications of the social control theory for positive youth development in general and for the promotion of bonding in particular are (1) attachment to parents as a result of the depth and quality of the parent–child interaction acts as a primary deterrent to engaging in delinquency, (2) attachment to school depends on how one appreciates the institution and how he/she is received by fellow peers and teachers, and (3) attachment to parents and school overshadows the bond formed with one's peers.

Social Development Model

The social development model of Catalano and Hawkins (1996) integrates perspectives from social control theory, social learning theory, and differential association theory that together also suggest a central role for bonding. According to this model, children and adolescents must learn patterns of behavior from their social environment through four processes: (1) perceived opportunities for involvement in activities and interactions with others, (2) actual involvement, (3) acquiring skills for involvement and interaction, and (4) perceived rewards from involvement and interaction (Catalano et al. 2004). Similar to social control theory, it hypothesizes that the predominant behavior, norms, and values held by those individuals or institutions will affect the behavior of the individual and influence them to become either prosocial or antisocial. Empirical support for the effects of bonding on both positive and problem behavior has also been found (Resnick et al. 1997; Hawkins et al. 1992; Hirschi 1969; Werner and Smith 1992).

The P.A.T.H.S. Project

Project P.A.T.H.S. (Fig. 1) goes beyond the view of bonding as being solely a stress-reducing system and aims at enabling adolescents to optimize bonding with peers in terms of emotional attachment and commitment during ordinary everyday circumstances. Attachment and commitment are built in the context of regular exchanges that include positive non-emergency situations that children enjoy (Posada and Lu 2011). Research points to important interrelations among adolescents' relationships with friends; secure bonding established in an adolescent's life with good friends will produce positive results in a number of ways.

What is friendship? Is it different from other kinds of relationships, like kinship, mutual aid, or romantic relationships? How does one recognize a real good friend?

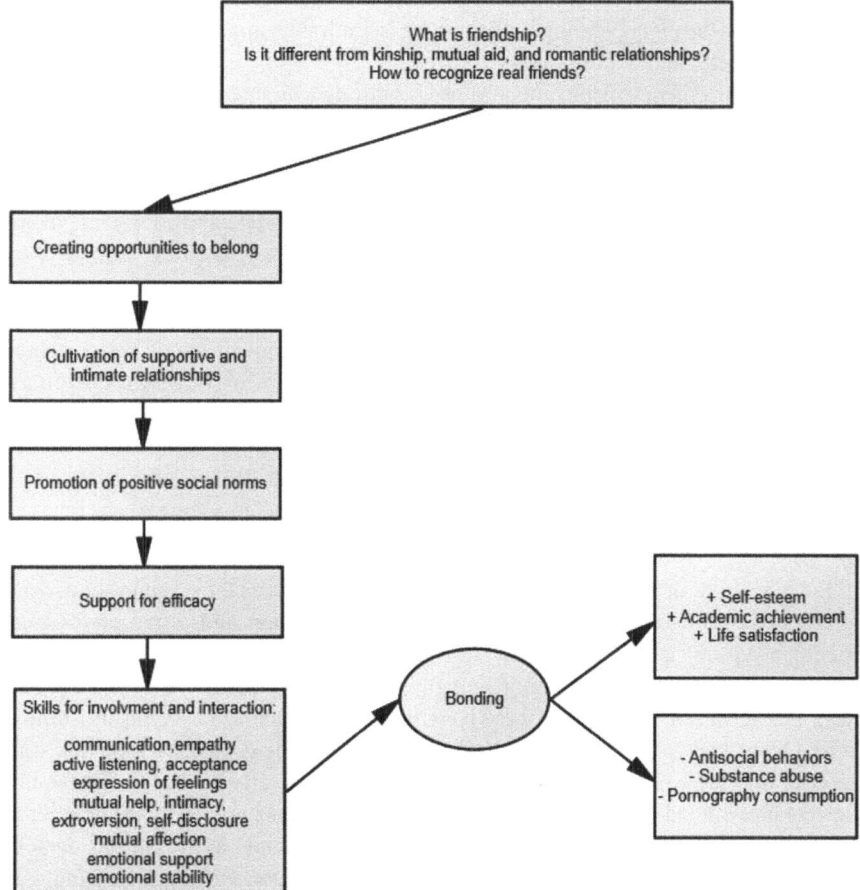

Fig. 1 Conceptual map for bonding

These are the starting questions for a reflection on friendship and for promoting positive bonding among peers.

Project P.A.T.H.S. aims at enhancing the process of this developmentally significant network of relationships through various steps:

1. *Creating opportunities to belong.* In bonding with peers and others in the community, opportunities for meaningful social inclusion (regardless of one's gender, ethnicity, sexual orientation, or disability status) are necessary conditions, while opportunities for sociocultural identity formation as well as support for cultural and bicultural competence should also be made available.
2. *Cultivation of supportive and intimate relationships.* Open and frequent communication with respect, feelings of warmth, caring and closeness, availability of supportive guidance, and responsiveness from family members, friends, and mature adults in social systems facilitate bonding and promote healthy intimate relationships.
3. *Promotion of positive social norms.* Adolescents need clear rules and behavioral expectations derived from prosocial values and morals. Prosocial norms can be reinforced through bonding to important socializing units, that is, the family, school, peers, and community.
4. *Support for efficacy.* Attachment to peers with undesirable behavior yields problem behavior and negative consequences. Positive youth development programs that promote self-efficacy will help adolescents counteract these negative influences. Youth-based empowerment practices or programs that support autonomy, making a real difference in one's community and being taken seriously, are major strategies. Practices that include enabling, responsibility granting, and involvement in meaningful challenges and focus on improvement rather than on current relative performance level can support adolescents to build their self-efficacy.
5. *Skills for involvement and interaction.* Good communication and relationships with others including trust, empathy, active listening, expression of feelings, mutual help, intimacy, self-disclosure, acceptance, mutual affection, emotional support, emotional stability, and extroversion all contribute to bonding (Berndt 2002; Choi et al. 2003; Schneider et al. 2001; Berndt 2004; Cheng et al. 1995; Weiss 1991). Hence, it is necessary to teach adolescents to acquire these positive features in order to bond with significant others in different systems.

Enhancement of bonding is at the same time a protective factor against antisocial behavior, substance abuse, and pornography consumption and a trigger for self-esteem, academic achievement, and life satisfaction.

Ten units are particularly significant for positive development of bonding with peers (Table 1). Of these units, some have been conceptualized specifically starting from a literature review of bonding. Indeed, bonding alone (BO) is an essential construct of the P.A.T.H.S. project. However, bonding is also an essential component of the modules on substance abuse prevention and sex education. For instance, drug consumption is highly related to peer influence (as explained in the chapter on substance abuse); likewise, as a part of the sex education program, students are encouraged to differentiate between friendship, love, and romantic relationships. Thus, these units (AD and SX) are informed by the construct of bonding (BO), and they may largely contribute to enhance a positive sense of bonding among students.

Table 1 Overview of the main units grounded in the construct of bonding (peer level)

Unit	Unit aims	Learning targets
Secondary One		
Be Both Friend and Tutor (BO 1.1)	To establish a sound relationship between instructors and students and among students so as to encourage active participation	1. To become acquainted with instructors
		2. To understand the importance of instructors and friends
		3. To know more about three classmates whom one does not know well or is not familiar with
The Power of Personality (BO 1.2)	To enhance students' understanding of their own personality and to investigate the effect of personality on interpersonal relationships	1. To learn about three main types of personality
		2. To understand the effect of personality on interpersonal relationships
Looking for Friend at the Crossroads (BO 1.3)	1. How to recognize desirable friends from undesirable ones and encourage students to choose the right friends and establish a healthy relationship	1. To identify the determinants for desirable and undesirable friends
	2. To show the required skills to resist temptation	2. To practice refusal principles and skills
Sail on Together (BO 1.4)	To establish trust among students	1. To understand the importance of trust in friendships
		2. To practice skills that establish or promote trust between classmates
Say No to Undesirable Friends (AD 1.7)	1. To show students how to recognize desirable friends from undesirable ones and encourage them to choose the right friends and establish a healthy relationship	1. To identify the determinants for desirable and undesirable friends
	2. To show students the required skills to resist temptation	2. To practice refusal principles and skills
Close Relationships? (SX 1.2)	To understand that opposite-sex and same-sex friendships require different attitudes and behavior	1. To understand that excessive intimacy with the opposite sex may lead to misunderstanding
		2. To learn about appropriate physical boundaries for getting along with the opposite sex
Sex and Peer Pressure (SX 1.4)	To understand how friends affect our decision-making and behavior	1. To know how peer pressure affects our decisions and behavior
		2. To think about the motives and attitudes before we face sexual behavior

(continued)

Table 1 (continued)

Unit	Unit aims	Learning targets
Find a Good Friend (AD 1.6)	To enhance students' understanding of their own personality and to investigate the effect of personality on interpersonal relationships	1. To learn about three main types of personality
		2. To understand the effect of personality on interpersonal relationships
Secondary Three		
Modern Love Stories (BO 3.1)	To understand the qualities of a healthy loving relationship	1. To examine one's attitude toward loving relationships
		2. To identify the essential elements of love
What Is Freedom of Love? (BO 3.2)	To construct the proper attitudes toward loving relationships	1. To differentiate the proper and improper attitudes that appear during the initial stage of loving relationships
		2. To generalize the do's and don'ts of dating

Rationale

Year 1

Year one is particularly important to the concept of bonding among peers (Fig. 1). The Secondary One curriculum focuses on building positive relationships with significant others by adolescents. There are four units in Secondary One: Bonding (BO), all of them aim to establish a trusting relationship between students, teachers, and desirable peers. Unit BO1.1 seeks to establish a sound relationship between instructors and students and among students so as to encourage active participation. Unit BO1.2 enhances students' understanding of their own personality and investigates the effect of personality on interpersonal relationships. In unit BO1.3, students are given an opportunity to learn to recognize desirable friends from undesirable ones, choose the right friend, and establish a supportive relationship, while unit BO1.4 aims to foster a trusting relationship among students and transfer such experience into daily life so as to develop close friendships with other peers (Fig. 2).

Year 2

Year two focuses on family bonding and is presented in the following chapter.

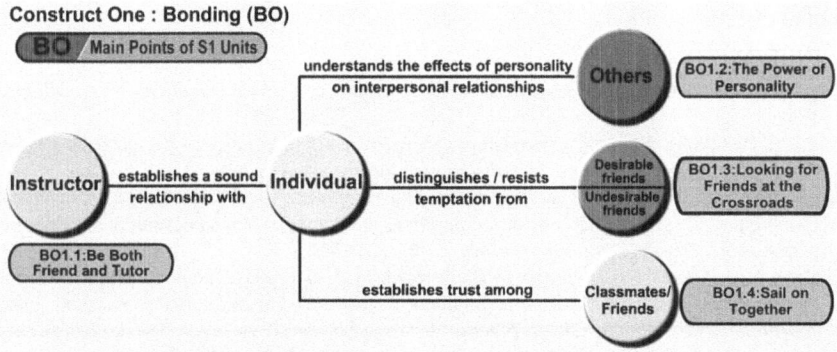

Fig. 2 S1 curriculum design

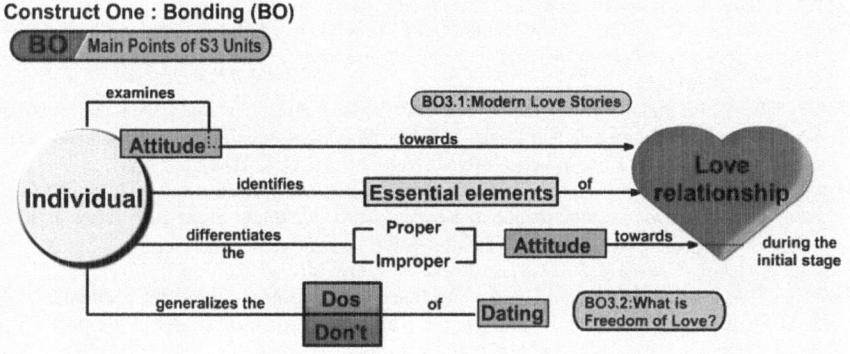

Fig. 3 S3 curriculum design

Year 3

Adolescents can easily access information about love, sexual, and romantic relationships from TV programs, magazines, and the Internet. However, some information can be inaccurate or misleading which in turn can affect the sexual perception of adolescents. Therefore, it is necessary to include the key topic of developing a healthy loving relationship in the curriculum. Students have the opportunity to apply and integrate the skills and principles about building positive relationships to develop loving relationships.

There are two units in Secondary Three curriculum (Fig. 3). Unit BO3.1 focuses on identifying the essential elements in a loving relationship, while Unit BO3.2 aims to construct proper attitudes toward loving relationships.

References

Berndt, T. J. (2002). Friendship quality and social development. *Current Directions in Psychological Science, 11*(1), 7–10.

Berndt, T. J. (2004). Children's friendships: Shifts over a half-century in perspectives on their development and their effects. *Merrill-Palmer Quarterly, 50*(3), 206–223.

Bronfenbrenner, U. (1979). *The ecology of human development*. Cambridge: Harvard University.

Bronfenbrenner, U. (1986). Ecology of the family as a context for human development: Research perspectives. *Developmental Psychology, 22*(6), 723–742.

Catalano, R. F., Oesterle, S., Fleming, C. B., & Hawkins, J. D. (2004). The importance of bonding to school for healthy development: Findings from the social development research group. *Journal of School Health, 74*(7), 252–261.

Catalano, R. F., & Hawkins, J. D. (1996). The social development model: A theory of antisocial behavior. In J. D. Hawkins (Ed.), *Delinquency and crime: Current theories* (pp. 149–197). New York: Cambridge University Press.

Cheng, C., Bond, M. H., & Chan, S. C. (1995). The perception of ideal best friends by Chinese adolescents. *International Journal of Psychology, 30*(1), 91–108.

Choi, P. Y. W., Au, C. K., Tang, C. W., Shum, S. M., Tang, S. Y., Choi, F. M., & Lee, T. C. (2003). *Making young tumblers: A manual of promoting resilience in schools and families*. Hong Kong: Breakthrough.

Collins, W. A., & Steinberg, L. (2006). Adolescent development in interpersonal context. In W. Damon, R. M. Lerner, & N. Eisenberg (Eds.), *Handbook of child psychology, social, emotional, and personality development* (6th ed., Vol. 3). New York: Wiley.

Hawkins, J. D., Catalano, R. F., & Miller, J. Y. (1992). Risk and protective factors for alcohol and other drug problems in adolescence and early adulthood: Implications for substance abuse prevention. *Psychological Bulletin, 112*(1), 64–105.

Hirschi, T. (1969). *Causes of delinquency*. Berkeley: University of California.

Posada, G., & Lu, T. (2011). Child–parent attachment relationships: A life-span phenomenon. In K. L. Fingerman, C. A. Berg, J. Smith, & T. C. Antonucci (Eds.), *Handbook of life-span development* (pp. 87–115). New York: Springer.

Resnick, M. D., Bearman, P. S., Blum, R. W., Bauman, K. E., Harris, K. M., Jones, J., Tabor, J., Beuhring, T., Sieving, R. E., Shew, M., Ireland, M., Bearinger, L. H., & Udry, J. R. (1997). Protecting adolescents from harm: Findings from the national longitudinal study on adolescent health. *Journal of the American Medical Association, 278*(10), 823–832.

Schneider, B. H., Atkinson, L., & Tardif, C. (2001). Child–parent attachment and children's peer relations: A quantitative review. *Developmental Psychology, 37*(1), 86–100.

Sebald, H. (1986). Adolescents' shifting orientation toward parents and peers: A curvilinear trend over recent decades. *Journal of Marriage and the Family, 48*, 5–13.

Weiss, R. S. (1991). The attachment bond in childhood and adulthood. In C. M. Parkes & J. Stevenson-Hinde (Eds.), *Attachment across the life cycle* (pp. 66–76). New York: Basic Books.

Werner, E. E., & Smith, R. S. (1992). *Overcoming the odds: High risk children from birth to adulthood*. Ithaca: Cornell University Press.

Wilks, J. (1986). The relative importance of parents and friends in adolescent decision making. *Journal of Youth and Adolescence, 15*(4), 323–334.

Promotion of Family Bonding: The P.A.T.H.S. Program

Tak Yan Lee and Diego Busiol

Abstract One of the most significant cultural heritages of Chinese society is that the core values of Confucianism place great emphasis on building harmonious inter-personal relationships. Project P.A.T.H.S. aims at helping students to build positive and healthy relationships with adults, teachers, and peers. It is intended that family bonding concerns both quantity and quality of the exchange between parents and children. The positive youth development (PYD) constructs inspiring the P.A.T.H.S. project and the activities implemented aim to promote adolescents thinking in terms of family, rather than selfish thinking. Improving family bonds has some other important consequences for adolescents that go beyond their relationship with their parents. Fourteen units are particularly significant to the development of family bonding; the rationale and the PYD constructs inspiring these units are presented with illustrations.

Introduction

Bonding refers to one's ability to relate, establish, and maintain good relations with others. Adolescents are required to develop different bonding skills when relating to friends, adults, and teachers.

One of the most significant cultural heritages of Chinese society is that the core values of Confucianism place great emphasis on building harmonious interpersonal relationships. Shek and Chan (1999) reported that Chinese parents consider bonding, especially the quality of the parent–child relationship and the obedience of the

The preparation for this work and the Project P.A.T.H.S. were financially supported by The Hong Kong Jockey Club Charities Trust.

This paper is based on an article originally published by *The Scientific World Journal*: Lee, T. Y., & Lok, D. P. (2012). Bonding as a positive youth development construct: A conceptual review. *The Scientific World Journal*, 11 pages.

T.Y. Lee (✉) • D. Busiol
Department of Applied Social Sciences, City University of Hong Kong,
Kowloon, Hong Kong, China
e-mail: ty.lee@cityu.edu.hk

© Springer Science+Business Media Singapore 2015
T.Y. Lee et al. (eds.), *Student Well-Being in Chinese Adolescents in Hong Kong*,
Quality of Life in Asia 7, DOI 10.1007/978-981-287-582-2_17

child, as the most important attribute of an "ideal child." Chao (1994) suggested that some aspects of Chinese "training" or guan might be interpreted as authoritarian control by non-Chinese. For instance, some aspects that might be experienced as domination, hostility, and mistrust by Western infants may be understood as concern by Chinese children. Stewart et al. (1998) tested this hypothesis in relation to 97 Hong Kong Chinese adolescents and found that parenting characteristics associated with guan or training showed coherence and correlated significantly with parental warmth and predicted well-being. However, and contrary to what is suggested by different authors, restrictive control is related negatively to self-esteem and well-being. Maternal control and parental warmth were shown to be primary parental variables in relating to adaptation, enhancing self-esteem, and relationship harmony. Liu et al. (2011) assessed the psychometric characteristics of the parental bonding instrument (PBI) in China. Normally the PBI is represented by a two-factor model (care and overprotection) or a three-factor model (care, overprotection, and autonomy); however, the authors suggested that a fourth factor may be needed to better represent some aspects of the parenting specifics of Chinese culture, which tend to value interdependence and group cohesion over independence: indifference. For example, the authors reported that participants in their study tended to classify items such as "Did not talk with me very much" or "Did not praise me" under indifference, whereas Western cultures have previously classified these as showing a lack of care. The authors suggest that Chinese children might not necessarily see these parents' responses as unloving behavior. Instead, they suggest that this might reflect Chinese values that tend to foster collectiveness and view the family as a singular unit and then as a priority to the individual.

Chen et al. (1992) suggested that the Chinese often form small well-defined "cliques" in contrast to Canadians. Chao and Tseng (2002) reported that Chinese mothers and fathers play very different roles in their parent–child relationships. Ho (1987) suggested that the difference between paternal and maternal parenting styles is well reflected in a traditional saying "strict father, kind mother." The role of the mother is to provide a secure and warm home environment and to develop a close and emotional relationship with children. On the other hand, the role of the father is to provide economic support and moral instruction, rather than an emotional relationship. A "traditional" father would love his child, but he seldom expresses his love verbally. However, a recent study by Shek (2007) found that the situation has been reversing – the notion has changed to "strict mother, kind father." Results also showed that the quality of parental control has declined and parent–child relational qualities have become poorer in early adolescent years in the contemporary Chinese culture of Hong Kong.

Project P.A.T.H.S.

Project P.A.T.H.S. aims at helping students to build positive and healthy relationships with adults, teachers, and peers (Fig. 1).

Construct One : Bonding (BO)

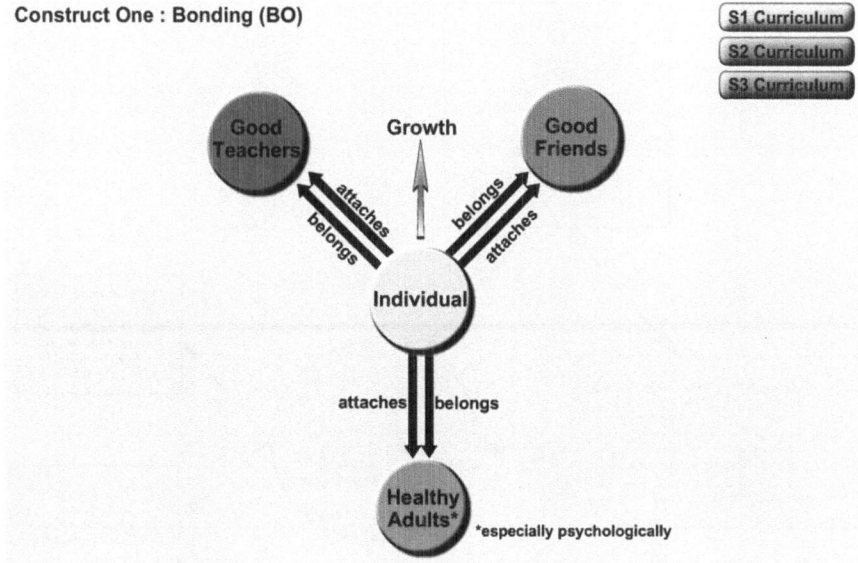

Fig. 1 Overview of bonding

As society changes and evolves, people become more isolated from one another. If young people are not provided a supportive environment in which they can grow up positively, they are more likely to participate in socially unacceptable behavior or activities. Promotion of bonding with adults and peers and living a positive lifestyle is crucial for the healthy development of adolescents.

The literature indicates that attachment with teachers and schoolmates promotes confidence and better involvement in school (Noller et al. 2013), while a sense of trust is an essential element to the establishment of relationships (Berndt 2002, 2004).

Thus, it is essential to teach students ways to enhance family relationships and positive communication, especially in their time of growth in a rapidly changing society. Otherwise, detached relationships or even conflicts are likely to occur within a family.

It is intended that family bonding (Fig. 2) concerns both quantity and quality of the exchange between parents and children. A positive relationship is when parents are able to listen, so that children can become gradually more open and trustworthy. On the other hand, children who feel accepted and perceive their parents as non-judgmental may learn to share their distress within the family and ask for parental support. They may learn to ask family members, and later they might be more willing to contribute as well, so that the relationship evolves into a more mutual one.

To reach this goal, it is important that children step into the shoes of their parents and understand their perspective, difficulties, limitations, and efforts. Only with this shift of perspective is it possible for a child to critically examine the concept and nature of the family as well as the relations among family members. The PYD con-

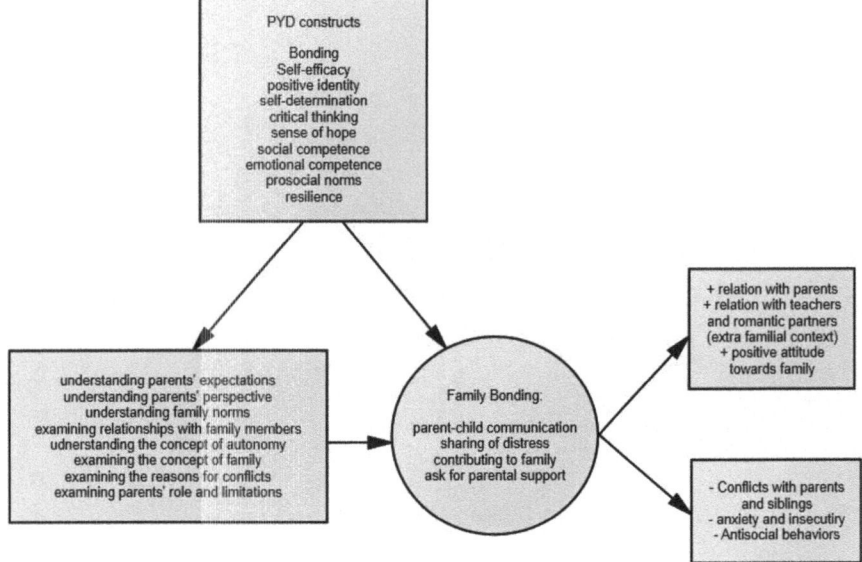

Fig. 2 Conceptual map for family bonding

structs inspiring the P.A.T.H.S. project and the activities implemented aim to promote adolescents thinking in terms of family, rather than selfish thinking. Adolescents need some help to recognize what characterizes positive and negative relationships in their lives. Also, they might need to understand what they may be feeling and how their behavior may have been understood by family members. Acquiring others' perspective might help to make relationships more equal and reciprocal and might help to create greater interdependence between family members (not just dependence or independence); furthermore, it helps youth to take responsibility for their own behavior in relationships.

Parents are normally the first significant persons children can relate to. However, improving family bonds has some other important consequences for adolescents that go beyond their relationship with their parents. For instance, a quality bond with family members may help them to face with less anxiety the multiple changes of early adolescence, as they might feel supported. Then they might have more skills and resources for avoiding or overcoming misunderstandings and conflicts (with family members but also with other people); it should be considered that children who feel that they can gain their parents' attention do not try to gain it in disruptive dangerous ways. Nurturing the parent–child relationship might lead to quality relations with parental figures like teachers as well as relationships with romantic partners later. In general, a positive experience within the family of origin might leave a better attitude toward the idea of forming one's own family.

Fourteen units are particularly significant to the development of family bonding (Table 1):

Table 1 Overview of the main units aimed at improving family bonding

Unit	Unit aims	Learning targets
Secondary one		
A Big Hand for Me (SE 1.3)	To enhance self-efficacy by understanding the feelings and intentions behind parents' discouraging words	1. To understand parental expectations and strengthen parent–child relationships 2. To enhance self-efficacy through self-affirmation
Rules Rule: Everyone Has to Get a Clue (PN 1.1)	To define social norms, to distinguish behavioral rules in daily life (in the family and at school), and to understand the moral rules in interpersonal relationships	1. To understand social norms, the importance of complying with rules and the reasons for observing social norms 2. To recognize that obeying the law, they have to pay attention to and follow certain behavioral rules in their daily lives
Those Were the Days (RE 1.1)	1. To learn to seek help from different people under different circumstances 2. To understand parents' communication style and to thus promote trust toward parents and a sense of belonging within the family	1. To learn to seek help from different people when encountering different types of problems 2. To recognize the potentially positive messages behind parents' words and actions
Autonomy License (SD 1.1)	To understand the meaning of autonomy and discover the degrees of autonomy approved by parents	1. To understand the meaning of autonomy 2. To comprehend the scope of autonomy and the prerequisites for exercising it
Know Yourself, Know Others (ID 1.2)	To enhance students' understanding of themselves, their family, and the people around them and encourage students to realize that their characters can be shaped by the people around them	1. To understand one's character 2. To understand that people who are important and close to you can influence the development of your character
Secondary two		
What Can I Do for My Family? (BO 2.1)	To make more contributions at home so as to strengthen relationships with the family	1. To recall the occasions on which students received care from their parents 2. To explore the roles played at home and to enhance motivations to contribute to families

(continued)

Table 1 (continued)

Unit	Unit aims	Learning targets
Parents' Messages (BO 2.2)	To learn the skills leading to better communication with one's parents and to strengthen parent–child relationships	1. To analyze parents' messages from people-oriented and task-oriented points of view 2. To demonstrate proper responses to parents' messages and establish a good relationship with one's parents
Two Are Better than One (EC 2.3)	To share distress with parents and family members	1. To identify the characteristics of parent–child communication 2. To list the appropriate skills for sharing with parents
Secondary three		
Marriage… Before and After (SX 3.4)	To examine the relationships among family, marriage, and sex	1. To understand the similarities and differences between dating relationships and marriage 2. To clarify one's values on sexual relationships in dating or before marriage
Who's Right? Who's Wrong? (SC 3.3)	To analyze the reasons for conflict among siblings and suggest solutions	1. To understand the reasons for conflict among siblings 2. To learn the proper attitude to get along with siblings
Believe It or Not (AD 3.3)	To use critical thinking for analyzing various causes of deviant behavior and help students enhance their empathy for parents	1. To enhance critical-thinking abilities 2. To reflect parents' role and limitations in improving teenagers' deviant behavior in order to empathize with parents
From Dream to Reality (RE 3.4)	To promote a sense of hope toward the future	1. To construct a vision of one's future family 2. To recognize that one needs to work hard and use resources properly in order to achieve his/her aspirations
Happily "Never" After (SX 3.5)	To cultivate positive views on marriage	1. To know the factors contributing to happy marriages and to divorces 2. To find out how one could be affected by the marriage of parents and close family
Let Me Say It! (SD 3.2)	To enhance students' ability to gain parental support for personal decisions	1. To discuss the proper way to seek parental support for personal decisions 2. To understand the ways in which different actions and tones of voice affect the outcome of a discussion

There are five units in Secondary One. Unit SE1.3 helps students to manage positively parental feedback that threatens self-efficacy, with the goal of self-affirmation. Unit PN1.1 guides students to define social norms and to realize that as well as obeying the law, they have to pay attention to and consider social norms in their daily lives. RE1.1 focuses on helping students learn the fact that they can seek help from different people in different circumstances and build up a positive attitude toward parents' way of expression. Unit SD1.1 targets at students' understanding of the meaning of self-determination and helps them comprehend the scope of the autonomy approved by their parents. Unit ID1.2 guides students to understand the influence of important people on them and to enhance their self-esteem and personal identity.

There are three units in Secondary Two. Secondary Two focuses mainly on bonding with family members. Unit BO2.1 seeks to encourage students to make more contribution at home so as to strengthen their relationship with the family, while Unit BO2.2 aims to teach the skills leading to better communications with parents. Unit EC2.3 aims to encourage youth to step into the shoes of their parents and understand the distress and limitations of parents, so that they can utilize opportunities for communication and help parents understand. It is hoped that the elements taught will enhance the family relationships of students.

As shown in the following conceptual map (Fig. 3), students are encouraged to reflect on parental care and learn to distinguish an order from a suggestion, a request, or a neglect. As a consequence, they are expected to make more contribution to their family and to make more effort to bond with their parents and family members.

Finally, Secondary Three includes six units. Unit SX3.4 helps students to reflect on the meaning of making a family and how it differs from dating and that a marriage also signifies the union of two families. Unit SX3.5 helps students to find out how one is affected by the marriages of their parents or close family members and aims at teaching students that a bad relationship between their parents does not necessarily mean that the children will repeat that status again. Unit SC3.3 analyzes reasons for conflict among siblings and provides solutions. Through a simulated

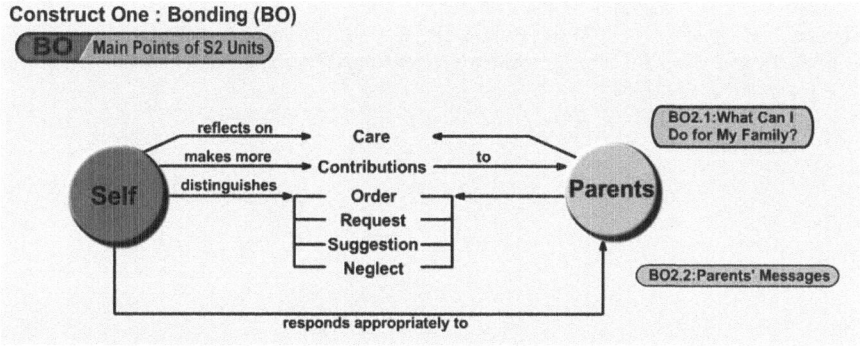

Fig. 3 S2 curriculum design

radio program, students are asked to play different sibling roles and simulate feelings after conflict. The goals of this activity are to encourage students to be more understanding and unselfish, to decrease conflict, to sensitize students toward the importance of positive family relations, and to establish cohesiveness and harmonious family relationships. Unit RE3.4 focuses on promoting a sense of hope toward the future and how to construct a positive vision of one's future family. Unit SD3.2 helps students to find the proper way to seek parental support for personal decisions. Unit AD3.3 aims at helping students to apply critical-thinking skills and analyze the responsibility of parents for a young person's drug use.

References

Berndt, T. J. (2002). Friendship quality and social development. *Current Directions in Psychological Science, 11*(1), 7–10.

Berndt, T. J. (2004). Children's friendships: Shifts over a half-century in perspectives on their development and their effects. *Merrill-Palmer Quarterly, 50*(3), 206–223.

Chao, R. K. (1994). Beyond parental control and authoritarian parenting style: Understanding Chinese parenting through the cultural notion of training. *Child Development, 65*(4), 1111–1119.

Chao, R. K., & Tseng, V. (2002). Parenting of Asians. In M. H. Bornstein (Ed.), *Handbook of parenting: Social conditions and applied parenting* (2nd ed., Vol. 4, pp. 59–93). Mahwah: Lawrence Erlbaum Associates Publishers.

Chen, X., Rubin, K. H., & Sun, Y. (1992). Social reputation and peer relationships in Chinese and Canadian children: A cross-cultural study. *Child Development, 63*(6), 1336–1343.

Ho, D. Y. (1987). Fatherhood in Chinese culture. In M. E. Lamb (Ed.), *The father's role: Cross-cultural perspectives* (pp. 227–245). Hillsdale: Erlbaum.

Liu, J., Li, L., & Fang, F. (2011). Psychometric properties of the Chinese version of the Parental Bonding Instrument. *International Journal of Nursing Studies, 48*(5), 582–589.

Noller, P., Feeney, J., & Peterson, C. (2013). *Personal relationships across the lifespan*. London: Routledge.

Shek, D. T. L. (2007). A longitudinal study of perceived differences in parental control and parent–child relational qualities in Chinese adolescents in Hong Kong. *Journal of Adolescent Research, 22*(2), 156–188.

Shek, D. T. L., & Chan, L. K. (1999). Hong Kong Chinese parents' perceptions of the ideal child. *The Journal of Psychology, 133*(3), 291–302.

Stewart, S. M., Rao, N., Bond, M. H., Fielding, R., & McBride-Chang, C. (1998). Chinese dimensions of parenting: Broadening western predictors and outcomes. *International Journal of Psychology, 33*, 345–358.

Promotion of Resilience: The P.A.T.H.S. Program

Tak Yan Lee and Diego Busiol

Abstract Project P.A.T.H.S. covers several areas as crucial elements in building resilience: bonding, self-efficacy, spirituality, clear and positive identity, and five core individual competencies of cognitive, emotional, moral, behavioral, and social competence. Few units of P.A.T.H.S. are expressly dedicated to the development of resilience; several others aim at enhancing resilience as part of anti-bullying, anti-drug use, cognitive competence, and sex education. The Secondary One program focuses on enhancing students' external protective factors (such as establishing a sense of belonging toward family) and internal protective factors (including problem solving, dealing with negative emotions, and conflict management). In the Secondary Two curriculum, the units focus on enhancing the belongingness to family and problem-solving skills as well as the competencies of emotional control and conflict management. Finally, units within the Secondary Three curriculum aim to promote optimism, cultivate the ability to face and handle crises, as well as promote a sense of hope toward the future. Concept maps of the curriculum for each school year are also presented.

Cultivating Adolescents' Resilience in Schools

There are several ways to foster students' resilience in schools. First, schools can arrange curriculum-based programs (Gillham and Reivich 2004; Shek and Ma 2012; Shek and Sun 2010) since many of these programs have been evidenced to enhance students' bonding, core competencies, and optimism through which students build up resilience. Project P.A.T.H.S. is a comprehensive program (Shek and

The preparation for this work and the Project P.A.T.H.S. were financially supported by The Hong Kong Jockey Club Charities Trust.

This paper is based on an article originally published by *The Scientific World Journal*: Lee, T. Y., Cheung, C. K., & Kwong, W. M. (2012). Resilience as a positive youth development construct: a conceptual review. *The Scientific World Journal, 2012*.

T.Y. Lee (✉) • D. Busiol
Department of Applied Social Sciences, City University of Hong Kong,
Kowloon, Hong Kong, China
e-mail: ty.lee@cityu.edu.hk

© Springer Science+Business Media Singapore 2015   221
T.Y. Lee et al. (eds.), *Student Well-Being in Chinese Adolescents in Hong Kong*,
Quality of Life in Asia 7, DOI 10.1007/978-981-287-582-2_18

Ma 2012; Shek and Sun 2010) that covers several areas as crucial elements in building resilience: bonding, self-efficacy, spirituality, clear and positive identity, and five core individual competencies of cognitive, emotional, moral, behavioral, and social competence. Moreover, these programs can incorporate positive social norms, cultural values and ideologies to cultivate adolescents' prosocial attitudes, and an optimistic outlook toward the future that are crucial for cultivating adolescents' resilience. Second, it has been found that attachment to adults other than a child's parents has positive effects on a child's resilience to adversity (Werner and Smith 1992; Dolan et al. 1989). Also, bonding with school teachers increases positive developmental outcomes (Catalano et al. 2004). Therefore, schools can develop a culture that promotes two primary and interdependent components of school bonding: (i) *attachment*, close affective relationships with teachers at school, and (ii) *commitment*, an investment in school and doing well in school because students will acquire teachers' values through a socialization process. Subsequently, these values will serve as a mediator of the effect of bonding on behavioral outcomes (Catalano et al. 2004). Third, extracurricular activities can be used to facilitate and maintain the healthy development of adolescents, but the effectiveness of these activities depends on the type, frequency, and quality of interchanges in the activity context (Mahoney et al. 2009). Besides, resilience-focused groups can be used for students who need more intensive intervention due to the severity of adversity (Greene 2008). In addition, specialized intervention programs such as adventure-based counseling can be used (Wong and Lee 2005). Finally, school social workers can collaborate with students' parents to encourage parental involvement and support in fostering the development of adolescents' resilience. Since adverse events affect the behavior of family members in terms of family rules, organizational structures, communication patterns, and belief systems, the ability to survive and recover from disruptive family life challenges is related to the family relationship network (Walsh 1999). In general, the school can adopt a whole-school approach to involve different stakeholders in the school, family, and community to nurture the development of adolescents' resilience.

Factors Influencing Resilience and Their Relevance in Hong Kong

Hong Kong is a society with immense pressure and competition. Many children and youths have already experienced many challenges and failures. In addition, although many students may have high academic performance, the values of the traditional Chinese continue to stress not only high academic performance but also an expectation of obedience toward parents. Often, the communication between family members is inadequate and a source of misunderstanding and conflict. Therefore, it is crucial to introduce proactive measures to cultivate resilience among youths.

In addition, two factors greatly influence the resilience of Hong Kong youth:

Coping Strategies Coping strategies can be an important protective factor against stressors and consequently can enhance resilience. Coping strategies are normally divided into emotion focused and problem oriented. The former are centered on emotions and are normally considered passive because they aim at reducing psychological discomfort by simply avoiding the stimulus, whereas the latter are centered on problem solving and aim at trying to change the stressful situation. Examples of emotion-focused coping strategies are wishful thinking (daydreaming, waiting for a miracle to happen), detachment (trying to forget or go along with fate), self-blame (criticizing oneself or promising that things would be different next time), tension reduction (taking a rest, drinking, or using drugs), and keeping to oneself (avoiding people or keep others from knowing how bad things are). Instead, active coping strategies include: seeking social support (talking to someone or asking someone for advice) and focusing on the positive (trying to look on the bright side, being creative). However, variability in the use of coping strategies has been reported, depending on age, gender, and cultural differences (Stern and Zevon 1990). Particularly, the use of avoidant coping strategies and keeping to oneself were found to be characteristic of Chinese contexts; Hong Kong Chinese normally consult professional help much less than Americans and Europeans, although they are not less willing to receive help (for a review, see Busiol 2015). This could also undermine the overall resilience of adolescents.

Impulsivity Impulsivity was found to be significantly related to several types of risky behavior, such as substance abuse, Internet addiction, gambling (Maccallum et al. 2007), bullying (Jolliffe and Farrington 2011), pornography consumption and sex-related issues (Park 2007), suicide, and materialistic orientation (Pham et al. 2012); furthermore, impulsivity was found to be stronger particularly at a young age (Loxton et al. 2008). For instance, it was found to be a predictor for suicide among Chinese in rural areas (Zhang et al. 2010); previous studies showed that sometimes even trivial quarrels and family conflicts could lead youth to behave in an extreme way following an impulse of the moment (Wu 2005). Finally, it has been suggested that in China many suicides are likely more impulsive acts than expression of a formal psychiatric diagnosis, as it is conceptualized in Western societies (Phillips et al. 2007). It may be that in a Chinese context, the weight of triggering life events is greater than some internal disposition.

In a study among drug users in Hong Kong (Loxton et al. 2008), impulsivity was significantly related to risky drug-related behavior; instead, there was no association between personality traits and preferred drug. Likely, this result indicates that addictive behavior (in general) and resilience might be negatively related; this was confirmed by other research on 348 secondary school students in China (Li et al. 2010), which showed that resilience was negatively associated with Internet addiction. Lastly, impulsivity is opposite not only to resilience but to positive development and good mental health in general. A study attempting to explore the risk and protective factors influencing the mental health of immigrant and local youth in Hong Kong (Wong 2008) showed that immigrant youths have better mental health and similar levels of stress than local youths. Particularly, it was shown that immigrant youths with a higher level of social competence like empathy, assertiveness, self-control, and self-esteem were less impulsive and more understanding of others' needs and problems.

The Conceptual Framework of P.A.T.H.S.

Resilience is a complex construct; it expresses the capacity of an individual to cope with stressful events (overcoming adversities) in a healthy way (good behavior and development). Resilience refers to the internal and external strengths (protective factors) against stress that an individual possesses. As a reintegration process, resilience allows an individual to go back to normal or even exhibit a better psychological condition than before (Fig. 1). Synonyms of resilience are flexibility and elasticity. Promoting a sense of optimism and giving, a contented heart, enhancing the belongingness toward healthy adults (in terms of psycho-social aspects), learning to solve conflicts with significant others, and learning from traditional cultural values can all contribute to higher levels of resilience (Choi et al. 2003; Wong and Lee 2005).

Resilience can be enhanced by several protective factors (Fig. 2), particularly by: bonding with peers and family members, cognitive competence, higher optimism and belief in the future, higher self-efficacy, perceived sense of control, and active coping strategies (rather than emotion-focused or passive strategies).

An improved resilience can have both a direct and indirect effect on risky behavior. On the one hand, higher resilience can make risky behavior (which often gives immediate pleasure or relief and might appear as quick and easy solutions at first) less attractive; youths with higher resilience have more tools for facing difficulties, can stand the uncertainties of life, and thus are less in need to find an immediate way out from problems.

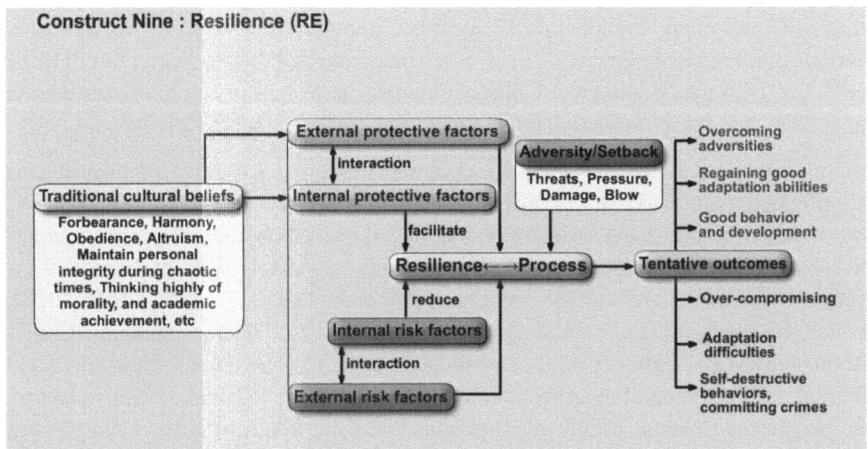

Fig. 1 Curriculum design for resilience

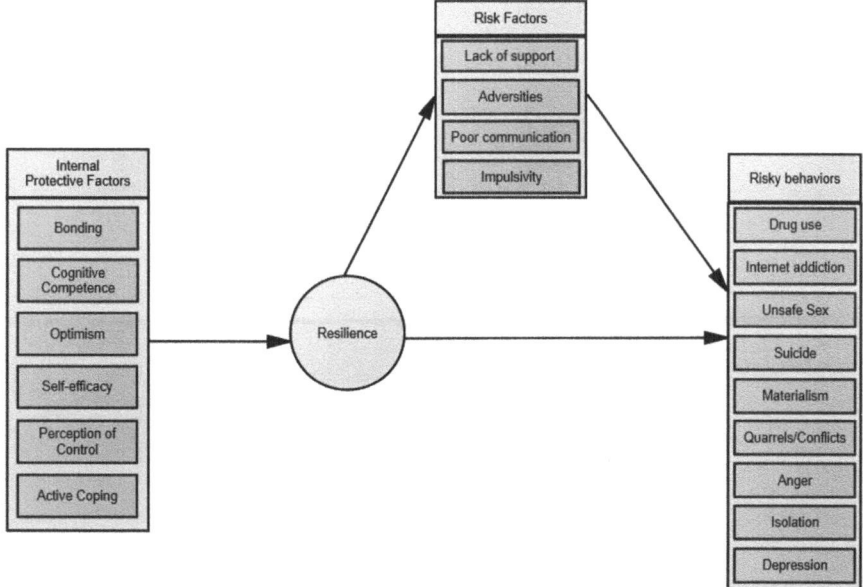

Fig. 2 Conceptual framework for resilience

Drug abuse, Internet addiction, anger, conflicts, quarrels, isolation, and depression are likely reactions to poor pain (or ambiguity or disappointment) tolerance.

On the other hand, higher resilience can help to tackle and reduce those risk factors which are also causes of risky behavior. For instance, higher resilience can have positive effects on social relations; it might reflect in more effective communication with peers, teachers, and family members and finally can lead to finding more support when difficulties arise. At the same time, resilience is important for reducing impulsivity and thus preventing dangerous *acting-out*, such as self-harm, suicide, anger responses, conflicts, and unsafe sex. Lastly, resilience is essential because it allows critical analysis of adversities from different perspectives; it is important to teach the youth that what is initially perceived as an adversity can also become an opportunity for growth and is not necessarily an obstacle. The way to positive youth development (and to prevent risky behavior) is providing the tools that open to different interpretations of reality. Thus, resilience is essential to make this process possible.

Few units of P.A.T.H.S. are expressly dedicated to the development of resilience; several others aim at enhancing resilience as part of anti-bullying, anti-drug use, cognitive competence, and sex education. When considering specifically the units on resilience, we see that:

The Secondary One program (Fig. 3) focuses on enhancing students' external protective factors (such as establishing a sense of belonging toward family) and internal protective factors (including problem solving, dealing with negative emotions, and conflict management). There are four units in this construct. RE 1.1 focuses on helping students learn the fact that they can seek help from different people in different

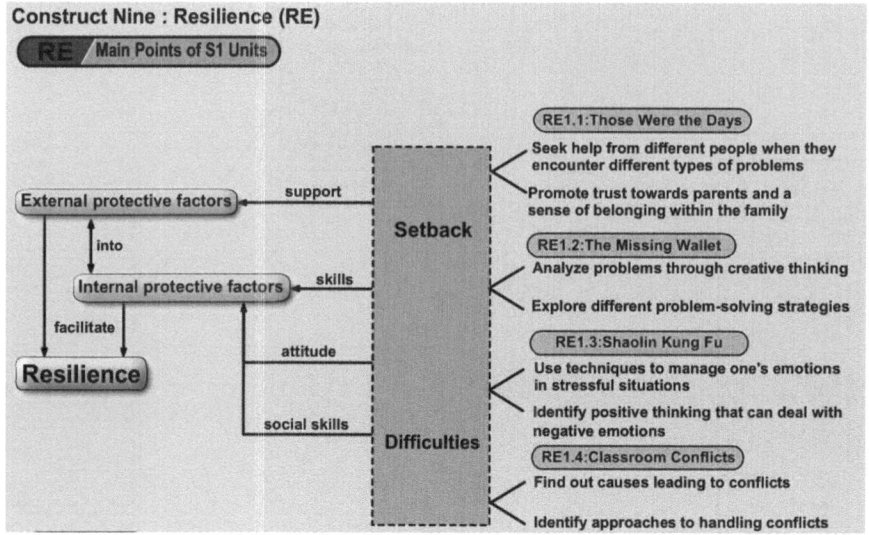

Fig. 3 S1 curriculum design

circumstances and build up a positive attitude toward parents' way of expression. In RE 1.2, students are guided to analyze problems from multiple perspectives and look for different solutions. RE 1.3 teaches students to use positive thinking to deal with negative emotions. Finally, in RE 1.4, students are guided to find out causes of conflicts by using different strategies and tackle them calmly, thus strengthening their resilience. They will also learn to identify what a bystander should do.

In the Secondary Two curriculum (Fig. 4), the units focus on enhancing the belongingness to family and problem-solving skills as well as the competencies of emotional control and conflict management. In the Secondary Two curriculum, there are four units which all aim to promote optimism. Unit RE 2.1 aims to rebuild the understanding of failures and learn from them; Unit RE 2.2 teaches students to face adversity with a sense of humor so that students confront difficulties in life optimistically; in Unit RE 2.3, students learn not to fall into avoidance traps when facing adversity, as avoidance will only lead to bigger difficulties, while in Unit RE 2.4, students learn to take significant life events as learning opportunities, even when facing difficulties and challenges in life.

There are four units within the Secondary Three curriculum (Fig. 5). Unit RE 3.1 aims to promote optimism through developing a contented heart. Unit RE 3.2 aims to cultivate the ability to face and handle crises. In unit RE 3.3, teachings from Mencius are introduced so as to enhance students' resilience. Finally, unit RE 3.4 focuses on promoting a sense of hope toward the future.

The following table details the units on resilience along the 3 years (Table 1). Although resilience alone (RE) is one of the 15 PYD constructs, resilience is also an essential component of the anti-drug program (AD), anti-bullying (AB), and sex education (SX), and it is significantly related to cognitive competence (CC).

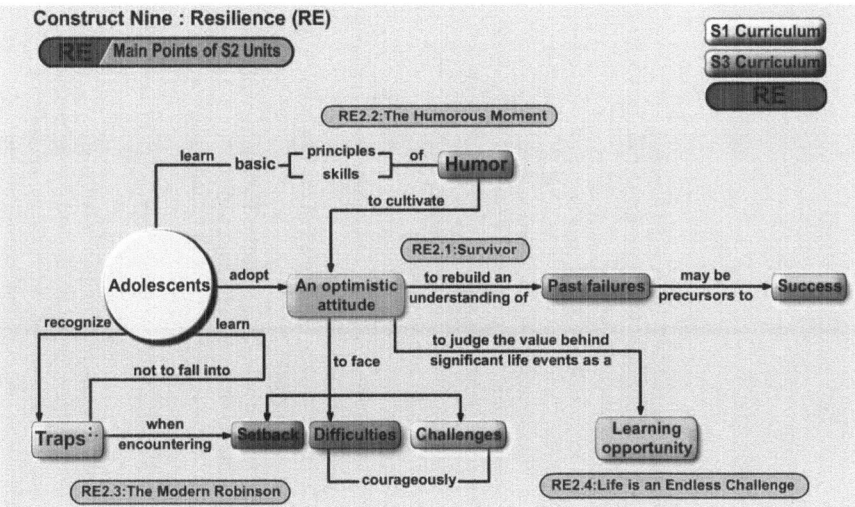

Fig. 4 S2 curriculum design

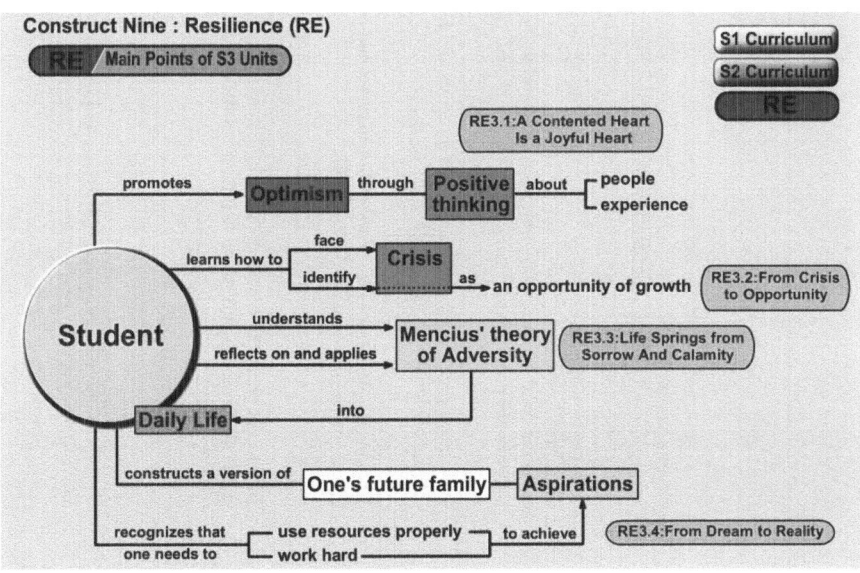

Fig. 5 S3 curriculum design

Table 1 Overview of the units on resilience

Unit	Unit aims	Learning targets
Secondary One curriculum		
Those Were the Days (RE 1.1)	To learn to seek help from different people under different circumstances To understand parents' communication style and to thus promote trust toward parents and a sense of belonging within the family	1. To learn to seek help from different people when encountering different types of problems 2. To recognize the potentially positive messages behind parents' words and actions
(RE 1.1U)	To understand that there are always some people who are willing to offer help when we are facing difficulties To understand parents' communication style and to thus promote trust toward parents and a sense of belonging within the family	1. To recognize the necessary conditions for overcoming difficulties: "maintaining good bonding," "enhancing problem-solving skills," and "having hope" 2. To understand that we should have hope and seek help from people around us whenever we have difficulties
The Missing Wallet (RE 1.2)	To analyze problems from multiple perspectives and look for different solutions to strengthen one's resilience	1. To practice the skill of "seeing into the core of the matter through creative thinking" 2. To explore different problem-solving strategies
Shaolin Kung Fu (RE 1.3)	To manage one's emotions in stressful situations and use positive thinking to deal with negative emotions	1. To identify five techniques to manage one's emotions in stressful situations 2. To identify positive thinking that can deal with negative emotions
Classroom Conflicts (RE 1.4)	To find out causes of conflicts by using different strategies and tackle them calmly and strengthen their resilience and ability to identify what a bystander should do	1. To find out at least three causes leading to conflicts or three factors that can aggravate conflicts 2. To understand the fact that a bystander plays an important role in conflicts 3. To identify the five common approaches to handling conflicts
Incidents of Bullying (AB 1.1)	To understand what is meant by bullying and its consequences and to avoid being a bully or a victim	1. To understand the definition of bullying 2. To investigate the behavioral and emotional reactions of the bully, the victim, and bystanders in bullying incidents and the consequences of bullying

Behind the Mask of Bullying (AB 1.2)	To understand the true needs of bullies and identify proper approaches to minimize bullying	1. To understand the reasons for bullying and the mentality of the bullies 2. To identify suitable approaches to fulfill the underlying needs of the bullies in order to reduce bullying
Choosing a Better Way (AD 1.1)	To understand that emotions may affect our ability to solve problems and thus lead to different consequences	1. To understand the relationship between coping methods and consequences 2. To analyze the influences of different coping methods
Emotion, Your Name Is… (CC 1.1)	To understand emotions, identify different emotional states caused by various conditions, and realize that individuals in certain emotional states are easily influenced by drugs	1. To enhance the ability to articulate and identify emotions through games 2. To identify various emotional states and their causes
At Sixes and Sevens (AD 1.5)	To encourage students to use critical thinking when they face peer pressure	1. To understand that people around us will try to influence our thinking, attitudes, and behavior through different techniques 2. To be aware of the necessity of using critical thinking when facing the above situations
Secondary Two curriculum		
Survivor (RE 2.1)	To rebuild the understanding of failures and learn from them	1. To demonstrate an understanding that failures may be precursors to success 2. To find out what one may learn from past failures
The Humorous Moment (RE 2.2)	To learn to face adversity with a sense of humor so that students can confront difficulties in life optimistically	1. To learn to face adversity with a sense of humor 2. To learn the basic principles and skills of humor
The Modern Robinson (RE 2.3)	To learn not to fall into avoidance traps when facing adversity, as avoidance will only lead to bigger difficulties	1. To demonstrate an understanding of why temptations are so tempting and learn skills to resist them 2. To stay away from short-term happiness that comes from avoidance of adversity
Life Is an Endless Challenge (RE 2.4)	To learn to take every moment as a learning opportunity and face difficulties and challenges in life courageously	1. To identify the difficulties and challenges that may help students become mature 2. To judge the value behind significant life events as a learning opportunity

(continued)

Table 1 (continued)

Unit	Unit aims	Learning targets
What Are Frustrations? (AD 2.3)	To reconstruct students' awareness of what frustrations are and to let them understand how to learn from the experience of frustrations	1. To understand how to face failures 2. To find out the learning points from the experience of frustrations
General's Choice (AD 2.4)	To learn that we should not accept any temptations when we are facing difficulties just to obtain excitement as we are creating greater problems for the future	1. To understand the luring effects of temptations and how to reject them 2. To learn that we should not accept any temptations and escape the real problems during adversity
Secondary Three curriculum		
A Contented Heart Is a Joyful Heart (RE 3.1)	To promote optimism through positive thinking	1. To describe experiences and that people can be our treasures 2. To develop an optimistic view of life among students
From Crisis to Opportunities (RE 3.2)	To cultivate the ability to face and handle crises	1. To demonstrate how to face crises 2. To identify crises as an opportunity for growth
Life Springs from Sorrow and Calamity (RE 3.3)	To introduce traditional values of the Chinese in relation to adversity so as to enhance students' resilience	1. To state how Mencius looked at adversity 2. To reflect upon oneself and how Mencius' teachings can be applied in daily life
From Dream to Reality (RE 3.4)	To promote a sense of hope toward the future	1. To construct a vision of one's future family 2. To recognize that one needs to work hard and use resources properly in order to achieve his/her aspirations
(RE 3.4)		1. To understand that we should have hope and act persistently in order to achieve our goals 2. To understand the impact of our current choices in life on achieving our goals

The New Biography of Sisyphus (AD 3.5)	To cultivate the ability to face and handle misery and adversity	1. To explore how to face misery and adversity 2. To understand that because our minds affect our behavior, positive thinking may help us to solve our problems
Unresolved (IT 3.1)	To enhance self-reflection on using the Internet is the only way to solve daily problems	1. To understand how to solve problems 2. To enhance self-reflection on using Internet is a good way or not to solve personal problems in daily life
Happily Never After (SX 3.5)	To cultivate positive views on marriage	1. To know the factors contributing to happy marriages and to divorces 2. To find out how one could be affected by the marriage of one's parents or close family members

References

Busiol, D. (2015). Cultural mediators in help-seeking behaviors and attitudes towards counseling: A qualitative study among Hong Kong Chinese University students. British Journal of Guidance & Counselling. In press.

Catalano, R. F., Oesterle, S., Fleming, C. B., & Hawkins, J. D. (2004). The importance of bonding to school for healthy development: Findings from the social development research group. *Journal of School Health, 74*(7), 252–261.

Choi, P. Y. W., Au, C. K., Tang, C. W., Shum, S. M., Tang, S. Y., Choi, F. M., & Lee, T. C. (2003). *Making young tumblers: A manual of promoting resilience in schools and families* (in Chinese). Hong Kong: Breakthrough.

Dolan, L. J., Kellam, S. G., & Brown, C. H. (1989). *Short-term impact of a mastery learning preventive intervention on early risk behaviors.* Baltimore: Johns Hopkins University.

Gillham, J., & Reivich, K. (2004). Cultivating optimism in childhood and adolescence. *The Annals of the American Academy of Political and Social Science, 591*(1), 146–163.

Greene, R. R. (2008). *Human behavior theory and social work practice* (3rd ed., pp. 315–343). New Brunswick: AldineTransaction.

Jolliffe, D., & Farrington, D. P. (2011). Is low empathy related to bullying after controlling for individual and social background variables? *Journal of Adolescence, 34*(1), 59–71.

Li, X., Shi, M., Wang, Z., Shi, K., Yang, R., & Yang, C. (2010). *Resilience as a predictor of internet addiction: The mediation effects of perceived class climate and alienation.* Proceedings 2010 IEEE 2nd Symposium on Web Society. Retrieved from http://cpfd.cnki.com.cn/Area/CPFDCONFArticleList-ZGAN201008001.htm

Loxton, N. J., Wan, V. L. N., Ho, A. M. C., Cheung, B. K. L., Tam, N., Leung, F. Y., & Stadlin, A. (2008). Impulsivity in Hong Kong-Chinese club-drug users. *Drug and Alcohol Dependence, 95*(1), 81–89.

Maccallum, F., Blaszczynski, A., Ladouceur, R., & Nower, L. (2007). Functional and dysfunctional impulsivity in pathological gambling. *Personality and Individual Differences, 43*(7), 1829–1838.

Mahoney, J. L., Vandell, D. L., Simpkins, S., & Zarrett, N. (2009). Adolescent out-of-school activities. In R. M. Lerner & L. Steinberg (Eds.), *Handbook of adolescent psychology* (3rd ed., pp. 228–269). Hoboken: Wiley.

Park, M. R. (2007). *Relationships among gender role attitudes, sexual attitudes, impulsivity, internet pornography addiction and sexual violence permissiveness.* Unpublished master's thesis, Kyungnam University, Masan.

Pham, T. H., Yap, K., & Dowling, N. A. (2012). The impact of financial management practices and financial attitudes on the relationship between materialism and compulsive buying. *Journal of Economic Psychology, 33*(3), 461–470.

Phillips, M. R., Shen, Q., Liu, X., Pritzker, S., Streiner, D., Conner, K., et al. (2007). Assessing depressive symptoms in persons who die of suicide in mainland China. *Journal of Affective Disorders, 98*(1), 73–82.

Shek, D. T. L., & Ma, C. M. S. (2012). Impact of the project P.A.T.H.S. in the junior secondary school years: Objective outcome evaluation based on eight waves of longitudinal data. *The Scientific World Journal, 2012*(2012), 1–12.

Shek, D. T. L., & Sun, R. C. F. (2010). Effectiveness of the tier 1 program of project P.A.T.H.S.: Findings based on three years of program implementation. *The Scientific World Journal, 10*, 1509–1519.

Stern, M., & Zevon, M. A. (1990). Stress, coping, and family environment: The adolescent's response to naturally occurring stressors. *Journal of Adolescent Research, 5*(3), 290–305.

Walsh, F. (1999). Families in later life: Challenges and opportunities. In B. Carter & M. McGoldrick (Eds.), *The expanded life cycle: Individual, family, and social perspectives* (3rd ed., pp. 307–324). Boston: Allyn and Bacon.

Werner, E. E., & Smith, R. S. (1992). *Overcoming the odds: High risk children from birth to adult-hood*. Ithaca: Cornell University Press.

Wong, D. F. K. (2008). Differential impacts of stressful life events and social support on the mental health of Mainland Chinese immigrant and local youth in Hong Kong: A resilience perspective. *British Journal of Social Work, 38*(2), 236–252.

Wong, K. Y., & Lee, T. Y. (2005). Professional discourse among social workers working with at-risk adolescents in Hong Kong. In M. Ungar (Ed.), *Pathways to resilience: A handbook of theory, methods, and intervention* (pp. 313–327). Thousand Oaks: Sage.

Wu, F. (2005). "Gambling for Qi": Suicide and family politics in a rural north China county. *The China Journal, 54*, 7–27.

Zhang, J., Wieczorek, W., Conwell, Y., Tu, X. M., Wu, B. Y. W., Xiao, S., & Jia, C. (2010). Characteristics of young rural Chinese suicides: A psychological autopsy study. *Psychological Medicine, 40*(4), 581–589.

Part III
Positive Youth Development and Adolescent Developmental Issues: Evidence of Success

Risk Factors and Protective Factors in Substance Abuse in Chinese Adolescents in Hong Kong

Daniel T.L. Shek and Jianqiang Liang

Abstract This chapter examines the effects of two risk factors (economic disadvantage and family non-intactness) and two protective factors (positive youth development and family functioning) on substance abuse among Chinese adolescents in Hong Kong. Based on four waves of data collected from Secondary 1 to Secondary 4 students in a longitudinal study (3328 students at Secondary 1), individual growth curve models demonstrated a growing trend of adolescents engaging in substance abuse across time. Gender, age, and family intactness were significantly related to the initial status of adolescent substance abuse, while economic disadvantage and family intactness were significantly related to the growth trajectory of substance abuse, with adolescents from poor and non-intact families having a higher risk of engaging in substance abuse. While positive youth development and family functioning at Wave 4 predicted substance abuse in Wave 4, positive youth development and family functioning at Wave 1 only predicted smoking but not overall substance abuse at Wave 4.

Introduction

Adolescent substance abuse is a growing global issue. Teenagers are not only taking conventional drugs such as tobacco and alcohol but also abusing other psychotropic substances (e.g., ketamine, cannabis, and ecstasy). Worse still, young people have a common myth that these substances are nonaddictive, harmless, and trendy (Shek et al. 2011). In Hong Kong, drinking and smoking were reported as the most frequent substance abuse behaviors among school adolescents (Shek 2007; Shek and Ma 2011a). Besides, adolescent substance abusers were getting younger (e.g., with

The preparation for this work and the Project PATHS were financially supported by The Hong Kong Jockey Club Charities Trust.

D.T.L. Shek (✉) • J. Liang
Department of Applied Social Sciences, The Hong Kong Polytechnic University,
11 Yuk Choi Road, Hung Hom, Kowloon, Hong Kong, China
e-mail: daniel.shek@polyu.edu.hk

© Springer Science+Business Media Singapore 2015   237
T.Y. Lee et al. (eds.), *Student Well-Being in Chinese Adolescents in Hong Kong*,
Quality of Life in Asia 7, DOI 10.1007/978-981-287-582-2_19

the youngest at the age of 12); they tended to have longer substance abuse history, and substance abuse was hidden in nature (such as taking drugs at home). Psychotropic substances also become more popular (Narcotics Division 2009, 2014). These changing trends bring a warning call for parents, school educators, social workers, and policy makers who are concerned about the healthy development of adolescents. Hence, it becomes necessary to develop a more accurate understanding of adolescent substance abuse in the individual, familial, community, and socioeconomic contexts. Against this background, this longitudinal study focused on personal and familial predictors of substance addiction among adolescents in the schools in Hong Kong.

Shek (2007) proposed to understand adolescent substance abuse in Hong Kong from an ecological perspective. Adolescent substance abuse is not only self-driven but also impacted by multiple risk and protective factors (Hemphill et al. 2011; Shek and Ma 2011a). On the one hand, adolescent substance abuse is correlated with some risk factors, such as familial economic disadvantage (Shek 2002), parental conflict and lack of parental care (Chilcoat and Anthony 1996; Shek 2003; Wagner et al. 2010), negative peer and social modeling (Garham et al. 1991), unstable and non-supportive community environment (Hemphill et al. 2011). On the other hand, assets of positive youth development and well family functioning are protective factors which protect adolescents from drug addiction. Studies showed that positive youth development programs could assist adolescents in preventing problem behaviors (Catalano et al. 2002; Shek 2010). Improvement of intrapersonal and interpersonal competencies (e.g., positive and healthy identity, cognitive, emotional, behavioral, and social competencies) also lowered the risk of adolescent substance abuse (Shek and Ma 2011a; Shek and Yu 2011a). Family functioning was also important to prevent adolescent substance abuse (Shek 2003; Shek and Ma 2011a), with mutual respect, good communication, and harmony inside the family help to create a caring and supportive environment for adolescents to discuss the harm of abusing drugs with their parents.

In particular, family attributes make a fundamental impact on adolescent substance abuse. These attributes can be described in three levels: economic status of the family (e.g., families on welfare), parental marital quality (e.g., divorce and separation), and parent–child relationship (e.g., mutual respect and communication). Adolescents from poor family may lack parental bonding because their parents need to work for a long time. As a result, they may have a higher risk of joining street gangs and developing addictive behaviors. Family intactness was also associated with adolescent substance abuse, with adolescents experiencing parental divorce having higher risk of substance abuse than did those who grow up in intact families (Shek and Yu 2011a). Parental modeling and parent–child relationship were considered more important than peer influence on adolescent's engagement in substance abuse (Feit and Wodarski 2014). However, few scholars have systematically examined the influence of multiple family attributes on adolescent substance abuse behavior in a single study.

A review of the scientific literature on adolescent substance abuse showed that most studies are cross-sectional studies, and there are few studies on the overtime effects of multiple predictors on substance abuse, especially in middle adolescence. Besides, research examining the influence of factors in the individual and family systems on adolescent substance abuse is urgently needed. Shek and his colleagues are filling this research gap through conducting a serious of systematic longitudinal studies based on the Project PATHS (Shek and Ma 2011a, c, 2012; Shek and & Yu 2011a, b, 2012). These studies utilized classical longitudinal data analyses methods (e.g., cross-sectional and longitudinal regression analyses) and multi-level linear modeling methods (e.g., individual growth curves). In this study, we continued to use such statistical analyses to explore the developmental trajectories as well as the effects of individual and family factors on adolescent substance abuse over a period of 4 years.

Method

Participants and Procedures

In 2009/2010 school year, 3328 students (Secondary 1 or Grade 7, mean age = 12.59, with 51.7 % males and 47.2 % females) from 28 schools were recruited to a 6-year longitudinal research project titled "A Longitudinal Study of Adolescent Development and Their Families in Hong Kong." Further details of the project can be seen elsewhere (Shek et al. 2014). The demographic characters of the students are shown in Table 1.

Table 1 Data profile across four waves

	Wave 1	%	Wave 2[a]	%	Wave 3[a]	%	Wave 4[a]	%
N (participants)	3328		2905		2858		2682	
Gender								
Male	1719	51.7	1445	49.7	1433	50.1	1335	49.8
Female	1572	47.2	1419	48.8	1405	49.2	1337	49.9
Economic disadvantage								
Not receiving CSSA	2606	78.3	2377	81.8	2339	81.8	2267	84.5
Receiving CSSA	225	6.8	160	5.5	147	5.1	132	4.9
Family intactness								
Intact families	2781	83.6	2415	83.1	2396	83.8	2211	82.4
Non-intact families	515	15.5	469	16.1	454	15.9	466	17.4

[a]The numbers were based on the participants whoever participated in Wave 1 assessment as only those joining Wave 1 assessment were included in LMM. The numbers of the students who did not report the corresponding information were not presented

They were invited to complete a questionnaire on adolescent development and the related psychosocial correlates in a self-administrated and voluntary manner. Written consent was obtained from all schools, parents, and participants. Enough time was given to the students to complete the questionnaire with the assistance of a well-trained research team (one research assistant for one class). Data cleaning and data matching were executed by well-trained research associates.

The present study utilized the data collected from Wave 1 to Wave 4. The attrition rates were acceptable, with 12.7 % of Wave 2, 14.1 % of Wave 3, and 19.4 % of Wave 4. Among those 3328 participants who had completed the questionnaire in Wave 1, 2682 students completed the questionnaires in all 4 years. Only those students who had took Wave 1 (N=3328) were included in the later longitudinal data analyses.

Instruments

Assessment of Substance Abuse The substance abuse scale contains eight questions which examine the frequency of different adolescent substance behaviors (such as tobacco, alcohol, and illicit drugs), on a six-point Likert scale (0=never, 1=1–2 times, 2=3–5 times, 3=more than 5 times, 4=several times a month, 5=several times a week, 6=everyday). Previous study showed that the scale had good psychometric properties (Shek and Ma 2011a). Table 2 shows eight items of adolescent substance abuse and the frequency of related behavior for each item.

Table 2 Frequencies of substance abuse in the past 12 months across four waves

	Wave 1		Wave 2[a]		Wave 3[a]		Wave 4[a]	
	N	%	N	%	N	%	N	%
Substance abuse								
1. Taking tobacco	32	0.96	47	1.62	53	2.03	42	1.71
2. Taking alcohol	80	2.42	121	4.19	139	7.90	131	8.38
3. Taking ketamine	2	0.06	5	0.17	4	0.15	3	0.12
4. Taking cannabis	1	0.03	3	0.10	1	0.04	3	0.12
5. Taking cough mixture	1	0.03	3	0.10	1	0.04	2	0.08
6. Taking organic solvent	9	0.27	4	0.14	3	0.11	6	0.23
7. Taking pills (including ecstasy and methaqualone)	2	0.06	2	0.07	2	0.07	3	0.12
8. Taking or injecting heroin	2	0.06	3	0.10	3	0.11	2	0.08
Total number	3328	100	2905	100	2858	100	2682	100

Note: All eight items in a six-point Likert scale (0=never; 1=1–2 times; 2=3–5 times; 3=more than 5 times; 4=several times a month; 5=several times a week; 6=everyday). N=who chose the responses 4–6, which considered as frequently abusing the substances
[a]The numbers were based on the participants whoever participated in Wave 1 assessment as only those joining Wave 1 assessment were included in LMM. The numbers of the students who did not report the corresponding information were not presented

A composite score was calculated for each wave by combining the scores of all items, with a higher score indicating a higher frequency of substance abuse. In multi-level modeling, substance abuse (SA) was a new variable which converted the measures (the above composite score at each wave) at Wave 1 to Wave 4 into a stacked format. In view of the prevalent use of tobacco and alcohol, additional analyses were also carried out by using Item 1 ("smoking") and Item 2 ("drinking") as separate indicators.

Assessment of Positive Youth Development Positive youth development was assessed by the Chinese Positive Youth Development Scale (CPYDS), which includes 15 key attributes assessing adolescent's holistic development. The scale was validated with good reliability and validity (Shek et al. 2007). In this study, the variable "positive youth development" was the mean score of the 15 constructs. Except spirituality (SP) which was a seven-point Likert scale, all other constructs were assessed on a six-point Likert scale.

Economic Disadvantage as a Family Attribute Economic disadvantage was operationalized in terms of whether the respondent's family received Comprehensive Social Security Assistance (CSSA), with "yes" as indicating economic difficulty. Missing data were removed from the analyses.

Family Intactness as a Family Attribute Different marital statuses of the parents were assessed in the questionnaire (1 = divorced but not remarried, 2 = separated but not remarried, 3 = married (first marriage), 4 = married (second or subsequent marriage), 5 = others). "Intact families" referred to those students whose parents were in their first marriage (with the response of answer 3), while "non-intact families" were defined by the rest of the responses.

Family Functioning as a Family Attribute Family functioning was assessed by the Chinese Family Assessment Instrument (CFAI) which assesses three major attributes: mutuality (mutual support, love, and concerns among family members), communication (frequency and nature of interaction among family members), and conflicts and harmony (the presence of conflicts and harmonious behavior in family). The variable "family functioning" was a combined score of the relevant items, with a higher score indicating a higher level of family functioning. Previous research showed that CFAI was a reliable and valid scale in the Chinese context (Shek and Ma 2010).

Research Questions and Hypotheses

Four observations were revealed in the previous studies. First, gender made a difference, with more male than female adolescents had substance abuse. Second, positive youth development constructs were inversely associated with substance abuse. Third, adolescents in non-intact families had more substance abuse than did intact families. Fourth, economic disadvantage was a risk factor of substance abuse behavior (Shek and Ma 2011a, c, 2012 Shek and Yu 2011a, b, 2012). On top of these findings, this study further explored the developmental trajectories and psychosocial predictors of adolescent substance abuse. The following research questions and several hypotheses were addressed in this study.

Research Question 1: Are Economic Disadvantage and Family Intactness Associated with the Initial Level and Growth Rate of Adolescent Substance Abuse? Based on the previous findings, the following hypotheses were proposed:

- Hypothesis 1: Consistent with the global scientific findings, the shape of the growth curves of substance abuse would show a rising trend across 4 years.
- Hypothesis 2a: Based on the literature on risk factors, adolescents from poor families would have a higher initial level and faster growth rate of substance abuse than did those from nonpoor families.
- Hypothesis 2b: Based on the literature on risk factors, adolescents from nonintact families would have a higher initial level and faster growth rate of substance abuse than did those from intact families.

Research Question 2: Do Family Functioning and Positive Youth Development Predict Substance Abuse Across Four Waves?

- Hypothesis 3a: Family functioning at Wave 4 would have a negative relationship with substance abuse at Wave 4.
- Hypothesis 3b: Positive youth development at Wave 4 would have a negative relationship with substance abuse at Wave 4.
- Hypothesis 4a: Family functioning at Wave 1 would predict decline in substance abuse across 4 years, particularly for drinking and smoking.
- Hypothesis 4b: Positive youth development at Wave 1 would predict decline in substance abuse across 4 years, particularly for drinking and smoking.

Data Analyses Strategies

Descriptive statistical analyses were performed to portray the sociodemographic statuses of the participants from Wave 1 to Wave 4, including percentages of economic disadvantage and family intactness (Table 1), frequencies of eight single substance abuse behaviors (Table 2), and means, standard deviations, as well as internal consistency of the scales (Table 3).

Linear mixed method (LMM) analyses were performed to understand the developmental trajectories of adolescent substance abuse in Hong Kong. We focused on the analyses of individual growth curves (IGC) which were generated by LMM through using SPSS 21 (IBM SPSS Statistics, IBM Corp, Somers, NY). The advantage of IGC and details of the method fitting the project can be found in Shek and Ma's paper (2011b).

Four waves of data were analyzed with maximum likelihood (ML) as the estimate method (Shek and Ma 2011b). A two-level hierarchical model that nested time (Level 1) within individuals (Level 2) was tested by using: (a) substance abuse (included intercepts and slopes) as the dependent variables (DVs), (b) time (four

Table 3 Descriptive statistics of key variables and internal consistency coefficients of scales (Waves 1–4)

| | Mean (SD) | | | | Reliability | | | |
	W1	W2	W3	W4	W1	W2	W3	W4
Family functioning [a]	3.73 (0.81)	3.65 (0.81)	3.65 (0.79)	3.66 (0.77)	.90	.90	.90	.91
Positive youth development [a]	4.51 (0.70)	4.43 (0.69)	4.44 (0.65)	4.45 (0.62)	.93	.96	.96	.96
Substance abuse [b]	0.09 (0.22)	0.11 (0.27)	0.12 (0.26)	0.13 (0.27)	.81	.89	.84	.90
Male	0.11 (0.25)	0.12 (0.21)	0.13 (0.22)	0.15 (0.33)	–	–	–	–
Female	0.08 (0.17)	0.10 (0.26)	0.11 (0.29)	0.11 (0.20)	–	–	–	–
Not receiving CSSA	0.09 (0.21)	0.11 (0.26)	0.11 (0.21)	0.12 (0.27)	–	–	–	–
Receiving CSSA	0.09 (0.20)	0.10 (0.20)	0.14 (0.28)	0.16 (0.31)	–	–	–	–
Intact families	0.08 (0.18)	0.11 (0.28)	0.11 (0.21)	0.12 (0.27)	–	–	–	–
Non-intact families	0.14 (0.29)	0.14 (0.24)	0.19 (0.38)	0.16 (0.26)	–	–	–	–

W1 Wave 1, *W2* Wave 2, *W3* Wave 3, *W4* Wave 4

[a]Mean score was used to indicate the level of family functioning and positive youth development

[b]Mean score was used to indicate the substance abuse (range = 1–6)

waves) as the Level 1 predictor, and (c) individual social-demographic characteristics (economic disadvantage and family intactness in Wave 1 as the main predictors, while initial age and gender as the control variables) as the Level 2 predictors. The first level of analyses were the repeated measures of within-person initial substance abuse behavior as well as the rate of change over time without taking account of the individual social-demographic characteristics. The second level of analyses examined the effects of the individual social-demographic characteristics on the initial level as well as the developmental patterns of substance abuse.

For the Level 1 predictor, "time" was recoded ($0 =$ Wave 1, $1 =$ Wave 2, $2 =$ Wave 3, and $3 =$ Wave 4). Dummy variables were used for the Level 2 predictors ("gender": female $= -1$, male $= 1$; "economic disadvantage": not receiving CSSA $= -1$, receiving CSSA $= 1$; "family intactness": non-intact family $= -1$, intact family $= 1$). "Initial age" was grand mean centered in order to simplify the interpretation of results (Kwok et al. 2008; Shek and Ma 2011b). Following the strategies suggested by other scholars (Singer and Willet 2003; Shek and Ma 2011b), there were three steps in the LMM analyses:

- Step 1: Unconditional mean model (Model 1) was conducted to measure individual substance abuse (intercepts only) without adding any level of predictors. It helped examine the total variance of substance abuse predicted by intrapersonal differences, which could indicate the need for further multi-level analyses.
- Step 2: Unconditional growth model (Model 2) was performed to examine the substance abuse trajectories of the participants by combining the individual trajectories into a collective one. This was a Level 1 model which examined the variation (both initial status and rate of change) among individual over time without adding the higher level of predictors.
- Step 3: Conditional growth model (Model 3) was a Level 2 model which evaluated the effects of interpersonal differences on initial substance abuse behavior as well as the rate of change (by adding both Level 1 predictor and Level 2 predictors). In this study, it focused on examining how the risk factors (economic disadvantage and non-intact family) predicted the initial status (intercepts) and rate of change (slopes) of adolescent substance abuse with initial age and gender controlled.

To further examine the longitudinal influences of protective factors (family functioning and positive youth development) on adolescent substance abuse, two multiple regression analyses were conducted. First, for the concurrent relationships among the variables, we tested whether Wave 4 family functioning and positive youth development would predict Wave 4 substance abuse behavior with gender, economic disadvantage, and family intactness controlled. Second, for the overtime effects, we tested whether Wave 1 family functioning and positive youth development would predict Wave 4 substance abuse behavior with gender, economic disadvantage, and family intactness from Wave 1 controlled. For both concurrent and overtime effects, we examined the predictions of the above two protective factors as a single predictor (Model A and Model B) and their predictions as simultaneous predictors (Model C).

Results

Adolescent Substance Abuse Across Time

Table 1 shows that percentages of adolescents from impoverished families or non-intact families were low, with the rate of receiving CSSA slightly deceased (from 6.8 % in Wave 1 to 4.9 % in Wave 4) and the rate of living in a non-intact family slightly increased (from 15.5 % in Wave 1 to 17.4 % in Wave 4). Table 2 reveals the percentages of frequently substance abuse in the past 12 months (for those who took the substance equal or more than several times a month) across four waves. Although some behaviors increased across time, overall substance abuse behavior in adolescents was not high. For example, there was an increasing trend of frequent smoking from 0.96 % in Wave 1 to 1.71 % in Wave 4. Similarly, the percentage of frequently taking alcohol increased consistently across four waves (from 2.42 % to 8.38 %). Drinking and smoking were the two most frequent substance abuse behaviors in all 4 years.

In Table 3, the mean scores of substance abuse increased consistently from Wave 1 to Wave 4 (0.09, 0.11, 0.12, 0.13), which indicated an increasing trend of substance abuse behavior in general over 4 years.

Male adolescents had higher mean score of substance abuse than did female adolescents (0.11 vs. 0.08, respectively, in Wave 1; 0.15 vs. 0.11, respectively, in Wave 4). Adolescents from non-intact families had higher mean abuse behavior than did those from intact families (0.14 vs. 0.08, respectively, in Wave 1; 0.16 vs. 0.12, respectively, in Wave 4). Adolescents who received CSSA (had economic disadvantage) had higher mean abuse behavior (0.16) than did those who did not receive CSSA (0.12) in Wave 4.

Linear mixed method was conducted to examine the developmental trajectories of adolescent substance abuse as well as the effects of economic disadvantage and family intactness on the initial status and rate of change of substance abuse behavior, while initial age and gender of the adolescents were controlled. The results of the three models were shown in Table 4.

Firstly, the unconditional mean model (Model 1) was tested to identify the total variance of adolescent substance abuse at different levels using intraclass correlation coefficient (ICC) as an indicator (Singer and Willet 2003). Results showed that about 43.02 % of total variance of adolescent substance abuse (ICC=0.4302) was due to interindividual differences. Therefore, the multi-level modeling analyses would be meaningful (Shek and Ma 2011b) to identify how different parameters relate to the development of adolescent substance abuse behavior. As we only had four points (W1 to W4), a linear trend would be sufficient.

Secondly, results showed that Model 2 had a better fit than Model 1 ($\Delta\chi2$ (3)=281.48; ΔAIC=275.48; ΔBIC=253.42; $p<.001$). In the unconditional growth model (Model 2), the initial level of substance abuse was very low ($\gamma00=.765$, $p<.001$). From the linear slope, the substance abuse behavior increased linearly by an average of 0.147 per year ($\gamma10=.147$, $p<.001$), which supported Hypothesis 1. On

Table 4 Results of individual growth curve of substance abuse for all models

		Model 1		Model 2		Model 3	
		Estimate	SE	Estimate	SE	Estimate	SE
Fixed effects							
Intercept	β_{0j}						
Initial status	γ_{00}	.947***	.028	.765***	.030	.848***	.062
Age	γ_{01}					.301***	.045
Gender	γ_{02}					.069*	.032
Economic disadvantage	γ_{03}					−.059	.064
Family intactness	γ_{04}					−.214***	.048
Linear slope	β_{1j}						
Initial status	γ_{10}			.147***	.014	.201***	.031
Age	γ_{11}					−.027	.023
Gender	γ_{12}					.033*	.016
Economic disadvantage	γ_{13}					.094**	.032
Family intactness	γ_{14}					.051*	.024
Random effects							
Level 1(within)							
Residual	r_{ij}	2.495***	.041	2.283***	.046	2.357***	.052
Level 2 (between)							
Intercept	u_{0j}	1.884***	.074	1.293***	.086	1.035***	.091
Time	u_{1j}			.062**	.019	.079**	.021
Fit statistics							
Deviance		47035.13		46753.65		39190.73	
AIC		47041.13		46765.65		39218.73	
BIC		47063.13		46809.71		39319.08	
df		3		6		14	

Note: Model 1 = unconditional mean model; Model 2 = unconditional growth model; Model 3 = conditional model

*p < .05; **p < .01; ***p < .001

average, adolescent substance abuse behavior increased over the years. In addition, significance of two between-subject random-effect variances (intercept, $p < .001$; linear slope, $p < .01$) indicated the potentials of some interpersonal factors (Level 2 predictors) to explain the developmental patterns of adolescent substance abuse.

Finally, when adding the Level 2 predictors, the conditional growth model (Model 3) showed a better model fit than the unconditional growth model (Model 2), ($\Delta\chi2$ (8) = 7562.92; ΔAIC = 7546.92; ΔBIC = 7490.63; $p < .001$). For the predictors (of both Level 1 and Level 2) of the intercept of substance abuse, results showed that family intactness was negatively associated with the initial level of substance abuse ($\gamma04 = -.214$, $p < .001$) above and beyond the effects of initial age ($\gamma01 = .301$, $p < .001$) and gender ($\gamma02 = .069$, $p < .05$). In the initial assessment, adolescents of non-intact families reported higher frequency of substance abuse; adolescents with older age reported a higher level of substance abuse than did those in younger age; male adolescents reported a higher level of substance abuse than did female adolescents. At the same time, family economic status had no significant association with the initial status of adolescent substance abuse. Around 20 % (from 1.293 in Model 2 to 1.035 in Model 3) of the variance of intercepts could be explained by Level 2 predictors.

For the predictors of slope, results of the fixed effects showed that both family intactness ($\gamma14=.051$, $p<.05$) and economic disadvantage ($\gamma13=.094$, $p<.01$) were significantly associated with the growth rate of substance abuse above and beyond the effects of gender ($\gamma12=.033$, $p<.05$). Adolescents from poor families showed faster increasing rate in substance abuse behavior than did those from nonpoor families. Although adolescents from non-intact families reported slower increasing rate of their substance abuse behavior than did those from intact families, adolescents from non-intact families still had a higher mean of substance abuse (0.16) than did those from intact families (0.12) in Wave 4. In terms of gender, male adolescents reported a faster growth of substance abuse than did female adolescents.

In short, the above findings partly supported Hypothesis 2a (e.g., adolescents from poorer families showed a faster growth rate of substance abuse) but fully support Hypothesis 2b (e.g., adolescents from non-intact families had a higher initial level and faster growth rate of substance abuse than did those growing up in intact families).

Concurrent and Longitudinal Effects of Family Functioning and Positive Youth Development on Prevention of Adolescent Substance Abuse

For the concurrent effects at Wave 4 (Table 5), multiple regression analyses showed that family functioning and positive youth development were inversely related to substance abuse behavior no matter they were examined separately or simultaneously.

Gender was positively related with substance abuse behavior, which echoed with the LMM results that male adolescents had a higher risk of substance abuse. Supporting Hypothesis 3a and 3b, these findings indicated that adolescents with better concurrent family functioning and positive youth development demonstrated lower risk of substance abuse. Family functioning and positive youth development had unique direct effects on reducing adolescent substance addiction.

For the longitudinal effects, when Wave 1 family functioning and positive youth development were examined separately, they did not have significant contribution to the substance abuse behavior at Wave 4, with their initial levels controlled. Similarly, when they were examined simultaneously, family functioning and positive youth development at Wave 1 did not significantly predict Wave 4 substance abuse behavior (see Table 6) as well as the drinking behavior (see Table 7). However, positive youth development at Wave 1 predicted smoking at Wave 4 (see Table 8). In short, there was partial support for Hypotheses 4a and 4b only.

Table 5 Multiple regression analyses on substance abuse at Wave 4

	Substance abuse					
	Model A		Model B		Model C	
Predictors	Beta	ΔR^2	Beta	ΔR^2	Beta	ΔR^2
Step 1		*.006****		*.006****		*.006****
Gender [a]	.066***		.066***		.065***	
Economic disadvantage [b]	−.016		.017		.016	
Family intactness [c]	−.005		−.015		−.007	
Step 2		*.015****				
Family functioning	−**.097*****					
Step 2				*.014****		
Positive youth development			−**.074*****			
Step 2						*.018****
Family functioning					−**.066****	
Positive youth development					−**.062****	

Model A includes family functioning, Model B includes positive youth development, and Model C includes both of them

*p<.05; **p<.01; ***p<.001

[a]Male = 1, female = 0

[b]Receiving CSSA = 1, not receiving CSSA = 0

[c]Intact = 1, non-intact = 0

Discussion

Compared with the previous longitudinal studies in the same research project (Shek and Ma 2011a; Shek and Yu 2011a), the study applied advanced multi-level analyses to further examine the trend and psychosocial correlates of adolescent substance abuse. Consistent with previous practice (Shek and Ma 2011b, c), individual growth curve modeling was applied to analyze the longitudinal data. By analyzing different models of individual trajectories and change of adolescent substance abuse, key constructs of risk factors (economic disadvantage and family intactness) and protective factors (positive youth development and family functioning) of adolescent substance abuse could be identified. The study provides rich information on the normative profile of adolescent substance abuse in Hong Kong over time, hence expanding our understanding of the objective picture of the developmental patterns of substance abuse from early adolescence to mid-adolescence.

Consistent with our expectation, adolescent substance abuse behavior increased in the adolescent years especially in the areas of smoking and drinking. This phenomenon may be partly associated with the addiction culture in young people and the relatively ease in getting tobacco and alcohol. Although the prevalence of adolescent substance abuse was not high, the rising rate of smoking and drinking

Table 6 Wave 1 variables predict Wave 4 substance abuse

Predictors	Substance abuse					
	Model A		Model B		Model C	
	Beta	ΔR^2	Beta	ΔR^2	Beta	ΔR^2
Step 1		*.081***		*.081***		*.081**
Initial behavior	.277***		.276***		.275***	
Step 2		*.086**		*.084**		*.086**
Gender[a]	.061**		.058**		.059**	
Economic disadvantage[b]	.035		.035		.035	
Family intactness[c]	.033		.030		.032	
Step 3		*.084*				
Family functioning	−.029					
Step 3				*.087*		
Positive youth development			−.034			
Step 3						*.087*
Family functioning					−.016	
Positive youth development					−.026	

Note: Model A includes family functioning, Model B includes positive youth development, and Model C includes both of them

$*p < .05; **p < .01; ***p < .001$

[a]Male = 1, female = 0

[b]Receiving CSSA = 1, not receiving CSSA = 0

[c]Intact = 1, non-intact = 0

suggests that there is a need to step up preventive education on adolescence substance abuse. Considering the risk factors of adolescent substance abuse, we examined how economic disadvantage and family intactness influenced the developmental patterns of adolescent substance abuse by controlling initial age and gender. We found that adolescents of non-intact families showed a higher risk of having substance abuse behavior initially. Although adolescent substance abuse of non-intact families increased slower than did the adolescents in intact families, they still had a higher mean abuse behavior at Wave 4 compared to those with parent staying in the first marriage. Consistent with our expectation, substance abuse behavior in adolescents from poor families increased faster than did those from nonpoor families. These findings echo the previous literature on the negative impacts of economic disadvantage and non-intact parental relationship on adolescent substance abuse (Feit and Wodarski 2014; Shek and Yu 2011a), and it enriches the related Chinese literature.

Furthermore, the positive attributes such as positive youth development and family function had positive effects on prevention of adolescent substance abuse. Both attributes had significant negative correlation with substance abuse behavior. However, the significant long-term effects of these two attributes were not

Table 7 Wave 1 variables predict Wave 4 substance abuse in drinking

	Substance abuse in drinking					
	Model A		Model B		Model C	
Predictors	Beta	ΔR^2	Beta	ΔR^2	Beta	ΔR^2
Step 1		*.152****		*.152****		*.152****
Initial behavior	.384***		.384***		.383***	
Step 2		*.156**		*.156**		*.156**
Gender[a]	.060**		.058**		.058**	
Economic disadvantage[b]	.011		.012		.011	
Family intactness[c]	.024		.022		.023	
Step 3		*.156*				
Family Functioning	−.021					
Step 3				*.156*		
Positive youth development			−.024			
Step 3						*.156*
Family Functioning					−.011	
Positive youth development					−.019	

Note: Model A includes family functioning, Model B includes positive youth development, and Model C includes both of them

*$p<.05$; **$p<.01$; ***$p<.001$

[a]Male = 1, female = 0

[b]Receiving CSSA = 1, not receiving CSSA = 0

[c]Intact = 1, non-intact = 0

established in this study. There are two possible explanations for these findings. First, as high-risk adolescents might dropout after Secondary 3, the sample at Wave 4 may be less at risk in terms of substance abuse, hence making the spread of scores in substance abuse less variable. Second, the influence of family functioning and positive youth development on substance abuse may weaken over time. Some research has shown that overconfidence and social maturity at an early age may in fact lead to more adolescent risk behavior (Lerner et al. 2005).

The study is not without limitations. First, the data were based on self-report format. Due to social desirability effect, they may not fully reflect the substance abuse situation in early adolescents. Therefore, replication studies with multiple methods of assessment (such as assessing the views of parents and teachers) are necessary to further examine the interrelationships among adolescent substance abuse and family attributes. Second, it will be helpful to explore other important potential determinants according to the ecological perspective (Shek 2002). Besides examination of the family environment, factors from the social environment, school environment, and peer environment should be examined in future analyses. In particular, as peer influence is important in early and middle adolescence, there is a

Table 8 Wave 1 variables predict Wave 4 substance abuse in smoking

	Substance abuse in smoking					
	Model A		Model B		Model C	
Predictors	Beta	ΔR^2	Beta	ΔR^2	Beta	ΔR^2
Step 1		*.114***		*.114***		*.144***
Initial behavior	.331***		.329***		.328***	
Step 2		*.120**		*.120**		*.120**
Gender[a]	.013		.009		.010	
Economic disadvantage[b]	.084***		.084***		.084***	
Family intactness[c]	.033		.031		.033	
Step 3		*.121*				
Family functioning	−.032					
Step 3				*.122**		
Positive youth development			**−.042***			
Step 3						*.122*
Family functioning					−.014	
Positive youth development					−.034	

Note: Model A includes family functioning, Model B includes positive youth development, and Model C includes both of them

*$p<.05$; **$p<.01$; ***$p<.001$

[a]Male = 1, female = 0

[b]Receiving CSSA = 1, not receiving CSSA = 0

[c]Intact = 1, non-intact = 0

need to take into account the related factors. Last but not least, family functioning as an important protective factor should be further explored. As parents are the live "models" of adolescents, it will be helpful to study the role of parenting style and parent–child relationship in the prevention of adolescent substance abuse.

References

Catalano, R. F., Berglund, M. L., Ryan, J. A., Lonczak, H. S., & Hawkins, J. D. (2002). Positive youth development in the United States: Research findings on evaluations of positive youth development programs. *Prevention & Treatment, 5*(1), 15a.

Chilcoat, H. D., & Anthony, J. C. (1996). Impact of parent monitoring on initiation of drug use through late childhood. *Journal of the American Academy of Child & Adolescent Psychiatry, 35*(1), 91–100.

Feit, M. D., & Wodarski, J. S. (2014). *Adolescent substance abuse: An empirical-based group preventive health paradigm*. New York: Routledge.

Graham, J., Mark, G., & Hansen, W. (1991). Social influence processes affecting adolescent substance abuse. *Journal of Applied Psychology, 16*(2), 291–298.

Hemphill, S. A., Heerde, J. A., Herrenkohl, T. I., Patton, G. C., Toumbourou, J. W., & Catalano, R. F. (2011). Risk and protective factors for adolescent substance use in Washington State, the United States and Victoria, Australia: A longitudinal study. *Journal of Adolescent Health, 49*(3), 312–320.

Kwok, O. M., Underhill, A. T., Berry, J. W., Luo, W., Elliott, T. R., & Yoon, M. (2008). Analyzing longitudinal data with multilevel models: An example with individuals living with lower extremity intra-articular fractures. *Rehabilitation Psychology, 53*(3), 370–386.

Lerner, R. M., Lerner, J. V., Almerigi, J. B., Theokas, C., Phelps, E., Gestsdottir, S., Naudeau, S., Jelicic, H., Alberts, A., Ma, L., Smith, L., Bobek, D. L., Richman-Raphael, D., Simpson, I., Christiansen, E. D., & von Eye, A. (2005). Positive youth development, participation in community youth development programs, and community contributions of fifth-grade adolescents findings from the first wave of the 4-H study of positive youth development. *The Journal of Early Adolescence, 25*(1), 17–71.

Narcotics Division of the Government of the Hong Kong Special Administrative Region. (2009). *Central registry of drug abuse: Fifty-eight report (1999–2008)*. Hong Kong.

Narcotics Division of the Government of the Hong Kong Special Administrative Region. (2014). *Local drug situation continues to show declining trend.* http://www.info.gov.hk/gia/general/201409/23/P201409230662.htm. Received 29 Sept 2014.

Shek, D. T. L. (2002). Family functioning and psychological well-being, school adjustment, and problem behavior in Chinese adolescents with and without economic disadvantage. *The Journal of Genetic Psychology, 163*(4), 497–502.

Shek, D. T. L. (2003). Family functioning and psychological well-being, school adjustment, and substance abuse in Chinese adolescents: Are findings based on multiple studies consistent. *Advances in Psychology Research, 20*, 163–184.

Shek, D. T. L. (2007). Tackling adolescent substance abuse in Hong Kong: Where we should go and should not go? *Scientific World Journal, 7*, 2021–2030.

Shek, D. T. L. (2010). Positive youth development and behavioral intention to gamble among Chinese adolescents in Hong Kong. *International Journal of Adolescent Medicine and Health, 22*(1), 163–172.

Shek, D. T. L., & Ma, C. M. S. (2010). The Chinese Family Assessment Instrument (C-FAI): Hierarchical confirmatory factor analyses and factorial invariance. *Research in Social Work Practice, 20*(1), 112–123.

Shek, D. T. L., & Ma, C. M. S. (2011a). Prevalence and psychosocial correlations. In D. T. L. Shek, R. C. F. Sun, & J. Merrick (Eds.), *Drug abuse in Hong Kong: Development and evaluation of a prevention program* (pp. 155–170). New York: Nova Science.

Shek, D. T. L., & Ma, C. M. S. (2011b). Longitudinal data analyses using linear mixed models in SPSS: Concepts, procedures and illustrations. *The Scientific World Journal: TSW Child Health & Human Development, 11*, 42–76.

Shek, D. T. L., & Ma, C. M. S. (2011c). Impact of the project P.A.T.H.S. in the junior secondary school years: Individual growth curve analyses. *The Scientific World Journal: TSW Child Health & Human Development, 11*, 253–266.

Shek, D. T. L., & Ma, C. M. S. (2012). Impact of the project P.A.T.H.S. on adolescent developmental outcomes in Hong Kong: Findings based on seven waves of data. *International Journal of Adolescent Medicine and Health, 24*(3), 231–244.

Shek, D. T. L., & Yu, L. (2011a). A longitudinal study of substance abuse in Hong Kong adolescents. In D. T. L. Shek, R. C. F. Sun, & J. Merrick (Eds.), *Drug abuse in Hong Kong: Development and evaluation of a prevention program* (pp. 171–196). New York: Nova Science.

Shek, D. T. L., & Yu, L. (2011b). Descriptive profiles and correlations of substance abuse in Hong Kong adolescents: A longitudinal study. *International Journal of Child Health and Human Development, 4*(4), 443–460.

Shek, D. T. L., & Yu, L. (2012). Longitudinal impact of the project P.A.T.H.S. on adolescent risk behavior: What happen after five years. *The Scientific World Journal, 2012*, 1–13.

Shek, D. T. L., Siu, A. M. H., & Lee, T. Y. (2007). The Chinese positive youth development scale: A validation study. *Research on Social Work Practice, 12*(3), 380–391.

Shek, D. T. L., Sun, R. C. F., & Merrick, J. (2011). Development and evaluation of a drug prevention program in Hong Kong. In D. T. L. Shek, R. C. F. Sun, & J. Merrick (Eds.), *Drug abuse in Hong Kong: Development and evaluation of a prevention program* (pp. 3–7). New York: Nova Science.

Shek, D. T. L., Sun, R. C. F., & Ma, C. M. S. (Eds.). (2014). *Chinese adolescents in Hong Kong: Family life, psychological well-being and risk behavior.* Singapore: Springer.

Singer, J. D., & Willett, J. B. (2003). *Applied longitudinal data analysis: Modeling change and event occurrence.* New York: Oxford University Press.

Wagner, K. D., Ritt-Olson, A., Chou, C. P., Pokhrel, P., Duan, L., Baezconde-Garbanati, L., Soto, D. W., & Unger, J. B. (2010). Associations between family structure, family functioning, and substance use among Hispanic/Latino adolescents. *Psychology of Addictive Behaviors, 24*(1), 98–108.

Sexual Behavior and Intention to Engage in Sexual Behavior Among Young Adolescents in Hong Kong: Findings Based on Four Waves of Data

Daniel T.L. Shek and Hildie Leung

Abstract This study examined the growth trajectories of sexual behavior and intention to engage in sexual behavior among young adolescents in Hong Kong across 4 years. Besides, the impact of family structure and economic disadvantage on the rate of change in adolescent sexual behavior and intention was studied, and the concurrent and longitudinal impact of family functioning and positive youth development on adolescent sexual behavior and intention was explored. Four waves of data were collected from adolescents ($n = 3328$ at Wave 1) in 28 secondary schools in Hong Kong. Individual growth curve models generally showed that adolescents from economically disadvantaged and non-intact families increased their sexual behavior at a faster rate than their counterparts, but they did not affect the rate of acceleration in intention to engage in sexual behavior. Multiple regression analyses revealed that family functioning and positive youth development influenced adolescent sexual behavior and intention.

Introduction

An important milestone of adolescence is sexual maturity. As such, acquisition of healthy skills to control the feelings of sexual arousal and manage consequences of sexual behavior is an important developmental task for adolescents (Rickert et al. 2002). This is particularly the case when worrying trends in adolescent sexual behavior are reported. A nationwide survey of students in grades 9–12 in the USA revealed that 47.4 % of them had had sexual intercourse and 33.7 % were sexually

The preparation for this work and the Project P.A.T.H.S. were financially supported by The Hong Kong Jockey Club Charities Trust.

D.T.L. Shek (✉) • H. Leung
Department of Applied Social Sciences, The Hong Kong Polytechnic University,
11 Yuk Choi Road, Hung Hom, Kowloon, Hong Kong, China
e-mail: daniel.shek@polyu.edu.hk

active (Eaton et al. 2012). According to the US "National Campaign to Prevent Teen Pregnancy," 2–4 % of adolescent boys and 6–8 % of adolescent girls reported having had sexual experience by the age of 12 (Albert et al. 2003). Early onset of sexual behaviors is a risk factor for HIV or other sexually transmitted diseases and pregnancy (Zabin and Hayward 1993). Sexual debut at early age is risky as youngsters are less likely than adults to use contraception at first sexual intercourse (Pedlow and Carey 2004). Although the situation appears to be less serious in different Chinese communities, startling trends have also been observed.

Shek and Leung (2013) examined problem behaviors among young adolescents in Hong Kong and reported worrying trends in adolescent sexual behavior. First, rates of premarital sex have increased over the years. From 1991 to 2011, rates of premarital sex have increased from 1.2 % to 9.8 % and 0.2 % to 7.4 % for adolescent boys and girls, respectively (Family Planning Association of Hong Kong 2012a). Second, 4.4 % adolescent boys and 3.0 % girls reported their first sexual intercourse under the age of 15 (Family Planning Association of Hong Kong 2012b). Third, adolescents are adopting more liberal attitudes toward sexual behaviors. For instance, 15 % and 11 % of adolescent boys and girls accepted multiple sex partners, respectively. Over 60 % of secondary school students accepted cohabitation rather than marriage (Family Planning Association of Hong Kong 2012b). These alarming figures indicate that "Hong Kong society will face a number of adolescent problems (e.g., teenage pregnancy and sexually transmitted diseases) shortly" (Shek et al. 2011, p. 2249). This calls for the need to investigate factors that influence adolescent sexual behavior and intention to engage in sexual behavior which may shed insight on possible interventions.

Family Influence on Adolescent Sexual Behavior

Guided by Bronfenbrenner's (1979) ecological systems theory, researchers have identified self, family, and community factors that contribute to adolescent sexual behaviors (Kotchick et al. 2001). Family influences on adolescent sexual behavior may be divided into two categories: (a) contextual and structural features of families (e.g., marital status, sibling composition) and (b) family processes or relationships (e.g., parental supervision, communication) (Miller 2002). Regarding family structure, it has been well established that adolescents of disrupted families are at a higher risk of engaging in sexual intercourse as compared with those from intact families (Santelli et al. 2000), and youngsters who live with two biological parents initiate sexual intercourse at a later stage than those from non-intact families (Albrecht and Teachman 2003; Moore 2001). Non-intact families may have underlying dysfunctional characteristics, such as parental mental health problems, marital discord, familial conflicts, and diminished quality of parent-child interactions which may account for adolescents' sexual behaviors (Flewelling and Bauman 1990). Thus, it is also important to examine the impact of family functioning on adolescent sexual behaviors.

Family functioning refers to "the quality of family life at the systemic and dyadic levels and concerns wellness, competence, strengths, and weaknesses of a family" (Shek 2002, p. 497) and may be operationalized in terms of family mutuality, communication, and harmony (Shek 2002). Most overseas research showed that perceived quality of parent-adolescent relationships was negatively related to young adult sexual risk behavior, such as lowered risk for sexuality transmitted infection diagnoses and healthy family interaction served as a promotive factor reducing early engagement in risky sexual behavior (Deptula et al. 2010). Family connectedness was also identified as a strong protective factor on postponing sexual intercourse among adolescents (Lammers et al. 2000). However, in Taris and Semin's (1997) study, positive parent-child relationships were not associated with delayed sexual initiation among adolescents. Parents' strong desire to maintain good relations with their children may dampen their willingness to clarify expectations of conduct and intensifies their worry that it may stir conflicts. In a comparative study of early adolescent sexual initiation in five nations (i.e., Finland, Scotland, France, Poland, and the USA), Madkour et al. (2010) found that respondents who reported higher levels of positive parental communication were at 50 % lower odds of sexual initiation. However, this was only found among adolescent girls in the USA.

Given the mixed findings in the scientific literature, it would be meaningful to examine the impact of family structure and functioning on adolescent sexual behavior in an Asian context like Hong Kong, where traditional Confucian values are eroded by rapid Westernization and modernization. Traditional Confucian values such as filial piety, self-cultivation of virtues, unequal gender roles, and restrictions on sexuality have been associated with less likelihood of premarital sexual intercourse among adolescents in Hanoi, Shanghai, and Taipei (Gao et al. 2012). The authors further argued that "different aspects of Confucian culture eroded unevenly might have different associations with adolescent and youths' sexual behaviors" and suggested future research to include "the moderating effects of individual socioeconomic status and parent-child communication" (p. 517) to gain a better understanding of adolescent sexual behaviors in other Asian countries.

Similarly, findings on the impact of socioeconomic status on adolescent sexual behavior are inconclusive. While some scholars argued that youngsters growing up in disadvantaged communities, with high poverty rates or residential instability, are more likely to initiate sex as teenagers and less likely to use contraception at first sex (Cubbin et al. 2005; Leventhal and Brooks-Gunn 2000), other researchers did not find any association between family income and adolescent sexual behaviors (Santelli et al. 2000).

Traditional research on adolescent sexual behavior adopts a risk perspective to examine negative influences that place youngsters at risk. In contrast, the strengths-based or promotion-focused approach has only been embraced recently (Vesely et al. 2004). Catalano et al. (2002) identified 15 positive youth development constructs, including bonding, resilience, social, cognitive, emotional, behavioral, moral competencies, belief in the future, self-efficacy, clear and positive identity, prosocial norms, spirituality, recognition for positive behavior, and self-determination. These constructs have been found to be associated with positive adolescent sexual behaviors. For intrapersonal competencies, more intelligent adolescents postponed the initiation of sexual activities (Halpern et al. 2000). Adolescents' cognitive immaturity may limit their ability to reason the consequences of risky sexual behavior. Youths may have difficulty in predicting or handling emotions associated with sexual activity (Pedlow and Carey 2004). Adolescents' self-esteem was negatively correlated with sexual attitudes and premarital intercourse experience (Miller 1987). More impulsive adolescents reported earlier age of first sexual intercourse and having more than one lifetime sexual partner (Kahn et al. 2002). Regarding interpersonal competencies, adolescents were highly susceptible to peer pressure to engage in sexual behavior (Berndt 1979). Adolescents who had confidence to say "no" to pressure exerted by their partners to have sex were less likely to try to engage in sexual behaviors (Guilamo-Ramos et al. 2008).

There are several limitations of the existing literature on adolescent sexual behavior. First, most studies focused on personal factors rather than familial and social factors as determinants. Second, little effort has been devoted to integrating personal, familial, social, and cultural factors to consider influence of multiple systems on adolescent sexual behaviors (Kotchick et al. 2001). Third, cross-sectional or short-term longitudinal studies were commonly conducted and few longer term longitudinal studies have examined the impact of different psychosocial factors on the growth rate of adolescent sexual behavior and intention, thus lacking sufficient basis for studying development (Willett et al. 1998).

To address the abovementioned gaps in the literature, the present chapter intends to integrate ecological and positive youth development theories to gain a better understanding of sexual behavior and intention in Chinese adolescents in Hong Kong. Particularly, we are interested to investigate: (a) the trajectories of adolescent sexual behavior and intention to engage in sexual behavior over 4 years, (b) the impact of economic disadvantage and family intactness on the rate of change of adolescent sexual behavior and intention, and (c) the concurrent and longitudinal impact of family functioning and positive youth development on adolescent sexual behavior and intention.

Method

Participants and Procedures

The present chapter reports data from the first four waves of a 6-year longitudinal study. A total of 3328 secondary 1 students (Mage $= 12.59 \pm 0.74$ years; 47.2 % female) were recruited from 28 local secondary schools in Hong Kong in the 2009/2010 academic year. Students were then assessed at intervals of 1 year. Demographic characteristics of the participants are shown in Table 1. Consent was obtained from schools, parents, and students who were fully informed about the study. Students completed the questionnaires in a classroom setting. A trained research assistant introduced the purpose of the study and emphasized the confidentiality of the collected data.

Table 1 Data profile across four waves

	Wave 1	%	Wave 2[a]	%	Wave 3[a]	%	Wave 4[a]	%
N (participants)	3328		2905		2858		2682	
Gender								
Male	1719	51.7	1445	49.7	1433	50.1	1335	49.8
Female	1572	47.2	1419	48.8	1405	49.2	1337	49.9
Economic disadvantage								
NOT receiving CSSA	2606	78.3	2377	81.8	2339	81.8	2267	84.5
Receiving CSSA	225	6.8	160	5.5	147	5.1	132	4.9
Family intactness								
Intact families	2781	83.6	2415	83.1	2396	83.8	2211	82.4
Non-intact families	515	15.5	469	16.1	454	15.9	466	17.4

[a]The numbers were based on the participants who ever participated in Wave 1 assessment as only those joining Wave 1 assessment were included in LMM. The numbers of the students who did not report the corresponding information were not presented

Instruments

Sexual Behavior Students were asked to indicate on a single item the number of times they had sexual intercourse in the past year with 7 options ranging from 0 (*never*) to 6 (*10 or more times*). A higher score represents more frequent past-year sexual intercourse.

Sexual Behavior Intention Sexual behavior intention was measured using one item. Students were asked to indicate on a 4-point Likert scale the likelihood of engaging in sexual intercourse in the next 2 years, ranging from 1 (*definitely will not*) to 4 (*definitely will*). Higher scores indicate a greater intention.

Family Functioning A simplified version of the Chinese Family Assessment Instrument (CFAI; Shek 2002) was administered to assess student perceptions of family functioning comprising of 9 items from 3 subscales assessing family mutuality, harmony, and communication. Respondents indicated their agreement to items describing their current family situation on a 5-point Likert scale anchored at 1 (*very dissimilar*) to 5 (*very similar*). A higher score indicated more positive family functioning. The scale was highly reliable (see Table 1).

Positive Youth Development The Chinese Positive Youth Development Scale (CPYDS; Shek et al. 2007; Shek and Ma 2010) was administered to assess positive youth development attributes including bonding, resilience, social competence, recognition for positive behavior, emotional competence, cognitive competence, behavioral competence, moral competence, self-determination, self-efficacy, clear and positive identity, beliefs in the future, prosocial involvement, prosocial norms, and spirituality. Students reported their agreement to the items on a 6-point Likert scale (with the exception of spirituality which was assessed using a 7-point scale).

Higher score indicates better positive youth development. A composite score was calculated by averaging the scores across the 15 subscales.

Assessment of Family Attributes Family economic status was assessed by whether participants' family was receiving Comprehensive Social Security Assistance (i.e., a financial aid provided by the Hong Kong Government for low-income families) at the time of assessment. Family intactness was indexed by the respondents' parental marital status. Intact families are families in which parents of respondents are legally married husband and wife in their first marriage at the time of study.

Data Analytic Plan

Latent growth curve analysis was used to systematically model intra- and interindividual differences in adolescent sexual behavior and intention to engage in sexual behavior over a period of 4 years. Advantages of latent growth curve analysis are well documented (Willett and Bub 2005; Shek and Ma 2011). Linear mixed model (LMM) with maximum likelihood (ML) as estimation method was conducted in SPSS22.0 (IBM SPSS Statistics, IBM Corp, Somers, NY). Three models were fitted for adolescent sexual behavior and intention, respectively. We first fitted the unconditional mean model (Model 1) to explore whether interindividual differences in change were present over time. Then, the unconditional linear growth curve model (Model 2) was fitted to examine the developmental trajectories. Third, the conditional growth curve model with gender, age, economic disadvantage, and family intactness as predictors was fitted (Model 3). Categorical variables were dummy coded (gender: female$=-1$, male$=1$; economic disadvantage: not receiving CSSA$=-1$, receiving CSSA$=1$; family intactness: non-intact family$=-1$, intact family$=1$) and continuous variable (i.e., initial age) was grand mean centered in order to simplify the interpretation of the results. Three indices were used for model evaluation including -2log likelihood (i.e., likelihood ratio test), Akaike information criterion (AIC), and Bayesian information criterion (BIC) (Shek and Ma 2011; Shek and Yu 2012) where lower values indicate better model fit. Multiple regression analyses were also conducted to examine the concurrent and longitudinal impact of family functioning and positive youth development on adolescent sexual behavior and intention to engage in sexual behavior.

Results

The prevalence rates of sexual behavior and intention to engage in sexual behavior among Hong Kong junior secondary school students across four waves are presented in Tables 2 and 3. The majority of participants had never had sexual intercourse at all four waves (ranging from 98.6 % to 99.3 %), nor do they have the intention to engage in sexual intercourse in the next 2 years (84.8–93.5 %). However, an increasing trend of sexual behavior and behavioral intention was observed over the 4 years.

Table 2 Prevalence of sexual behavior and intention to engage in sexual behavior across four waves

	Wave 1		Wave 2		Wave 3		Wave 4	
	N	%	N	%	N	%	N	%
Sexual contacts in the preceding year								
Never	3293	99.3	2862	98.9	2730	98.9	2546	98.6
1–2 times	18	0.5	13	0.4	13	0.5	10	0.4
3–4 times	2	0.1	6	0.2	3	0.1	7	0.3
5–6 times	0	0.0	6	0.2	2	0.1	1	0.0
7–8 times	0	0.0	0	0.0	2	0.1	1	0.0
9–10 times	0	0.0	1	0.0	1	0.0	1	0.0
Over 10 times	2	0.1	7	0.2	8	0.3	17	0.7
Intention to engage in sexual behaviors in the next 2 years								
Absolutely no	3104	93.5	2612	90.2	2436	88.5	2185	84.8
Probably no	137	4.1	176	6.1	167	6.1	194	7.5
Probably yes	59	1.8	89	3.1	122	4.4	164	6.4
Absolutely yes	19	0.6	20	0.7	29	1.1	33	1.3

Note: One school (*N*= 124) declined to report sexual behavior and intention to engage in sexual behavior since Wave 3

Table 3 Descriptive statistics of key variables and internal consistency coefficients of scales (Waves 1–4)

	Mean (SD)				Cronbach's α			
	W1	W2	W3	W4	W1	W2	W3	W4
Family functioning[a]	3.73 (.81)	3.65 (.81)	3.65 (.79)	3.66 (.77)	.90	.90	.90	.91
Positive youth development	4.51 (.70)	4.43 (.69)	4.44 (.65)	4.45 (.62)	.93	.96	.96	.96
Sexual behavior								
Male	.00 (.08)	.01 (.20)	.04 (.41)	.05 (.50)	–	–	–	–
Female	.01 (.10)	.04 (.37)	.02 (.28)	.05 (.53)	–	–	–	–
NOT receiving CSSA	.01 (.08)	.02 (.30)	.03 (.36)	.04 (.45)	–	–	–	–
Receiving CSSA	.02 (.14)	.04 (.35)	.01 (.12)	.27 (1.2)	–	–	–	–
Intact families	.00 (.07)	.02 (.28)	.02 (.32)	.03 (.40)	–	–	–	–
Non-Intact families	.01 (.14)	.04 (.40)	.05 (.48)	.16 (.91)	–	–	–	–
Intention to engage in sexual behavior					–	–	–	–
Male	1.12 (.44)	1.18 (.52)	1.24 (.63)	1.36 (.73)	–	–	–	–
Female	1.06 (.31)	1.09 (.39)	1.10 (.42)	1.11 (.44)	–	–	–	–
NOT receiving CSSA	1.09 (.38)	1.13 (.45)	1.17 (.54)	1.23 (.60)	–	–	–	–
Receiving CSSA	1.09 (.37)	1.21 (.60)	1.18 (.52)	1.34 (.75)	–	–	–	–
Intact families	1.08 (.36)	1.13 (.44)	1.16 (.53)	1.21 (.59)	–	–	–	–
Non-Intact families	1.13 (.47)	1.20 (.56)	1.22 (.59)	1.34 (71)	–	–	–	–

W1 Wave 1, *W2* Wave 2, *W3* Wave 3, *W4* Wave 4

[a]Mean score was used to indicate the level of family functioning and positive youth development

Table 4 Results of individual growth curve of past sexual behavior

		Model 1		Model 2		Model 3	
		Estimate	SE	Estimate	SE	Estimate	SE
Fixed effects							
Intercept	β_{0j}						
Initial status	γ_{00}	.031***	.004	.011**	.004	.004	.008
Age	γ_{01}					.008	.006
Gender	γ_{02}					−.004	.004
Economic disadvantage	γ_{03}					−.000	.009
Family intactness	γ_{04}					.005	.006
Linear slope	β_{1j}						
Initial status	γ_{10}			.016***	.003	.040***	.007
Age	γ_{11}					.003	.005
Gender	γ_{12}					.003	.004
Economic disadvantage	γ_{13}					.017*	.007
Family intactness	γ_{14}					−.013*	.006
Random effects							
Level 1 (within)							
Residual	r_{ij}	.109***	.002	.076***	.001	.066***	.001
Level 2 (between)							
Intercept	u_{0j}	.025***	.002	.00	.00	.00	.00
Time	u_{1j}			.016***	.001	.018***	.001
Fit statistics							
Deviance		9157.90		7500.13		4905.35	
AIC		9163.90		7512.13		4933.35	
BIC		9185.96		7556.26		5033.84	
df		3		6		14	

Note: Model 1 = unconditional mean model; Model 2 = unconditional growth model; Model 3 = conditional model (with age, gender, economic disadvantage, and family intactness as predictors) *$p < .05$; **$p < .01$; ***$p < .001$

To examine the trajectories of adolescent sexual behavior and intention to engage in sexual behavior, as well as the impact of economic disadvantage and family intactness on the initial status and rate of change of the two variables, individual growth curve analyses were conducted (see Tables 4 and 5).

Results from Model 1 (i.e., the unconditional mean model) yielded ICCs of 0.187 for sexual behavior and 0.832 for intention to engage in sexual behavior, indicating that 18.7 % and 83.2 % of the total variance were attributed to differences between individuals. Thus, individual growth curve analysis was employed to explore these other interindividual factors.

Model 2 (i.e., the unconditional linear growth curve model) examined the individual rate of change over time. Significant values were yielded for both the intercept and linear slope parameters for sexual behavior and intention to engage in sexual behavior, indicating that the initial status and linear growth rate were not

Table 5 Results of individual growth curve of intention to engage in sexual behavior

		Model 1		Model 2		Model 3	
		Estimate	SE	Estimate	SE	Estimate	SE
Fixed effects							
Intercept	β_{0j}						
Initial status	γ_{00}	1.164***	.007	1.092***	.007	1.097***	.014
Age	γ_{01}					.048***	.010
Gender	γ_{02}					.017*	.007
Economic disadvantage	γ_{03}					−.005	.014
Family intactness	γ_{04}					−.020	.011
Linear slope	β_{1j}						
Initial status	γ_{10}			.055***	.004	.069***	.009
Age	γ_{11}					.017**	.006
Gender	γ_{12}					.033***	.004
Economic disadvantage	γ_{13}					.007	.009
Family intactness	γ_{14}					−.009	.007
Random effects							
Level 1(within)							
Residual	r_{ij}	.177***	.003	.143***	.003	.138***	.003
Level 2 (between)							
Intercept	u_{0j}	.088***	.004	.037***	.004	.031***	.004
Time	u_{1j}			.018***	.001	.017***	.001
Fit statistics							
Deviance		16027.75		14996.92		12125.71	
AIC		16033.75		15008.92		12153.71	
BIC		16055.81		15053.05		12254.19	
df		3		6		14	

Note: Model 1=unconditional mean model; Model 2=unconditional growth model; Model 3=conditional model (with age, gender, economic disadvantage, and family intactness as predictors)
*p<.05; **p<.01; ***p<.001

constant over time. For sexual behavior, Model 2 showed a better model fit than Model 1 ($\Delta\chi^2_{(3)}=1657.77$; ΔAIC=1651.77; ΔBIC=1629.70). The mean estimated initial status of sexual behavior was .011 (SE=.004, $p<.01$) and had a significant linear increase by .016 unit per year ($\beta=.016$, SE=.003, $p<.001$). Furthermore, the random error term associated with the linear effect was significant ($p<.001$), indicating that the variability could be explained by between-factor individual predictors. For intention to engage in sexual behavior, Model 2 was also a better fit than Model 1 ($\Delta\chi^2_{(3)}=1030.83$; ΔAIC=1024.83; ΔBIC=1002.76). The mean estimated initial status of sexual behavior was 1.092 (SE=.007, $p<.001$) and had a significant linear increase by .055 unit per year ($\beta=.055$, SE=.004, $p<.001$).

Model 3 (i.e., the conditional growth curve model with age, gender, economic disadvantage, and family intactness as predictors) of the intercepts and slopes was tested. Regarding sexual behavior, Model 3 resulted in a better fit than Model 2 ($\Delta\chi^2_{(8)}=2594.78$; ΔAIC$=2578.78$; ΔBIC$=2522.42$). For the intercepts, age, gender, economic disadvantage, and family intactness were non-significant predictors. This means that whether adolescents received CSSA or lived in non-intact families did not impact on their initial assessment of sexual behavior. However, for the linear slopes of past sexual behavior, both economic disadvantage and family intactness were associated with the growth rate of sexual behavior. Particularly, adolescents receiving CSSA ($\beta=.017$, $SE=.007$, $p<.01$) increased their sexual behaviors at a faster rate than their counterparts without receiving CSSA. Adolescents from intact families ($\beta=-.013$, $SE=.006$, $p<.01$) increased their sexual behaviors at a slower rate than those from non-intact families.

Regarding intention to engage in sexual behavior, Model 3 also resulted in a better fit than Model 2 ($\Delta\chi^2_{(8)}=2871.21$; ΔAIC$=2855.21$; ΔBIC$=2798.86$). For the intercepts, age and gender were significant predictors of initial status of intention to engage in sexual behavior, with older ($\beta=.048$, $SE=.010$, $p<.001$) and male ($\beta=.017$, $SE=.007$, $p<.05$) adolescents reporting higher intention. Yet, both economic disadvantage and family intactness were non-significant predictors.

Similarly, for the linear slopes of sexual behavior, both age and gender were significant predictors. Older adolescents increased their intention of sexual behavior at a faster rate than younger adolescents ($\beta=.017$, $SE=.006$, $p<.01$). Male adolescents ($\beta=.033$, $SE=.004$, $p<.001$) also accelerated intention at a faster rate than females. Yet, neither economic disadvantage nor family intactness was a significant predictor, implying that economic and family background of the adolescent did not impact on the rate of growth in adolescents' intention to engage in sexual behavior.

To investigate the concurrent impact of family functioning and positive youth development on sexual behavior and intention to engage in sexual behavior at Secondary 4, hierarchical multiple regression analyses were conducted as reported in Table 6.

For sexual behaviors, results revealed that beyond demographic factors, family functioning ($p<.01$) and positive youth development ($p<.01$) were significant predictors of adolescent sexual behaviors when examined in separate models. Adolescents with better family functioning and positive youth development reported lower levels of sexual behaviors. However, family functioning and positive youth development did not predict sexual behaviors in the simultaneous model. Regarding intention to engage in sexual behavior, results showed that family functioning and positive youth development were both significant predictors of sexual behavior intention in separate ($p<.001$) and simultaneous models ($p<.01$). Specifically, adolescents from better functioning families and high positive youth development had lower intention to engage in sexual behavior.

Table 7 shows results from hierarchical multiple regression analyses examining the longitudinal impact of family functioning and positive youth development on adolescent past sexual behavior and intention to engage in sexual behavior.

Regarding sexual behavior, when examining the predictors in separate models, both family functioning and positive youth development were significant predictors

Table 6 Multiple regression analyses on sexual behavior and intention to engage in sexual behavior at Wave 4

Predictors	Sexual behavior						Intention to engage in sexual behavior					
	Model A		Model B		Model C		Model A		Model B		Model C	
	Beta	ΔR2	Beta	ΔR2	Beta	ΔR2	Beta	ΔR2	Beta	ΔR2	Beta	ΔR2
Step 1		.015***		.017***		.018***		.047***		.048***		.046***
Gender[a]	.006		-.010		-.009		.203***		.201***		.198***	
Economic disadvantage[b]	.082***		.091***		.096***		.019		.033		.030	
Family intactness[c]	-.056*		-.066**		-.060**		-.062**		-.070**		-.060**	
Step 2		.004**						.011***				
Family functioning	-.067**						-.108***					
Step 2				.003**						.014***		
Positive youth development			-.059**						-.118***			
Step 2						.005**						.019***
Family functioning					-.042						-.076**	
Positive youth development					-.041						-.089***	

Note: Model A includes family functioning, Model B includes positive youth development, and Model C includes both variables

*p<.05; **p<.01; ***p<.001

[a]Male=1, female=0

[b]Receiving CSSA=1, not receiving CSSA=0

[c]Intact=1, non-intact=0

Table 7 Multiple regression analyses on Wave 1 variables predicting sexual behavior and intention to engage in sexual behavior at Wave 4

| | Sexual behavior | | | | | | Intention to engage in sexual behavior | | | | | |
| | Model A | | Model B | | Model C | | Model A | | Model B | | Model C | |
Predictors	Beta	$\Delta R2$	Beta	$\Delta R2$	Beta	$\Delta R2$	Beta	$\Delta R2$	Beta	$\Delta R2$	Beta	$\Delta R2$
Step 1		.015***		.012***		.013***		.042***		.046***		.043***
Gender[a]	.007		.004		.008		.199***		.202***		.203***	
Economic disadvantage[b]	.072**		.074**		.077**		.014		−.001		.003	
Family intactness[c]	−.060*		−.051*		−.040		−.044		−.053*		−.038	
Step 2		.007***						.013***				
Family functioning	−.086***						−.115***					
Step 2				.006**						.011***		
Positive youth development			−.075**						−.105***			
Step 2						.009***						.014***
Family functioning					−.070*						−.062*	
Positive youth development					−.039						−.075**	

Note: Model A includes family functioning, Model B includes positive youth development, and Model C includes both variables
*p<.05; **p<.01; ***p<.001
[a]Male = 1, female = 0
[b]Receiving CSSA = 1, not receiving CSSA = 0
[c]Intact = 1, non-intact = 0

($p < .001$). In the simultaneous model, however, only family functioning ($p < .05$) significantly impacted past sexual behavior among youngsters, where those from healthier families reported lower intention. In terms of sexual behavior intention, both family functioning and positive youth development at Wave 1 predicted sexual behavior intention at Wave 4 in both the separate ($p < .001$) and simultaneous models ($p < .05$). Similar patterns were yielded for longitudinal effects when controlling initial assessment of past sexual behavior and intention to engage in sexual behavior (see Table 8).

Discussion

Our study was the first to describe the trajectories of sexual behavior and intention among young adolescents in Hong Kong. Over the course of 4 years, we examined the influence of economic disadvantage and family intactness on adolescent initial levels and trajectories of change in sexual behavior and intention and the influence of family functioning and positive youth development on adolescent sexual behavior and intention.

In line with earlier studies (Shek 2013), results showed that adolescent sexual behavior and intention increased with time. However, novel findings regarding the factors that impact on their growth rates were revealed. First, gender and age had no influence on the rate of increase in sexual behaviors. Similar findings have been reported in previous studies in that growth rates in problem behaviors are quite similar for boys and girls (Deković et al. 2004). However, older and male adolescents tended to accelerate their sexual behavior intention at a faster rate than their counterparts. An explanation may operate in terms of change in perception of risk. Steinberg (2004) reported that young adolescents (aged 11–13) were more likely than other age groups to rate risk behaviors such as unprotected sex as risky, scary, dangerous, and harmful, whereas adolescents over the age of 14 perceived the same amount of risk as young adults would. A decrease in perceived risks associated with sexual behaviors may contribute to its increasing intention among older adolescents.

Second, economic disadvantage and family intactness had no influence on the rate of change in the intention to engage in sexual behavior. These findings suggest that factors that affecting the development of adolescents' sexual intention are not primarily family factors. One's intentions are influenced by subjective norms, i.e., the perceived social pressure to engage in certain behaviors (Ajzen 1991). Therefore, it is likely that peer influence may impact the growth of adolescent sexual behavioral intention more so than family factors.

However, adolescents from disadvantaged and non-intact families increased their sexual behaviors at a faster rate. This observation is in line with overseas studies. Scholars in the USA and UK reported that poorer adolescent girls were more likely to initiate sexual activity before the age of 20, as compared to more well-off counterparts (Singh et al. 2001). Higher socioeconomic status was associated with postponing

Table 8 Multiple regression analyses on Wave 1 variables predicting sexual behavior and intention to engage in sexual behavior at Wave 4 controlling initial behavior

Predictors	Sexual behavior						Intention to engage in sexual behavior					
	Model A		Model B		Model C		Model A		Model B		Model C	
	Beta	ΔR2	Beta	ΔR2	Beta	ΔR2	Beta	ΔR2	Beta	ΔR2	Beta	ΔR2
Step 1		.006**		.007***		.007***		.061***		.069***		.071***
Initial behavior	.067**		.080**		.077**		.222***		.242***		.244***	
Step 2		.015***		.011***		.012***		.036***		.040***		.038***
Gender[a]	.009		.008		.012		.183***		.190***		.188***	
Economic disadvantage[b]	.070**		.070**		.073**		.012		.004		.008	
Family intactness[c]	−.062*		−.053*		−.043		−.046*		−.053*		−.041	
Step 3		.007***						.006***				
Family functioning	−.082***						−.079***					
Step 3				.005**						.005**		
Positive youth development			−.073**						−.072**			
Step 3						.008**						.006**
Family functioning					−.067*						−.039	
Positive youth development					−.039						−.053*	

Note: Model A includes family functioning, Model B includes positive youth development, and Model C includes both variables
*p < .05; **p < .01; ***p < .001
[a]Male = 1, female = 0
[b]Receiving CSSA = 1, not receiving CSSA = 0
[c]Intact = 1, non-intact = 0

sexual intercourse in adolescents (Lammers et al. 2000). Several factors may account for these findings, including limited access to social services and support, lack of positive role models, risky environments, lowered personal competence, skills, and motivation (Singh et al. 2001), and difficulties in providing on-site and off-site supervision to children (Hogan and Kitagawa 1985). In a study of parenting characteristics of economically disadvantaged parents in Hong Kong, Leung and Shek (2013) found that low educational standards, physically demanding nature of jobs, and nonstandard working hours may pose difficulties on parenting. Indeed, poorer parents are often preoccupied with the adverse effect of economic disadvantage and may be less sensitive to the problem behavior of their children or lack parenting skills (Conger et al. 2000; Shek 2005) which are likely to impact on adolescents' sexual behavior.

Our findings also converge with earlier research showing the impact of family structure on adolescent sexual behaviors. Adolescents growing up in non-intact families often reported higher risks of ever having had sex (Cubbin et al. 2005), earlier sexual activity, and higher number of sexual partners (Feldman and Brown 1993) than those who live with both biological parents. The different sexual behavior trajectories of adolescents from non-intact families may be due to the lack of protective factors on the familial level. Specifically, restrictive parenting (Wight et al. 2006), family connectedness, and parent-adolescent communication reduce risky sexual behavior, early sexual debut, and frequency of sex in adolescents (Markham et al. 2010), yet these are often lacking in non-intact families. For instance, James and colleagues (2012) reported that father absence in disrupted families had a significant indirect effect on earlier sexual debut through lower quality of family relationships. Young et al. (1991) reasoned that intact families have two adult role models to provide guidance and emotional support which lack in disrupted families. Moreover, adult models of nonmarital sexual behavior are more common or salient for teenagers from single-parent homes.

The present study also shows concurrent and longitudinal impact of family functioning and positive youth development on adolescent sexual behavior and intention. The present findings coincide with overseas studies and support the importance of family functioning on healthy adolescent development universally. Specifically, scholars found that adolescents who perceived their parents to be warm reported less risky sexual behavior and had lower odds of adolescent onset of sexual intercourse or having multiple sexual partners (Rodgers and McGuire 2012). Adolescents who perceived their parents to be friendly in communication reported lower levels of sexual activity (Mueller and Powers 1990).

A survey of existing research reveals that while sexual behavior among youth is consistently framed as being problematic, little empirical attention is put on investigating the developmental processes involved in becoming a healthy sexual adult (Kotchick et al. 2001). Our findings contribute to the literature by adopting a more positive approach in identifying positive youth development as a protective factor for adolescent sexual behavior and intention. Our results coincide with the findings showing that adolescent developmental assets (e.g., future aspirations, participation in religious activities, ability to make responsible choices, positive peer role models, emotional control, self-esteem) can help to avoid potentially harmful sexual behaviors (Miller 1987; Mueller et al. 2010; Pedlow and Carey 2004).

The present study has both theoretical and practical implications. "Developmental theories are extremely vague about what produces change, and efforts to explain stability or to predict change in problem behavior have not been particularly successful" (Deković et al. 2004, p. 11). Theoretically, our findings contribute to the existing literature in identifying family structure and economic disadvantage as factors that impact change in adolescent sexual behavior and intention. Furthermore, our findings provide support to the protective role of family functioning and positive youth development for delaying sexual behavior and lessening intention, particularly in the Chinese context. Practically, the trajectories of sexual behavior may guide practitioners to intervene earlier to provide enhanced intervention to slow the rate of growth in sexual risk behavior among adolescents from disrupted or economically disadvantaged families. Positive youth development programs may be developed to provide a more holistic set of skills, motivations, and confidence needed to complement the skills taught in traditional sexuality education (Gavin et al. 2010). Also, as pointed out by Santelli et al. (2000), "increasing life opportunities and fostering aspirations for young adolescents may contribute to delaying the onset of intercourse" (p. 1587).

Despite the pioneer nature of the study, it has several limitations. First, measures are of self-report nature and studies have found that males tended to overreport sexual behaviors whereas females underreport (Stevenson et al. 2007). However, taking into consideration ethical and practical concerns and the sensitivity of the topic especially for young adolescents, self-report measures are most appropriate. Second, as this study was conducted in Hong Kong, the findings may not be generalizable to other Chinese communities such as China or Taiwan. Future studies should be conducted to further examine the growth patterns of older adolescents and those in other Chinese contexts. Third, as sexual behavior and intention were measured using two single items in this study, subsequent research should include additional items to measure students' attitudes, beliefs, perceived risks, or norms related to sexual behavior which may further shed light on the issue.

References

Ajzen, I. (1991). The theory of planned behavior. *Organizational Behavior and Human Decision Processes, 50*(2), 179–211.

Albert, W., Brown, S., & Flanigan, C. (2003). *Fourteen and younger: The sexual behavior of young adolescents*. Washington, DC: The National Campaign to Prevent Teen Pregnancy.

Albrecht, C., & Teachman, J. D. (2003). Childhood living arrangements and the risk of premarital intercourse. *Journal of Family Issues, 24*(7), 867–894.

Berndt, T. J. (1979). Developmental changes in conformity to peers and parents. *Developmental Psychology, 15*(6), 608–616.

Bronfenbrenner, U. (1979). *The ecology of human development: Experiments by nature and design*. Cambridge, MA: Harvard University Press.

Catalano, R. F., Berglund, M. L., Ryan, J. A., Lonczak, H. S., & Hawkins, J. D. (2002). Positive youth development in the United States: Research findings on evaluations of positive youth development programs. *Prevention & Treatment, 5*(1). Retrieved from http://journals.apa.org/prevention/volume5/pre0050015a.html

Conger, K. J., Rueter, M. A., & Conger, R. D. (2000). The role of economic pressure in the lives of parents and their adolescents: The family stress model. In L. J. Crockett & R. K. Silbereisen (Eds.), *Negotiating adolescence in times of social change* (pp. 201–233). New York: Cambridge University Press.

Cubbin, C., Santelli, J., Brindis, C. D., & Braveman, P. (2005). Neighborhood context and sexual behaviors among adolescents: Findings from the national longitudinal study of adolescent health. *Perspectives on Sexual and Reproductive Health, 37*(3), 125–134.

Deković, M., Buist, K. L., & Reitz, E. (2004). Stability and changes in problem behavior during adolescence: Latent growth analysis. *Journal of Youth and Adolescence, 33*(1), 1–12.

Deptula, D. P., Henry, D. B., & Schoeny, M. E. (2010). How can parents make a difference? longitudinal associations with adolescent sexual behavior. *Journal of Family Psychology, 24*(6), 731–739.

Eaton, D. K., Kann, L., Kinchen, S., Shanklin, S., Flint, K. H., Hawkins, J., Harris, W. A., Lowry, R., McManus, T., Chyen, D., Whittle, L., Lim, C., & Wechsler, H. (2012). Youth risk behavior surveillance: United States, 2011. *Morbidity and Mortality Weekly Report. Surveillance Summaries, 61*(4), 1–162.

Family Planning Association of Hong Kong. (2012a). *Youth sexuality study 2011: Age 18–27 survey* (in Chinese) [Electronic version]. Retrieved from http://www.famplan.org.hk/fpahk/zh/press/press/20120626-press-chi.ppt

Family Planning Association of Hong Kong. (2012b). *Youth sexuality study 2011: Secondary school survey* (in Chinese) [Electronic version]. Retrieved from http://www.famplan.org.hk/fpahk/zh/press/press/20120619-press-chi.ppt

Feldman, S. S., & Brown, N. L. (1993). Family influences on adolescent male sexuality: The mediational role of self-restraint. *Social Development, 2*(1), 15–35.

Flewelling, R. L., & Bauman, K. E. (1990). Family structure as a predictor of initial substance use and sexual intercourse in early adolescence. *Journal of Marriage and the Family, 52*(1), 171–181.

Gao, E., Zuo, X., Wang, L., Lou, C., Cheng, Y., & Zabin, L. S. (2012). How does traditional Confucian culture influence adolescents' sexual behavior in three Asian cities? *Journal of Adolescent Health, 50*(3), S12–S17.

Gavin, L. E., Catalano, R. F., David-Ferdon, C., Gloppen, K. M., & Markham, C. M. (2010). A review of positive youth development programs that promote adolescent sexual and reproductive health. *Journal of Adolescent Health, 46*(3), S75–S91.

Guilamo-Ramos, V., Jaccard, J., Dittus, P., Gonzalez, B., & Bouris, A. (2008). A conceptual framework for the analysis of risk and problem behaviors: The case of adolescent sexual behavior. *Social Work Research, 32*(1), 29–45.

Halpern, C. T., Joyner, K., Udry, J. R., & Suchindran, C. (2000). Smart teens don't have sex (or kiss much either). *Journal of Adolescent Health, 26*(3), 213–225.

Hogan, D. P., & Kitagawa, E. M. (1985). The impact of social status, family structure and neighborhood on fertility of black adolescents. *American Journal of Sociology, 90*(4), 825–855.

James, J., Ellis, B. J., Schlomer, G. L., & Garber, J. (2012). Sex-specific pathways to early puberty, sexual debut, and sexual risk taking: Tests of an integrated evolutionary-developmental model. *Developmental Psychology, 48*(3), 687–702.

Kahn, J. A., Kaplowitz, R. A., Goodman, E., & Emans, S. J. (2002). The association between impulsiveness and sexual risk behaviors in adolescent and young adult women. *Journal of Adolescent Health, 30*(4), 229–232.

Kotchick, B. A., Shaffer, A., Miller, K. S., & Forehand, R. (2001). Adolescent sexual risk behavior: A multi-system perspective. *Clinical Psychology Review, 21*(4), 493–519.

Lammers, C., Ireland, M., Resnick, M., & Blum, R. (2000). Influences on adolescents' decision to postpone onset of sexual intercourse: A survival analysis of virginity among youths aged 13 to 18 years. *Journal of Adolescent Health, 26*(1), 42–48.

Leung, J. T. Y., & Shek, D. T. L. (2013). Parental beliefs and parenting characteristics of Chinese parents experiencing economic disadvantage in Hong Kong. *International Journal on Disability and Human Development, 12*(2), 139–149.

Leventhal, T., & Brooks-Gunn, J. (2000). The neighborhoods they live in: The effects of neighborhood residence on child and adolescent outcomes. *Psychological Bulletin, 126*(2), 309–337.

Madkour, A. S., Farhat, T., Halpern, C. T., Godeau, E., & Gabhainn, S. N. (2010). Early adolescent sexual initiation as a problem behavior: A comparative study of five nations. *Journal of Adolescent Health, 47*(4), 389–398.

Markham, C. M., Lormand, D., Gloppen, K. M., Peskin, M. F., Flores, B., Low, B., & House, L. D. (2010). Connectedness as a predictor of sexual and reproductive health outcomes for youth. *Journal of Adolescent Health, 46*(3), S23–S41.

Miller, B. C. (1987). Adolescent self-esteem in relation to sexual attitudes and behavior. *Youth and Society, 19*(1), 93–111.

Miller, B. C. (2002). Family influences on adolescent sexual and contraceptive behavior. *Journal of Sex Research, 39*(1), 22–26.

Moore, M. R. (2001). Family environment and adolescent sexual debut in alternative household structures. In R. T. Michael (Ed.), *Social awakening: Adolescent behavior as adulthood approaches* (pp. 109–136). New York: Russell Sage.

Mueller, K. E., & Powers, W. G. (1990). Parent-child sexual discussion: Perceived communicator style and subsequent behavior. *Adolescence, 25*(98), 469–482.

Mueller, T., Gavin, L., Oman, R., Vesely, S., Aspy, C., Tolma, E., & Rodine, S. (2010). Youth assets and sexual risk behavior: Differences between male and female adolescents. *Health Education & Behavior, 37*(3), 343–356.

Pedlow, C. T., & Carey, M. P. (2004). Developmentally appropriate sexual risk reduction interventions for adolescents: Rationale, review of interventions, and recommendations for research and practice. *Annals of Behavioral Medicine, 27*(3), 172–184.

Rickert, V. I., Sanghvi, R., & Wiemann, C. M. (2002). Is lack of sexual assertiveness among adolescent and young adult women a cause for concern? *Perspectives on Sexual and Reproductive Health, 34*(4), 178–183.

Rodgers, K. B., & McGuire, J. K. (2012). Adolescent sexual risk and multiple contexts: Interpersonal violence, parenting, and poverty. *Journal of Interpersonal Violence, 27*(11), 2091–2107.

Santelli, J. S., Lowry, R., Brener, N. D., & Robin, L. (2000). The association of sexual behaviors with socioeconomic status, family structure, and race/ethnicity among US adolescents. *American Journal of Public Health, 90*(10), 1582–1588.

Shek, D. T. L. (2002). Assessment of family functioning in Chinese adolescents: The Chinese version of the family assessment device. *Research on Social Work Practice, 12*(4), 502–524.

Shek, D. T. L. (2005). Paternal and maternal influences on the psychological well-being, substance abuse, and delinquency of Chinese adolescents experiencing economic disadvantage. *Journal of Clinical Psychology, 61*(3), 219–234.

Shek, D. T. L. (2013). Sexual behavior and intention to engage in sexual behavior in junior secondary school students in Hong Kong. *Journal of Pediatric and Adolescent Gynecology, 26*, S33–S41.

Shek, D. T. L., & Leung, J. T. Y. (2013). Adolescent developmental issues in Hong Kong: Phenomena and implications for youth service. In D. T. L. Shek & R. C. F. Sun (Eds.), *Development and evaluation of Positive Adolescent Training through Holistic Social Programs (PATHS)* (pp. 1–13). Singapore: Springer.

Shek, D. T. L., & Ma, C. M. S. (2010). Dimensionality of the Chinese positive youth development scale: Confirmatory factor analyses. *Social Indicators Research, 98*(1), 41–59.

Shek, D. T. L., & Ma, C. M. S. (2011). Longitudinal data analyses using linear mixed models in SPSS: Concepts, procedures and illustrations. *The Scientific World Journal, 11*, 42–76.

Shek, D. T. L., & Yu, L. (2012). Longitudinal impact of the project PATHS on adolescent risk behavior: What happened after five years? *The Scientific World Journal*, Article ID 316029, 13 pages. doi: 10.1100/2012/316029s

Shek, D. T. L., Siu, A. M. H., & Lee, T. Y. (2007). The Chinese positive youth development scale: A validation study. *Research on Social Work Practice, 12*(3), 380–391.

Shek, D. T. L., Ma, H. K., & Sun, R. C. F. (2011). A brief overview of adolescent developmental problems in Hong Kong. *The Scientific World Journal, 11*, 2243–2256.

Singh, S., Darroch, J. E., & Frost, J. J. (2001). Socioeconomic disadvantage and adolescent women's sexual and reproductive behavior: The case of five developed countries. *Family Planning Perspectives, 33*(6), 251–289.

Steinberg, L. (2004). Risk taking in adolescence: What changes, and why? *Annals of the New York Academy of Sciences, 1021*(1), 51–58.

Stevenson, F., Zimmerman, M. A., & Caldwell, C. H. (2007). Growth trajectories of sexual risk behavior in adolescence and young adulthood. *American Journal of Public Health, 97*(6), 1096–1101.

Taris, T. W., & Semin, G. R. (1997). Parent-child interaction during adolescence and the adolescent's sexual experience: Control, closeness, and conflict. *Journal of Youth and Adolescence, 26*(4), 373–398.

Vesely, S. K., Wyatt, V. H., Oman, R. F., Aspy, C. B., Kegler, M. C., Rodine, S., Marshall, L., & McLeroy, K. R. (2004). The potential protective effects of youth assets from adolescent sexual risk behaviors. *Journal of Adolescent Health, 34*(5), 356–365.

Wight, D., Williamson, L., & Henderson, M. (2006). Parental influences on young people's sexual behavior: A longitudinal analysis. *Journal of Adolescence, 29*(4), 473–494.

Willett, J. B., & Bub, K. L. (2005). Structural equation modeling: Latent growth curve analysis. In B. S. Everitt, D. C. Howell (Eds.), & D. Rindskopf (Section Ed.), *Encyclopedia of statistics in behavioral science* (pp. 772–779). Chichester: Wiley.

Willett, J. B., Singer, J. D., & Martin, N. C. (1998). The design and analysis of longitudinal studies of development and psychopathology in context: Statistical models and methodological recommendations. *Development and Psychopathology, 10*(2), 395–426.

Young, E. W., Jensen, L. C., Olsen, J. A., & Cundick, B. P. (1991). The effects of family structure on the sexual behavior of adolescents. *Adolescence, 26*(104), 977–986.

Zabin, L. S., & Hayward, S. C. (1993). *Adolescent sexual behavior and childbearing*. Newbury Park: Sage.

Family Attributes, Family Functioning, and Positive Youth Development as Predictors of Adolescent Self-Harm: A Longitudinal Study in Hong Kong

Daniel T.L. Shek and Li Lin

Abstract Utilizing four waves of longitudinal data ($N=3{,}328$ at Wave 1), the present study examined the influence of family attributes (family intactness and economic disadvantage), family functioning, and positive youth development on self-harm and suicidal behavior of Chinese adolescents in Hong Kong. While 17.1–24.7 % of students had deliberately harmed themselves at least once, there were decreasing trends of deliberate self-harm behavior and suicidal signs over 4 years. For sociodemographic correlates, family intactness but not economic disadvantage was related to initial deliberate self-harm and suicidal behavior. Besides, suicidal behaviors in adolescents from non-intact families decreased faster than those from intact families. At Wave 4, family functioning and positive youth development negatively predicted deliberate self-harm behavior and suicidal behavior. While Wave 1 positive youth development predicted Wave 4 deliberate self-harm without controlling the initial level of deliberated self-harm, Wave 1 family functioning predicted Wave 4 suicidal signs even after controlling the initial level of suicidal signs.

Introduction

Adolescent self-harm, including both suicidal behavior and deliberate self-harm without suicidal intent, has become a global concern (Hawton et al. 2012). For young people aged from 10 to 24, self-inflicted injury has become the second most common cause of death globally (Patton et al. 2009). The prevalence rate of suicidal attempt among Hong Kong nonclinical adolescents ranged from 3.3 % to 8.4 % (Cheung et al. 2013; Lee et al. 2005; Shek and Yu 2012; Stewart et al. 2006; Wan

This work and the Project PATHS are financially supported by the Hong Kong Jockey Club Charities Trust.

D.T.L. Shek (✉) • L. Lin
Department of Applied Social Sciences, The Hong Kong Polytechnic University,
11 Yuk Choi Road, Hung Hom, Kowloon, Hong Kong, China
e-mail: daniel.shek@polyu.edu.hk

© Springer Science+Business Media Singapore 2015
T.Y. Lee et al. (eds.), *Student Well-Being in Chinese Adolescents in Hong Kong*,
Quality of Life in Asia 7, DOI 10.1007/978-981-287-582-2_21

275

and Leung 2010; Yip et al. 2004). Though it is comparatively lower than the prevalence rate among Western adolescents (see Shek et al. 2005; Stewart et al. 2006; Yip et al. 2004), suicide has become a leading cause of death for youth in Hong Kong (Yip et al. 2004).

Deliberate self-harm (i.e., non-suicidal self-injury) is a distinct form of self-harm which refers to the purposeful, self-inflicted, socially unsanctioned destruction or alteration of body tissue without conscious suicidal intent (Nock and Favazza 2009). On the one hand, deliberate self-harm can co-occur with suicidal attempts (Cheung et al. 2013). On the other hand, deliberate self-harm is differentiated from suicidal behavior in function (Andover et al. 2012). While adolescents attempting suicide hold a purpose to end their lives, adolescents with a history of deliberate self-harm often report to use this approach to regulate negative affect such as relieving anxiety or elicit other's attention (Jacobson and Gould 2007; Messer and Fremouw 2008).

In Hong Kong, 1-year prevalence among adolescents was around 14 % when five primary forms of deliberate self-harm behavior (i.e., self-cutting, self-burning, punching, reckless and risky behavior, and others) were assessed (Cheung et al. 2013). If more behaviors were included, the rate was even higher, with 24.9 % in You et al.'s (2012) study (11 forms) and 23.5 % in Law and Shek's (2013) study (17 forms).

Several observations can be highlighted from previous studies on adolescent deliberate self-harm and suicidal behavior. First, although some studies have been conducted to understand the prevalence of adolescent deliberate self-harm and suicide (e.g., Cheung et al. 2013; Law and Shek 2013; Skegg 2005), there are few studies on the changes of such behavior across the adolescent years (for an exception about deliberate self-harm over two late-adolescent years, see Barrocas et al. 2014). Some research suggests that self-harm behavior increases in adolescence because puberty and challenge of developmental tasks render adolescents more vulnerable to negative life events (see Conner and Goldston 2007; Shek et al. 2005). In Lee and Tsang's (2004) research, the 1-year prevalence of suicidal behavior of 15–19 age group was higher than that of the 10–14 age group. Yet, dissimilar patterns were observed in other studies (Lee et al. 2009; You and Leung 2012). As such, it is necessary to directly examine the developmental course of adolescent self-harm, which possibly helps to identify the critical period for prevention and intervention.

Second, although some studies have examined the impact of family adversity on adolescent self-harm (see Greydanus and Shek 2009; Skegg 2005), few studies have studied how it influences the developmental trend of self-harm over adolescent years. For example, although broken families may increase the risk of adolescent self-harm (e.g., Laye-Gindhu and Schonert-Reichl 2005; Shek and Yu 2012) and adolescents living in families with financial difficulties are more likely to report self-harm (e.g., Baetens et al. 2014; Shek and Yu 2012), their influences on the developmental trends are not clear.

Third, compared to risk factors, protective factors in adolescent self-harm and suicidal behavior are not well understood. Family functioning and positive youth development as protective factors have been considered to be relevant in previous literature (Law and Shek 2013, 2014; Shek and Yu 2012). Adolescents without self-harm often experienced better family relationship and family climate than those with self-harm (Lai and McBride-Chang 2001; Wan and Leung 2010; Wong et al. 2007; Yip et al. 2004). In addition to the direct link between family functioning and adolescent self-harm, Law and Shek (2014) found that Year 1 family functioning influenced Year 3 deliberate self-harm and suicide through Year 2 positive youth development among Hong Kong adolescents.

Positive youth development perspective posits that optimizing adolescent positive youth development would help to diminish their problems (Benson et al. 2006; Lerner et al. 2012). Nevertheless, whether this argument is valid in the case of deliberate self-harm and suicide is far from clear, since the majority of the research on adolescent problems includes externalizing problems like delinquent behavior and substance use as well as internalizing problems like depression (Arbeit et al. 2014; Geldhof et al. 2014; Shek and Lin 2014) without inclusion of self-harm thoughts and behavior. The only exception was the study conducted by Shek and colleagues who found that positive youth development was associated with these self-harm behaviors concurrently in Secondary 1 (Shek and Yu 2012) and Secondary 2 students (Law and Shek 2013) and longitudinally with one year interval (Law and Shek 2014).

Against this background, we examined deliberate self-harm and suicidal behavior with a large sample of Hong Kong adolescents using four waves of data. Three research questions were addressed in this study as follows:

- Research question 1: What are the developmental trajectories of deliberate self-harm behavior and suicidal signs during adolescence?
- Research question 2: Do adverse family attributes (family non-intactness and economic disadvantage) affect the initial levels and developmental patterns of self-harm and suicidal behavior?

  - Hypothesis 1a: Adolescents in non-intact families would show higher initial levels of deliberate self-harm behavior and suicidal signs than those in intact families.
  - Hypothesis 1b: Adolescents in poor families would show higher initial levels of deliberate self-harm behavior and suicidal signs than those in nonpoor families.

- Research question 3: What are the concurrent and longitudinal relationships of family functioning and positive youth development with self-harm behavior and suicidal behavior? Based on the previous literature (e.g., Greydanus and Shek 2009; Law and Shek 2013, 2014; Skegg 2005), the following hypotheses were tested:

  - Hypothesis 2a: Family functioning would be negatively associated with deliberate self-harm behavior and suicidal signs at Wave 4.
  - Hypothesis 2b: Positive youth development would be negatively associated with deliberate self-harm behavior and suicidal signs at Wave 4.
  - Hypothesis 3a: Family functioning at Wave 1 predicted lower levels of deliberate self-harm behavior and suicidal signs at Wave 4.
  - Hypothesis 3b: Positive youth development at Wave 1 predicted lower levels of deliberate self-harm behavior and suicidal signs at Wave 4.

Method

Participants and Procedure

A total of 3,328 Secondary 1 students (Mage = 12.59 ± 0.74 years; 47.2 % female) from 28 local secondary schools were recruited to join our ongoing 6-year longitudinal study. They were assessed approximately annually on multiple domains of adjustment and family processes. This study included four waves of data with acceptable attrition rates: 12.7 % (Wave 2), 14.1 % (Wave 3), and 19.4 % (Wave 4). The characteristics of participants were presented in Table 1.

During regular school hours, students completed a battery of questionnaires. Study purpose was explained and the confidentiality of the data was emphasized to all the participating students before the administration.

Instruments

Students responded to items and questions assessing deliberate self-harm behavior, suicidal signs, positive youth development, family functioning, and demographic information on four occasions. The scales have good psychometric properties in previous studies (Law and Shek 2013; Shek and Lin 2014; Shek and Tsui 2012) and this study (see Table 2).

Self-Harm Adolescents reported on whether they had engaged in 17 forms of deliberate self-harm behavior without suicidal ideation using a checklist (0 = no; 1 = yes). The forms of deliberate self-harm behavior were presented in Table 3. A

Table 1 Data profile across four waves

	Wave 1	%	Wave 2[a]	%	Wave 3[a]	%	Wave 4[a]	%
N (participants)	3,328		2,905		2,858		2,682	
Gender								
Male	1,719	51.7	1,445	49.7	1,433	50.1	1,335	49.8
Female	1,572	47.2	1,419	48.8	1,405	49.2	1,337	49.9
Economic disadvantage								
Not receiving CSSA	2,606	78.3	2,377	81.8	2,339	81.8	2,267	84.5
Receiving CSSA	225	6.8	160	5.5	147	5.1	132	4.9
Family intactness								
Intact families	2,781	83.6	2,415	83.1	2,396	83.8	2,211	82.4
Non-intact families	515	15.5	469	16.1	454	15.9	466	17.4

[a]The numbers were based on the participants who participated in the Wave 1 assessment as only those joining Wave 1 assessment were included in LMM. The numbers of the students who did not report the corresponding information were not presented

Table 2 Descriptive statistics of key variables and internal consistency coefficients of scales

	Mean		(SD)			Reliability			
	W1	W2	W3	W4		W1	W2	W3	W4
Family functioning[a]	3.73 (0.81)	3.65 (0.81)	3.65 (0.79)	3.66 (0.77)		0.90	0.90	0.90	0.91
Positive youth development[a]	4.51 (0.70)	4.43 (0.69)	4.44 (0.65)	4.45 (0.62)		0.93	0.96	0.96	0.96
Deliberate self-harm behavior[b]	0.65 (1.66)	0.65 (1.67)	0.51 (1.37)	0.36 (1.08)		0.83	0.83	0.79	0.75
Male	0.59 (1.67)	0.46 (1.50)	0.37 (1.20)	0.28 (0.87)		–	–	–	–
Female	0.73 (1.64)	0.84 (1.81)	0.67 (1.52)	0.45 (1.25)		–	–	–	–
Not receiving CSSA	0.62 (1.53)	0.64 (1.66)	0.51 (1.36)	0.34 (1.03)		–	–	–	–
Receiving CSSA	0.66 (1.69)	1.08 (2.26)	0.68 (2.26)	0.50 (1.19)		–	–	–	–
Intact families	0.60 (1.56)	0.61 (1.62)	0.50 (1.37)	0.34 (1.05)		–	–	–	–
Non-intact families	0.95 (2.10)	0.89 (1.92)	0.61 (1.42)	0.53 (1.24)		–	–	–	–
Suicidal signs[b]	0.23 (0.62)	0.22 (0.61)	0.19 (0.55)	0.14 (0.47)		0.68	0.69	0.66	0.63
Male	0.17 (0.54)	0.15 (0.52)	0.12 (0.45)	0.10 (0.41)		–	–	–	–
Female	0.29 (0.69)	0.29 (0.69)	0.25 (0.64)	0.17 (0.52)		–	–	–	–
Not receiving CSSA	0.22 (0.60)	0.22 (0.60)	0.19 (0.55)	0.13 (0.44)		–	–	–	–
Receiving CSSA	0.33 (0.73)	0.32 (0.74)	0.30 (0.71)	0.22 (0.64)		–	–	–	–
Intact families	0.21 (0.59)	0.21 (0.60)	0.17 (0.53)	0.13 (0.46)		–	–	–	–
Non-intact families	0.35 (0.76)	0.28 (0.67)	0.29 (0.69)	0.14 (0.49)		–	–	–	–

W1 Wave 1, *W2* Wave 2, *W3* Wave 3, *W4* Wave 4

[a]Mean scores were used for indicate the levels of family functioning and positive youth development

[b]Sum scores were used to indicate the levels of deliberate self-harm behavior (range = 1–17) and suicidal behavior (range = 1–3) for easy interpretation

sum score was taken with higher numbers indicating more serious deliberate self-harm. Suicidal signs were assessed by suicidal ideation, plan, and attempt using a checklist (0 = no; 1 = yes). A sum score was adopted with higher numbers indicating stronger suicidal signs.

Table 3 Percentages of students with deliberate self-harm behavior and suicidal signs in the past 12 months across 4 waves

	Wave 1		Wave 2		Wave 3		Wave 4	
	N	%	N	%	N	%	N	%
Deliberate self-harm behavior								
1. Wrist cutting	277	8.3	254	8.7	188	6.8	118	4.6
2. Burn with cigarette	26	0.8	27	0.9	20	0.7	5	0.2
3. Burn with fire	42	1.3	35	1.2	22	0.8	9	0.3
4. Carving word on body	161	4.8	143	4.9	97	3.5	63	2.4
5. Carving marks on body	169	5.1	127	4.4	98	3.5	70	2.7
6. Self-scratching	343	10.3	310	10.7	243	8.8	160	6.2
7. Biting	244	7.3	200	6.9	160	5.8	97	3.7
8. Rubbing sandpaper	30	0.9	20	0.7	8	0.3	7	0.3
9. Acid dripping	10	0.3	9	0.3	6	0.2	3	0.1
10. Bleach scrubbing	16	0.5	15	0.5	4	0.1	6	0.2
11. Sharp objects into body	103	3.1	70	2.4	40	1.4	25	1.0
12. Rub glass into skin	52	1.6	36	1.2	16	0.6	9	0.3
13. Break bones	20	0.6	13	0.4	8	0.3	4	0.2
14. Head banging	138	4.1	101	3.5	68	2.5	46	1.8
15. Self-punching	184	5.5	150	5.2	120	4.3	72	2.8
16. Prevent wound from healing	272	8.2	276	9.6	261	9.4	213	8.2
17. Other forms of self-harm	148	4.4	98	3.4	78	2.8	48	1.9
At least one self-harm behavior	830	24.7	686	23.6	605	21.9	433	17.1
Suicidal signs								
1. Suicidal thoughts	446	13.4	385	13.3	316	11.4	230	8.9
2. Suicidal plans	158	4.7	145	5.0	111	4.0	76	2.9
3. Suicidal attempts	152	4.6	118	4.1	95	3.4	49	1.9
Total number	3,328	100	2,905	100	2,764	100	2,588	100

Note: One school ($N=124$) declined to report deliberate self-harm behavior and suicidal signs since Wave 3, and thus its students were recovered from calculating prevalence on Wave 3 and 4

Family Functioning Family functioning was assessed by the simplified version of the Chinese family assessment instrument (Shek 2002). Mutuality (mutual support, love, and concern among family members), communication (frequency and nature of interaction among family members), conflicts, and harmony (presence of conflicts and harmonious behavior in the family) were assessed with three items each in a 5-point scale. After reversing the appropriate items, nine items were averaged with higher scores indicating better family functioning.

Positive Youth Development Positive youth development was evaluated with the trimmed version of the Chinese positive youth development scale (CPYDS; Shek et al. 2007; Sun and Shek 2013), which covered the 15 developmental assets proposed by Catalano et al. (2004). Two to three items were made to measure these developmental assets in a 6-point scale except spirituality (7-point scale). All items were averaged to yield a positive youth development variable.

Family Attributes (Economic Disadvantage and Family Intactness) Economic disadvantage was categorized in terms of receiving comprehensive social security assistance (CSSA) or not. In Hong Kong, families receiving CSSA were considered to have financial difficulties (Wong 2005). Therefore, adolescents who reported receiving CSSA were categorized as poor group while those who reported not receiving CSSA were categorized as nonpoor group (see Table 1). This way of defining families experiencing economic disadvantage has been used in the prior studies (Shek and Lin 2014; Shek and Tsui 2012). For family intactness, we referred to the marital status of adolescents' parents. Only adolescents with parents in the first marriage were regarded as living in intact families, while those with parents separated, divorced, remarried, or in other marital status were identified as living in non-intact families (see Table 1). Adolescents who did not report the information of family attributes were excluded from the corresponding analyses.

Data Analysis Plan

In order to understand the developmental patterns of deliberate self-harm behavior and suicidal signs, two-level individual growth curve modeling was performed with time (Level 1) being nested within individual (Level 2). We coded time as $0 =$ Wave 1, $1 =$ Wave 2, $2 =$ Wave 3, and $3 =$ Wave 4. The first level describes the aggregated developmental trajectory, which includes the average within-person initial level and rate of change over time without other predictors. The second level tests how individual characteristics influence the initial status and the rate of change. We primarily examined the effects of economic disadvantage (i.e., receiving CSSA or not) and family intactness while controlling gender and initial age.

Individual growth curve was conducted by using the linear mixed model (LMM) in SPSS 22.0 statistical software (IBM SPSS Statistics, IBM Corp, Somers, NY) with maximum likelihood (ML) as estimation method. Three steps were taken for LMM. Firstly, we estimated an unconditional mean model (Model 1) to identify the proportion of between-person variance of self-harm over the sum of the variances (i.e., intraclass correlation coefficient or ICC; Singer and Willett 2003). Secondly, we estimated an unconditional growth model (Model 2), in which the aggregated developmental trajectories of these participants were investigated. Lastly, we estimated a conditional model with economic disadvantage and family intactness as major level 2 predictors while controlling for initial age and gender (Model 3).

For the level 2 predictors, dummy codes were given to categorical variables (gender, female $=-1$, male $= 1$; economic disadvantage, not receiving CSSA $=-1$, receiving CSSA $= 1$; family intactness, non-intact family $=-1$, intact family $= 1$), while grand mean centering was taken for continuous variable (i.e., initial age) for the simplification in interpreting results (Shek and Ma 2011). Three indexes that have been commonly used in previous research were used to evaluate models: $-2\log$ likelihood (i.e., likelihood ratio test), Akaike information criterion (AIC), and Bayesian information criterion (BIC) (Shek and Ma 2011; Kwok et al. 2008) with smaller numbers representing better model fit. The proposed final models for self-harm, denoted by the term, Y_{tj}, were as follows:

$$\text{Level 1:} \quad Y_{tj} = \beta_{0j} + \beta_{1j}(\text{Time}) + r_{tj}$$

where β_{0j} is the initial level of self-harm for jth individual, β_{1j} is the rate of change for jth individual, r_{tj} is the within-person random error in the self-harm for jth individual at time t, and Y_{tj} is the repeated measure of self-harm for jth individual at time t.

$$\begin{aligned} \text{Level 2:} \quad \beta_{0j} &= \gamma_{00} + \gamma_{01}(\text{age}) + \gamma_{02}(\text{gender}) + \gamma_{03}(\text{economic disadvantage}) \\ &\quad + \gamma_{04}(\text{family intactness}) + u_{0j} \\ \beta_{1j} &= \gamma_{10} + \gamma_{11}(\text{age}) + \gamma_{12}(\text{gender}) + \gamma_{13}(\text{economic disadvantage}) \\ &\quad + \gamma_{14}(\text{family intactness}) + u_{1j} \end{aligned}$$

where γ_{01}, γ_{02}, γ_{03}, and γ_{04} represent whether the demographic factors (i.e., age, gender, economic disadvantage, and family intactness) are associated with the initial level of self-harm; γ_{11}, γ_{12}, γ_{13}, and γ_{14} represent the extent to which demographic factors influence developmental change of self-harm; γ_{00} is the initial level of self-harm for the whole sample; γ_{10} is the linear slope of change relating to the self-harm for the whole sample; and u_{0j} and u_{1j} are the between-person random error that are not explained by level 2 predictors for the intercept and slope, respectively.

For concurrent effects, we used the Wave 4 data to examine whether family functioning and positive youth development were associated with deliberate self-harm behavior and suicidal signs, respectively, above and beyond the effects of demographic predictors (i.e., gender, economic disadvantage, and family intactness). For overtime effects, we used Wave 1 family functioning and positive youth development to predict Wave 4 deliberate self-harm behavior and suicidal behavior, respectively. We examined their overtime effects in two regression models, including one with initial levels controlled and the other without inclusion of initial levels.

Results

While the prevalence of each deliberate self-harm behavior was not high, the proportion of students who ever conducted at least one deliberate self-harm behavior was notably high across four waves of assessment (17.1–24.7 %; Table 3). In particular, quite a significant proportion of students engaged in self-scratching (6.2–10.7 %), preventing wound from healing (8.2–9.6 %), and wrist cutting (4.6–8.7 %). Meanwhile, while suicidal plans and attempts were not prevalent, the proportion of adolescents who had suicidal ideation was quite remarkable (8.9–13 %). However, decreasing trends of deliberate self-harm behavior and suicidal behavior over 4 years were also observed.

The results of individual growth curve models are presented in Table 4. Firstly, unconditional mean models (Model 1) of deliberate self-harm behavior and suicidal behavior showed that about 42.1 % (ICC=0.421) and 39.2 % (ICC=0.392) of the total variation were due to interindividual differences, which indicated a need for further multilevel analyses (Lee 2000; Shek and Ma 2011).

Secondly, the unconditional growth model (Model 2) of deliberate self-harm behavior fitted the data better than Model 1 ($\Delta\chi^2_{(3)}=430.89, p<0.001$; ΔAIC=424.89; ΔBIC=402.98). According to Model 2, the initial level of deliberate self-harm behavior was not high, and it decreased linearly by an average of 0.092 unit per year. The unconditional growth model (Model 2) of suicidal behavior also improved the model fit as compared to Model 1 ($\Delta\chi^2_{(3)}=263.10$, $p<0.001$; ΔAIC=257.10; ΔBIC=235.06). According to Model 2, the initial level of suicidal signs was not strong, and it decreased linearly by an average of 0.028 unit per year.

Finally, as significant between-person random errors were found in the intercepts and slopes for deliberate self-harm behavior and suicidal signs, economic disadvantage and family intactness were added as level 2 predictors of the intercepts and the slopes with gender and initial age as covariates. The conditional models (Model 3) of deliberate self-harm behavior ($\Delta\chi^2_{(8)}=6,458.75$, $p<0.001$; ΔAIC=6,442.75; ΔBIC=6,386.78) and suicidal behavior ($\Delta\chi^2_{(8)}=3,306.14$, $p<0.001$; ΔAIC=3,284.14; ΔBIC=3,205.82) fitted the data better than corresponding Model 2. For the predictors of the intercept of deliberate self-harm, results showed that the effect of family intactness was significant above and beyond the effects of initial age and gender. Specifically, as compared to adolescents from intact families, adolescents from non-intact families reported more deliberate self-harm behavior at the initial assessment. However, no significant association was detected between economic disadvantage and the initial level of deliberate self-harm behavior, which indicates initial deliberate self-harm behavior did not differ by receiving CSSA or not. Level 2 predictors explained 14.2 % of the intercept variance of deliberate self-harm behavior. For the predictors of the intercept of suicidal signs, the effect of family intactness was significant above and beyond the effects of initial age and gender. Similar to the case of deliberate self-harm behavior, adolescents from non-intact families demonstrated more suicidal signs than those from intact families at the initial assessment.

For the predictors of slopes, results revealed that neither family intactness nor economic disadvantage was associated with the change rate of deliberate self-harm behavior above and beyond the effects of initial age and gender. Level 2 predictors explained 57.0 % of the slope variance in deliberate self-harm behavior, which was possibly owing to the age effect. In the model of suicidal signs, family intactness was associated with the change rate above and beyond the effects of initial age and gender, with adolescents from non-intact families decreasing faster than those from intact families. Level 2 predictors explained 20 % of the slope variance of suicidal

Table 4 Results of individual growth curve of deliberate self-harm and suicidal signs for all models

		Deliberate self-harm behavior						Suicidal signs					
		Model 1		Model 2		Model 3		Model 1		Model 2		Model 3	
		Estimate	SE	Estimate	SE	Estimate	SE	Estimate	SE	Estimate	SE	Estimate	SE
Fixed effects													
Intercept	β_{0j}												
Initial status	γ_{00}	0.584***	0.001	0.707***	0.029	0.823***	0.059	0.243***	0.010	0.242***	0.010	0.308***	0.022
Age	γ_{01}					0.028	0.042					0.012	0.016
Gender	γ_{02}					−0.138***	0.030					−0.071***	0.011
Economic disadvantage	γ_{03}					0.027	0.061					0.021	0.023
Family intactness	γ_{04}					−0.141**	0.046					−0.062***	0.017
Linear slope	β_{1j}												
Initial status	γ_{10}			−0.092***	0.011	−0.088***	0.022			−0.028**	0.004	−0.036***	0.009
Age	γ_{11}					−0.034*	0.016					0.000	0.006
Gender	γ_{12}					0.005	0.011					0.009*	0.004
Economic disadvantage	γ_{13}					0.022	0.017					0.003	0.009
Family intactness	γ_{14}					0.018	0.023					0.014*	0.007

Random effects		Est.	SE	Est.	SE	Est.	SE	Est.	SE	Est.	SE	Est.	SE
Level 1 (within)													
Residual	r_{ij}	1.320***	0.021	1.188***	0.024	1.202***	0.026	0.203***	0.003	0.178***	0.004	0.180***	0.004
Level 2 (between)													
Intercept	u_{0j}	0.958	0.037	1.748***	0.071	1.500***	0.071	0.131***	0.005	0.222***	0.009	0.210***	0.010
Time	u_{1j}			0.086***	0.011	0.037***	0.011			0.015***	0.002	0.012***	0.002
Fit statistics													
Deviance		38,237.66		37,806.76		31,348.01		18,031.331		17,768.234		14,725.19	
AIC		38,243.66		37,818.76		31,376.01		18,037.331		17,780.234		14,753.19	
BIC		38,265.57		37,862.59		31,475.82		18,059.364		17,824.300		14,853.54	
df		3		6		14		3		6		14	

Note: Model 1 = unconditional mean model; Model 2 = unconditional growth model; Model 3 = conditional model

*$p < 0.05$; **$p < 0.01$; ***$p < 0.001$

Table 5 Predictors of deliberate self-harm and suicidal signs at Wave 4

Predictors	Deliberate self-harm behavior		Suicidal signs	
	Beta	ΔR^2	Beta	ΔR^2
Step 1		*0.008***		*0.006**
Gender[a]	−0.077***		−0.073**	
Economic disadvantage[b]	−0.015		0.011	
Family intactness[c]	−0.032		0.008	
Step 2		*0.044****		*0.054****
Family functioning	**−0.093***		**−0.137***	
Positive youth development	**−0.152***		**−0.141***	

*$p < 0.05$; **$p < 0.01$; ***$p < 0.001$
[a]Male = 1, female = 0
[b]Receiving CSSA = 1, not receiving CSSA = 0
[c]Intact = 1, non-intact = 0

signs. However, suggested by the gamma coefficients, the faster decrease rate in the adolescents from non-intact families did not offset the higher initial levels of suicidal signs. Therefore, those from non-intact families (vs. intact families) had higher overall levels of suicidal signs throughout the course of study.

For concurrent effects at Wave 4 (see Table 5), multiple regression analyses demonstrated that beyond the effects of demographic factors, family functioning and positive youth development were inversely related with deliberate self-harm behavior and suicidal signs, which accounted for additional 4.4 % and 5.4 % of the variances, respectively.

For the longitudinal effects of deliberate self-harm behavior, Wave 1 positive youth development predicted Wave 4 deliberate self-harm behavior. However, when the initial level was controlled, neither family functioning nor positive youth development had longitudinal effects on Wave 4 deliberate self-harm (see Table 6). Additionally, Wave 1 family functioning predicted Wave 4 suicidal behavior even after the initial level was controlled.

Discussion

Our findings showed that the prevalence rate of having at least one deliberate self-harm behavior was quite high across 4 years of investigation. Although prevalence rates of suicidal plan and attempt were not high, quite a proportion of students reported having suicidal thoughts. Together with previous research examining the prevalence rate among Hong Kong adolescents (e.g., Cheung et al. 2013; You et al. 2012), these results underscore the importance of investigating Hong Kong adolescents' self-harm with a goal of facilitating prevention and intervention. Our investigation on developmental courses of deliberate self-harm and suicidal behavior could suggest a critical period for prevention and intervention. Also, our

Table 6 Wave 1 variables predict Wave 4 deliberate self-harm and suicidal signs

Predictors	Deliberate self-harm behavior				Suicidal signs			
	Controlling initial level		Not controlling initial level		Controlling initial level		Not controlling initial level	
	Beta	ΔR²	Beta	ΔR²	Beta	ΔR²	Beta	ΔR²
Step 1								
Initial level	0.290***	0.095***			0.199***	0.054***		
Step 2		0.003		0.007**		0.004*		0.008**
Gender[a]	−0.028		−0.056*		−0.016		−0.037	
Economic disadvantage[b]	0.011		0.021		0.066*		0.074**	
Family intactness[c]	−0.037		−0.035		0.039		0.041	
Step 3		0.003		0.016***		0.010***		0.027***
Family functioning	−0.005		−0.055		**−0.088****		**−0.133*****	
Positive youth development	−0.055		**−0.089****		−0.030		−0.051	

Note: Standardized beta weights in the final regression model are shown above

$*p<0.05$; $**p<0.01$; $***p<0.001$

[a]Male = 1, female = 0

[b]Receiving CSSA = 1, not receiving CSSA = 0

[c]Intact = 1, non-intact = 0

investigation on family attributes, family functioning, and positive youth development as predictors of self-harm also suggests risk and protective factors for deliberate self-harm and suicidal behavior.

To our best knowledge, the present study is the first study to track the developmental course of adolescent self-harm in a community sample over 4 years. We found that there were declining trends in both deliberate self-harm and suicidal behavior. Transition into secondary school typically coincides with pyramid changes and challenges in individual, school, peer, and family contexts (Eccles and Midgley 1989). A wealth of research has indicated this period as a vulnerable time for the onset of multiple psychological difficulties, such as increased depression and psychological distress (e.g., Chung et al. 1998; Hankin et al. 1998), which are associated with engagement in self-harm (Conner and Goldston 2007; Wong et al. 2007). With adjustment to secondary school life, self-harm problem becomes less severe, which is consistent with a decreasing trend of anxiety over secondary school year in the extant literature (e.g., Benner and Graham 2009). These findings indicate that transition into secondary school may be a critical period for prevention and intervention, while more investigation is needed over the transition process from primary school to secondary school for a better understanding of the changes of adolescents' related mental states.

While extant literature suggests that family attributes were related to adolescent engagement in self-harm (Greydanus and Shek 2009; Skegg 2005), this study only found the effects of family intactness. Consistent with some previous research (e.g., Laye-Gindhu and Schonert-Reichl 2005; Wan and Leung 2010; Yip et al. 2004), adolescents living in non-intact families (vs. intact families) reported higher initial levels of deliberate self-harm and suicidal behavior. Fortunately, over the 4 years, they reduced suicidal signs faster than those from intact families, which is in line with the previous finding that the negative impact of family disruption might be minimized over time (Malone et al. 2004). Nevertheless, it should be noted that the overall levels of both deliberate self-harm and suicidal behavior among adolescents from non-intact families were consistently higher than their counterparts from intact families, as the higher decrease rate in adolescents from non-intact families cannot offset their higher initial levels. In contrast, the absence of poverty effects in this study and previous studies (e.g., Shek and Lin 2014) implies a need to investigate the resilience of poor adolescents in Hong Kong (e.g., positive self-concept, parental support, positive peer relationship; Everall et al. 2006).

Positive youth development was linked to deliberate self-harm while family functioning was linked to suicidal signs 3 years later. In particular, the effect of family functioning on suicidal behavior was significant even after using a stringent approach by controlling the initial level of suicidal behavior. On the one hand, these results suggest that promoting positive youth development and improving family functioning may be helpful to prevent adolescents from self-harm. In particular, this study goes beyond previous research documenting the concurrent relations of family functioning and positive youth development attributes, including social competence (Baetens et al. 2012), self-esteem (Hawton et al. 2002), and parental bonding (Hsu and Chen 2013), with adolescent self-harm by investigating their overtime associations. Results suggest that positive youth development and adaptive family functioning are protective antecedents of adolescent deliberate self-harm and suicidal signs, respectively. On the other hand, given that the effect sizes of positive youth development and family functioning were small, other influential proactive factors probably take a role in reducing adolescent self-harm, such as peer support (e.g., Kerr et al. 2006).

This study has several limitations. First, this study did not regard family attributes as dynamic variables but families might experience changes of economic status and family structure during the 4 years. Previous studies also have suggested that fluctuation of family economic status rather than family poverty itself makes a difference in adolescent problem (Pagani et al. 1999), and the negative impact of family disruption might fade out with time (Malone et al. 2004). It is thus necessary to consider duration when relating family poverty and family disruption to adolescent self-harm. Moreover, we examined the severity of self-harm in terms of the number of self-harm behavior. However, the severity could be manifested in the frequency and recurrence of self-harm as well (Lloyd-Richardson et al. 2007; You and Leung 2012), which should be examined in future studies. Besides, the findings are confined to adolescents in Hong Kong only. Hence, replications of the findings in other adolescent populations are necessary. Finally, we only used self-report without the involvement of any other informants for all the variables. Admittedly, self-harm is a private or even hidden behavior (Greydanus and Shek 2009), which is thus often examined by self-report. Nonetheless, parents and teachers may be helpful to provide other information like positive youth development and family functioning.

References

Andover, M. S., Morris, B. W., Wren, A., & Bruzzese, M. E. (2012). The co-occurrence of non-suicidal self-injury and attempted suicide among adolescents: Distinguishing risk factors and psychosocial correlates. *Child and Adolescent Psychiatry and Mental Health, 6*(11). doi:10.1186/1753-2000-6-11

Arbeit, M. R., Johnson, S. K., Champine, R. B., Greenman, K. N., Lerner, J. V., & Lerner, R. M. (2014). Profiles of problematic behaviors across adolescence: Covariations with indicators of positive youth development. *Journal of Youth and Adolescence, 43*(6), 971–990.

Baetens, I., Claes, L., Muehlenkamp, J., Grietens, H., & Onghena, P. (2012). Differences in psychological symptoms and self-competencies in non-suicidal self-injurious Flemish adolescents. *Journal of Adolescence, 35*(3), 753–759.

Baetens, I., Claes, L., Martin, G., Onghena, P., Grietens, H., Van Leeuwen, K., & Griffith, J. W. (2014). Is nonsuicidal self-injury associated with parenting and family factors? *The Journal of Early Adolescence, 34*(3), 387–405.

Barrocas, A. L., Giletta, M., Hankin, B. L., Prinstein, M. J., & Abela, J. R. (2014). Nonsuicidal self-injury in adolescence: Longitudinal course, trajectories, and intrapersonal predictors. *Journal of Abnormal Child Psychology, 43*(2), 369–380.

Benner, A. D., & Graham, S. (2009). The transition to high school as a developmental process among multiethnic urban youth. *Child Development, 80*(2), 356–376.

Benson, P. L., Scales, P. C., Hamilton, S. F., & Sesma, A. (2006). Positive youth development: Theory, research, and applications. In R. M. Lerner (Ed.), & W. Damon & R. M. Lerner

(Editors-in-chief), *Handbook of child psychology: Theoretical models of human development* (Vol. 1, pp. 894–941). Hoboken: Wiley.

Catalano, R. F., Berglund, M. L., Ryan, J. A. M., Lonczak, H. S., & Hawkins, J. D. (2004). Positive youth development in the United States: Research findings on evaluations of positive youth development programs. *The Annals of the American Academy of Political Social Science, 591*, 98–124.

Cheung, Y. T. D., Wong, P. W. C., Lee, A. M., Lam, T. H., Fan, Y. S. S., & Yip, P. S. F. (2013). Non-suicidal self-injury and suicidal behavior: Prevalence, co-occurrence, and correlates of suicide among adolescents in Hong Kong. *Social Psychiatry and Psychiatric Epidemiology, 48*(7), 1133–1144.

Chung, H., Elias, M., & Schneider, K. (1998). Patterns of individual adjustment changes during middle school transition. *Journal of School Psychology, 36*(1), 83–101.

Conner, K. R., & Goldston, D. B. (2007). Rates of suicide among males increase steadily from age 11 to 21: Developmental framework and outline for prevention. *Aggression and Violent Behavior, 12*(2), 193–207.

Eccles, J. S., & Midgley, C. (1989). Stage-environment fit: Developmentally appropriate class-rooms for young adolescents. In R. E. Ames & C. Ames (Eds.), *Research on motivation in education* (Vol. 3, pp. 139–186). San Diego: Academic.

Everall, R. D., Altrows, K. J., & Paulson, B. L. (2006). Creating a future: A study of resilience in suicidal female adolescents. *Journal of Counseling & Development, 84*(4), 461–470.

Geldhof, G. G., Bowers, E., Mueller, M., Napolitano, C., Callina, K., & Lerner, R. (2014). Longitudinal analysis of a very short measure of positive youth development. *Journal of Youth and Adolescence, 43*(6), 933–949.

Greydanus, D. E., & Shek, D. (2009). Deliberate self-harm and suicide in adolescents. *The Keio Journal of Medicine, 58*(3), 144–151.

Hankin, B. L., Abramson, L. Y., Moffitt, T. E., Silva, P. A., McGee, R., & Angell, K. E. (1998). Development of depression from preadolescence to young adulthood: Emerging gender differences in a 10-year longitudinal study. *Journal of Abnormal Psychology, 107*(1), 128–140.

Hawton, K., Rodham, K., Evans, E., & Weatherall, R. (2002). Deliberate self harm in adolescents: Self report survey in schools in England. *BMJ, 325*(7374), 1207–1211.

Hawton, K., Saunders, K. E., & O'Connor, R. C. (2012). Self-harm and suicide in adolescents. *The Lancet, 379*(9834), 2373–2382.

Hsu, Y. F., & Chen, P. F. (2013). Parental bonding and personality characteristics of first episode intention to suicide or deliberate self-harm without a history of mental disorders. *BMC Public Health, 13*, 421. doi:10.1186/1471-2458-13-421.

Jacobson, C. M., & Gould, M. (2007). The epidemiology and phenomenology of non-suicidal self-injurious behavior among adolescents: A critical review of the literature. *Archives of Suicide Research, 11*, 129–147.

Kerr, D. C., Preuss, L. J., & King, C. A. (2006). Suicidal adolescents' social support from family and peers: Gender-specific associations with psychopathology. *Journal of Abnormal Child Psychology, 34*(1), 99–110.

Kwok, O. M., Underhill, A. T., Berry, J. W., Luo, W., Elliott, T. R., & Yoon, M. (2008). Analyzing longitudinal data with multilevel models: An example with individuals living with lower extremity intra-articular fractures. *Rehabilitation Psychology, 53*(3), 370–386.

Lai, K. W., & McBride-Chang, C. (2001). Suicidal ideation, parenting style, and family climate among Hong Kong adolescents. *International Journal of Psychology, 36*(2), 81–87.

Law, B. M. F., & Shek, D. T. L. (2013). Self-harm and suicide attempts among young Chinese adolescents in Hong Kong: Prevalence, correlates, and changes. *Journal of Pediatric and Adolescent Gynecology, 26*(3), 26–32.

Law, B. M., & Shek, D. T. (2014). A longitudinal study on deliberate self-harm and suicidal behaviors among Chinese adolescents. In D. T. L. Shek, R. C. F. Sun, & C. M. S. Ma (Eds.), *Chinese adolescents in Hong Kong – Family life, psychological well-being and risk behavior* (pp. 155–172). Singapore: Springer.

Laye-Gindhu, A., & Schonert-Reichl, K. A. (2005). Nonsuicidal self-harm among community adolescents: Understanding the "whats" and "whys" of self-harm. *Journal of Youth and Adolescence, 34*(5), 447–457.

Lee, V. E. (2000). Using hierarchical linear modeling to study social contexts: The case of school effects. *Educational Psychologist, 35*(2), 125–141.

Lee, A., & Tsang, C. K. K. (2004). Youth risk behaviour in a Chinese population: A territory-wide youth risk behavioural surveillance in Hong Kong. *Public Health, 118*(2), 88–95.

Lee, A., Lee, N., Tsang, C. K. K., Wong, W. C. W., Cheng, K. F. F., Wong, S. Y. S., et al. (2005). Youth risk behaviour survey, Hong Kong (2003/04). *Journal of Primary Care and Health Promotion.* Retrieved from http://www.cuhk.edu.hk/med/hep/research/pdf/reports/YRBS%20 2003.pdf

Lee, A., Wong, S. Y. S., Tsang, K. K., Ho, G. S. M., Wong, C. W., & Cheng, F. (2009). Understanding suicidality and correlates among Chinese secondary school students in Hong Kong. *Health Promotion International, 24*(2), 156–165.

Lerner, J. V., Bowers, E. P., Minor, K., Lewin-Bizan, S., Boyd, M. J., Mueller, M. K., ... & Lerner, R. M. (2012). Positive youth development: Processes, philosophies, and programs. In R. M. Lerner, M. A. Easterbrooks & J. Mistry (Eds.), & I. B. Weiner (Editor-in-Chief), *Comprehensive handbook of psychology: Developmental psychology* (Vol. 6, pp. 365–392). New York: Wiley.

Lloyd-Richardson, E. E., Perrine, N., Dierker, L., & Kelley, M. L. (2007). Characteristics and functions of non-suicidal self-injury in a community sample of adolescents. *Psychological Medicine, 37*(08), 1183–1192.

Malone, P. S., Lansford, J. E., Castellino, D. R., Berlin, L. J., Dodge, K. A., Bates, J. E., & Pettit, G. S. (2004). Divorce and child behavior problems: Applying latent change score models to life event data. *Structural Equation Modeling, 11*(3), 401–423.

Messer, J. M., & Fremouw, W. J. (2008). A critical review of explanatory models for self-mutilating behaviors in adolescents. *Clinical Psychology Review, 28*(1), 162–178.

Nock, M. K., & Favazza, A. R. (2009). Nonsuicidal self-injury: Definition and classification. In M. K. Nock (Ed.), *Understanding nonsuicidal self-injury: Origins, assessment, and treatment.* Washington, DC: American Psychological Association.

Pagani, L., Boulerice, B., Vitaro, F., & Tremblay, R. E. (1999). Effects of poverty on academic failure and delinquency in boys: A change and process model approach. *Journal of Child Psychology and Psychiatry, 40*(8), 1209–1219.

Patton, G. C., Coffey, C., Sawyer, S. M., Viner, R. M., Haller, D. M., Bose, K., & Mathers, C. D. (2009). Global patterns of mortality in young people: A systematic analysis of population health data. *The Lancet, 374*(9693), 881–892.

Shek, D. T. L. (2002). Assessment of family functioning in Chinese adolescents: The Chinese Family Assessment Instrument. *International Perspectives on Child and Adolescent Mental Health, 2*, 297–316.

Shek, D. T. L., & Lin, L. (2014). Development of delinquent behavior in early adolescents in Hong Kong. In D. T. L. Shek, R. C. F. Sun, & C. M. S. Ma (Eds.), *Chinese adolescents in Hong Kong – Family life, psychological well-being and risk behavior* (pp. 111–132). Singapore: Springer.

Shek, D. T. L., & Ma, C. M. S (2011). Longitudinal data analyses using linear mixed models in SPSS: Concepts, procedures and illustrations. *The Scientific World Journal, 11*, 42–76.

Shek, D. T. L., & Tsui, P. F. (2012). Family and personal adjustment of economically disadvantaged Chinese adolescents in Hong Kong. *The Scientific World Journal.* doi:10.1100/2012/142689.

Shek, D. T. L., & Yu, L. (2012). Self-harm and suicidal behaviors in Hong Kong adolescents: Prevalence and psychosocial correlates. *The Scientific World Journal.* doi:10.1100/2012/932540.

Shek, D. T. L., Lee, B. M., & Chow, J. (2005). Trends in adolescent suicide in Hong Kong for the period 1980 to 2003. *The Scientific World Journal, 5*, 702–723.

Shek, D. T. L., Siu, A. M. H., & Lee, T. Y. (2007). The Chinese positive youth development scale: A validation study. *Research on Social Work Practice, 17*(3), 380–391.

Singer, J. D., & Willett, J. B. (2003). *Applied longitudinal data analysis: Modeling change and event occurrence*. London: Oxford University Press.

Skegg, K. (2005). Self-harm. *The Lancet, 366*(9495), 1471–1483.

Stewart, S. M., Felice, E., Claassen, C., Kennard, B. D., Lee, P. W., & Emslie, G. J. (2006). Adolescent suicide attempters in Hong Kong and the United States. *Social Science & Medicine, 63*(2), 296–306.

Sun, R. C., & Shek, D. T. L. (2013). Longitudinal influences of positive youth development and life satisfaction on problem behaviour among adolescents in Hong Kong. *Social Indicators Research, 114*(3), 1171–1197.

Wan, G. W., & Leung, P. W. (2010). Factors accounting for youth suicide attempt in Hong Kong: A model building. *Journal of Adolescence, 33*(5), 575–582.

Wong, H. (2005). The quality of life of Hong Kong's poor households in the 1990s: Levels of expenditure, income security and poverty. *Social Indicators Research, 71*(1–3), 411–440.

Wong, J. P., Stewart, S. M., Ho, S. Y., & Lam, T. H. (2007). Risk factors associated with suicide attempts and other self – Injury among Hong Kong adolescents. *Suicide and Life-Threatening Behavior, 37*(4), 453–466.

Yip, P. S., Liu, K. Y., Lam, T. H., Stewart, S. M., Chen, E., & Fan, S. (2004). Suicidality among high school students in Hong Kong, SAR. *Suicide and Life-Threatening Behavior, 34*(3), 284–297.

You, J., & Leung, F. (2012). The role of depressive symptoms, family invalidation and behavioral impulsivity in the occurrence and repetition of non-suicidal self-injury in Chinese adolescents: A 2-year follow-up study. *Journal of Adolescence, 35*(2), 389–395.

You, J., Leung, F., & Fu, K. (2012). Exploring the reciprocal relations between nonsuicidal self-injury, negative emotions and relationship problems in Chinese adolescents: A longitudinal cross-lag study. *Journal of Abnormal Child Psychology, 40*(5), 829–836.

Internet Addiction in Hong Kong Adolescents Based on Four Waves of Longitudinal Data

Daniel T.L. Shek, Xinli Chi, and Lu Yu

Abstract Using longitudinal data with four waves from Secondary 1 to Secondary 4, the study investigated Internet addiction and its related psychosocial correlates (economic disadvantage, family intactness, family functioning, and positive youth development) among adolescents in Hong Kong. Results showed that although Internet addiction generally declined throughout the adolescent years, around one-fourth to one-fifth of students were classified as Internet addicts in this period. Adolescents from non-intact families reported higher initial levels of Internet addiction, and those from non-intact and nonpoor families reported faster decreasing rate in Internet addiction. Concurrently, family functioning and positive youth development negatively predicted Internet addictive behavior at Wave 4. Longitudinally, economic disadvantage experience and low positive youth development at Wave 1 positively predicted Internet addictive behavior at Wave 4. Findings suggest that while economic disadvantage and family non-intactness are risk factors, family functioning and positive youth development are protective factors in the development of adolescent Internet addiction.

Introduction

Internet addiction has been conceived as an individual's unregulated use of the Internet which leads to the development of symptoms such as cognitive and behavioral preoccupation with the Internet (Shek et al. 2012; Van den Eijnden et al. 2008). A vast literature has found that adolescent addiction to the Internet has resulted in academic failure, impaired social functioning, emotional problems, and psychiatric problems (Beard 2005; Kaltiala-Heino et al. 2004; Kuss et al. 2014; Yen et al. 2007a). Although adolescent Internet addition has become a significant public

The preparation for this paper and the Project P.A.T.H.S. were financially supported by The Hong Kong Jockey Club Charities Trust.

D.T.L. Shek (✉) • X. Chi • L. Yu
Department of Applied Social Sciences, The Hong Kong Polytechnic University,
11 Yuk Choi Road, Hung Hom, Kowloon, Hong Kong, China
e-mail: daniel.shek@polyu.edu.hk

health concern, longitudinal studies on Internet addiction are sparse, especially in the Asian context. As such, this study attempted to investigate Internet addiction in Hong Kong adolescents over a period of 4 years.

Many studies have been conducted to examine Internet addiction among adolescents around the world. In a study involving 11,956 adolescents in 11 European countries, the overall prevalence of Internet addiction was 4.4 % (Durkee et al. 2012). Based on a systematic review on 18 empirical studies of problematic Internet use among US youth, prevalence rates reported ranged from 0 % to 26.3 % (Moreno et al. 2011). A more recent study in Iran showed that 2.1 % of the participants were at risk and 5.2 % were Internet addicted (Salehi et al. 2014).

In the Asian contexts, some important prevalence studies have been carried out. Based on 1573 high school students in Korea, Kim et al. (2006) reported that 1.6 % of the participants were diagnosed as Internet addicts, while 38.0 % were classified as possible Internet addicts. In another study using nationally representative sample of college students in Taiwan ($N=3616$), 15.3 % of the students were diagnosed as having Internet addiction (Lin et al. 2011). A more recent study based on 755 adolescents in Wuhan, China, revealed that the prevalence rate of Internet addiction was 6.0 % among adolescent Internet users (Tang et al. 2014). In a nationally representative sample study based on middle school students recruited from 100 counties in 31 provinces in China, it was found the percentage of Internet addicts was 11.9 % (Li et al. 2014). Regarding Hong Kong, one study based on 3328 secondary school students found that 26.4 % of the participants may be classified as Internet addicts (Shek and Yu 2012a). Using longitudinal data in the same project, Yu and Shek (2013) further tracked the development of Internet addiction in this group of students and found that the prevalence rates of Internet addiction were 26.7 % and 22.5 % at Wave 2 (1 year after the first survey) and Wave 3 (2 years after the first survey), respectively.

Although these studies provide valuable information, most of them are cross-sectional studies in nature and there is a dearth of study on how Internet addiction develops as a function of time or age. Investigating the developmental pattern of Internet addiction over time can help develop theoretical models and intervention strategies on Internet addiction (Kraut et al. 1998; Yellowless and Marks 2007). Based on longitudinal data collected in 4 years, the present study intended to investigate the developmental trajectory of Internet addiction among Hong Kong adolescents.

Adolescents who are addicted to the Internet often displayed various psychosocial problems such as suicide ideation, depression, loneliness, and substance dependence (Muusses et al. 2014; Van den Eijnden et al. 2008), which negatively affected their personal development, academic performance, daily life, as well as relationship with others (Muusses et al. 2014). With regard to risk factors associated with Internet addiction, economic disadvantage and family non-intactness deserve our attention. According to Lempers et al. (1989)'s research, family financial difficulties influenced parents' parenting that eventually created distress in adolescents. Similarly, based on the model of family stress, financial difficulties lead to parents' pressure, which reduces their marital relationship, psychological well-being, and effective child-rearing (Conger and Conger 2008). The maladaptive family environment, especially negative child-rearing styles, further put poor adolescents at greater risk of problem behavior involvement, such as problematic Internet use. Hur (2006) showed that disadvantaged socioeconomic status surrounding the teenagers predicted higher prevalence of Internet addiction disorder. As such, it was hypothesized that family economic disadvantage would predict higher prevalence of Internet addiction concurrently and longitudinally in adolescents.

Apart from economic disadvantage, family non-intactness is considered another potential risk factor contributing to Internet addiction. Compared to adolescents in intact families, adolescents from non-intact families are more likely to lack physical and psychological regulations from parents and experience interparental conflict which predisposes them to risk behavior (Lansford 2009). Empirical research has demonstrated that family structure (e.g., divorce, separation, or remarriage) correlated with adolescents' Internet addiction (Shek and Yu 2012a). A more recent study conducted on 5122 high school adolescents in Shanghai, China, found that parental separation and family structure of "left-behind adolescents" were significantly correlated with some symptoms of Internet addiction (Xu et al. 2014). In the present study, we speculated that family non-intactness (e.g., divorce or separation) would be related to higher level of Internet addiction concurrently and longitudinally.

On the other hand, protective factors related to Internet addiction have been examined by researchers (Kuss et al. 2013; Liu et al. 2013; Shek and Yu 2012a; Yu and Shek 2013). Among them, healthy family functioning and positive youth development are two essential factors preventing or reducing adolescent Internet addiction. Healthy family functioning is defined by strong bonding, mutuality, open communication, interpersonal harmony, absence of conflicts, as well as good parent–child relationship (Quatman 1997; Shek 2002). Previous research consistently showed that healthy family functioning predicted less likelihood of having Internet addiction among adolescents (Park et al. 2008; Yen et al. 2007b). For example, data from 3662 middle school students in Taiwan suggested that lower parent–adolescent conflict was related to less Internet addictive behavior (Yen et al. 2007b). A recent survey on 1744 adolescents aged between 14 and 17 years in Germany showed that self-perceived positive family functioning (e.g., good family involvement, open affective expression and communication in family) significantly predicted lower occurrence of problematic Internet use (Wartberg et al. 2014). Hence, it was predicted that family functioning would have negative concurrent and longitudinal relationships with Internet addictive behavior among adolescents in Hong Kong.

Concerning positive youth development, many researchers have argued that the related attributes reduce the likelihood of risk behavior (Catalano et al. 2012; Shek and Yu 2012b) and contribute to psychological well-being among adolescents (Flay 2002; Rutter 1987). Despite the importance of positive youth development in reducing adolescent problem behavior, scientific literature on the relationship between these attributes and Internet addiction is not abundant. Among the few related studies conducted, some studies showed that positive youth development indicators significantly predicted pathological use of the Internet concurrently and over time

(Shek and Yu 2012a; Yu and Shek 2013). Based on the existing literature, it was hypothesized that positive youth development would have negative concurrent and longitudinal predictive relations with Internet addictive behavior among adolescents in Hong Kong.

Against the research background, the present study was designed to explore the profiles of Internet addictive behaviors and the changes in a period of 4 years among Hong Kong adolescents. The study also examined four psychosocial correlates (family economic disadvantage, family intactness, family functioning, and positive youth development) of Internet addictive behaviors concurrently and longitudinally.

Method

Participants and Procedure

The present study is part of an ongoing 6-year longitudinal project. A total of 3328 Secondary 1 students (52.7 % male and 47.2 % female; age = 12.59 ± 0.74 years) from 28 local secondary schools in Hong Kong were recruited in the longitudinal project. The participants were evaluated on multiple aspects of adolescent development (i.e., family process, positive youth development attributes, and risk behaviors) every year. The study included four waves of data with acceptable attrition rates: 12.7 %, 14.1 %, and 19.4 % at Wave 2, Wave 3, and Wave 4, respectively. The demographic profiles of participants are presented in Table 1. All participants were repeatedly informed that the personal information would be kept in strict confidentiality. Researchers were present throughout the assessment process to answer questions.

Table 1 Demographic profiles of the participants across four waves

	Wave 1	%	Wave 2[a]	%	Wave 3[a]	%	Wave 4[a]	%
N (participants)	3328		2905		2858		2682	
Gender								
Male	1719	51.7	1445	49.7	1433	50.1	1335	49.8
Female	1572	47.2	1419	48.8	1405	49.2	1337	49.9
Economic disadvantage								
Not receiving CSSA	2606	78.3	2377	81.8	2339	81.8	2267	84.5
Receiving CSSA	225	6.8	160	5.5	147	5.1	132	4.9
Family intactness								
Intact families	2781	83.6	2415	83.1	2396	83.8	2211	82.4
Non-intact families	515	15.5	469	16.1	454	15.9	466	17.4

[a]The numbers were based on the participants who ever participated in Wave 1 assessment as only those joining Wave 1 assessment were included in LMM. The numbers of the students who did not report the corresponding information were not presented

Instruments

Internet Addiction The Chinese version of Young's 10-item Internet Addiction Test (IAT) validated by Shek and colleagues (2008) was used to measure participants' Internet addiction. The 10-item IAT asks respondent to answer "Yes" or "No" as to whether they had the listed Internet addictive behaviors in the past 1 year. A person is classified as "Internet addicted" if he/she shows four or more of the listed behaviors. Cronbach's alpha of IAT for the present sample was 0.79, 0.79, 0.80, and 0.79 at Wave 1, Wave 2, Wave 3, and Wave 4, respectively (see Table 2).

Family Functioning Family functioning was investigated by the refined version of the Chinese Family Assessment Instrument (CFAI; Shek and Ma 2010) with nine items assessing mutuality, communication, as well as conflicts and harmony. Means of the nine items were computed and higher scores indicated healthier family functioning, after reversing the appropriate items. Previous research has showed that the CFAI has good psychometric properties (Shek and Lin 2014; Shek and Yu 2012a). In the current study, Cronbach's alpha coefficients for the CFAI at each wave are presented in Table 2.

Positive Youth Development Positive youth development attributes identified by Catalano et al. (2004) were assessed by the refined version of the Chinese Positive Youth Development Scale (CPYDS; Shek et al. 2007; Sun and Shek 2010). Global positive youth development was reflected by the mean scores across the different

Table 2 Descriptive statistics of key variables and internal consistency coefficients of scales (Waves 1–4)

	Mean	(SD)			Reliability			
	W1	W2	W3	W4	W1	W2	W3	W4
Family functioning[a]	3.73 (.81)	3.65 (.81)	3.65 (.79)	3.66 (.77)	.90	.90	.90	.91
Positive youth[a] development	4.51 (.70)	4.43 (.69)	4.44 (.65)	4.45 (.62)	.93	.96	.96	.96
Internet addictive behavior[b]	2.31 (2.40)	2.36 (2.40)	2.08 (2.32)	1.94 (2.22)	.79	.79	.80	.79
Male	2.43 (2.49)	2.47 (2.53)	2.21 (2.51)	2.18 (2.43)	–	–	–	–
Female	2.19 (2.29)	2.26 (2.27)	1.95 (2.10)	1.72 (1.97)	–	–	–	–
Not receiving CSSA	2.24 (2.37)	2.36 (2.38)	2.03 (2.26)	1.95 (2.21)	–	–	–	–
Receiving CSSA	2.56 (2.31)	2.37 (2.33)	2.19 (2.26)	2.11 (2.12)	–	–	–	–
Intact families	2.23 (2.38)	2.33 (2.39)	2.08 (2.32)	1.93 (2.22)	–	–	–	–
Non-intact families	2.74 (2.48)	2.45 (2.41)	2.12 (2.29)	2.02 (2.26)	–	–	–	–

W1 Wave 1, *W2* Wave 2, *W3* Wave 3, *W4* Wave 4
[a]Mean score was used to indicate the level of family functioning and positive youth development
[b]Sum scores were used to indicate the levels of Internet addictive behaviors (range = 0–10) for easy interpretation

subscales. The CPYDS has been widely used in previous studies with good psychometric properties (Shek and Lin 2014; Shek and Tsui 2012). Cronbach's alpha coefficients for the CPYDS in this study at each wave are presented in Table 2.

Family Economic Disadvantage Economic disadvantage was measured in terms of whether the participant family receives Comprehensive Social Security Assistance (CSSA) or not. Families receiving CSSA were regarded financially difficult in Hong Kong (Shek and Lin 2014; Shek and Tsui 2012). At the initial assessment, 78.3 % of all respondents reported not receiving CSSA and 6.8 % reported receiving CSSA (see Table 1). The rest of the cases with no response to this question (14.9 %) were removed from the corresponding analyses.

Family Intactness Family intactness was defined based on the marital status of participants' parents (*1 = divorced but not remarried, 2 = separated but not remarried, 3 = married (first marriage), 4 = married (second or above marriage), 5 = others*). Only respondents with parents who are married in the first marriage were regarded as living in intact families. At the initial survey, among all respondents, 83.6 % of students reported living in intact families and 15.5 % of students reported living in non-intact families. Those participants who did not report this information (0.9 %) were not included in the study (see Table 1).

Data Analytic Plan

There were three parts in the analyses. First, frequency analyses were carried out to look at the profiles of students' Internet addictive behaviors in four waves. Second, in order to understand the developmental patterns of Internet addiction, individual growth curve modeling was performed by using linear mixed model (LMM) in SPSS 22.0 statistical software with maximum likelihood (ML) as estimation method. Hierarchical model with two levels that nested time (Level 1) within individual (Level 2) was created. Time was coded as 0 = Wave 1, 1 = Wave 2, 2 = Wave 3, and 3 = Wave 4. Level 1 described the normative developmental patterns of adolescent Internet addiction, which included the average within-person initial level and changing rate in a long term without other predictor variables. Level 2 tested how demographic factors influenced the initial levels and the changing rate. The effects of economic disadvantage and family intactness were mainly examined with initial age and gender controlled. Three steps were taken for LMM. Firstly, to identify the variance of Internet addiction over time, Model 1 (unconditional mean model) was estimated (i.e., intraclass correlation coefficient or ICC; Singer and Willett 2003). Secondly, Model 2 (unconditional growth model) was estimated in which the developmental patterns of the participants were examined. Lastly, Model 3 (conditional model) was estimated with economic disadvantage and family intactness as predictors at Level 2 after controlling the effects of initial age and gender. The specific procedure of LMM can be seen elsewhere (Shek and Ma 2011; Shek and Yu 2012b). Third, multiple regression analyses were conducted to explore concurrent and over-time effects of positive youth development and family functioning on Internet addiction after controlling the predictions of demographic predictors (i.e., gender, family intactness, and economic disadvantage).

Results

Several observations can be highlighted from the frequencies and percentages of participants showing Internet addictive behaviors across the four waves of data (Table 3).

First, Internet addictive behaviors were quite common among Hong Kong adolescents across 4 years (7.0–48.9 %). For example, nearly half of the students agreed that they "stay online longer than originally intended" in 4 years (42.4 % in Wave 1, 46.9 % in Wave 2, 47.8 % in Wave 3, and 48.9 % in Wave 4). Second, according to Young's criterion, nearly one-fourth to one-fifth of the students can be classified as having Internet addiction (26.2 % in Wave 1, 25.5 % in Wave 2, 22.3 % in Wave 3, and 19.4 % in Wave 4) in 4 years. Third, 19.2 %, 19.7 %, 20.8 %, and 20.1 % of the students reported "go online to escape problems or relieve feelings, such as helplessness, guilt, anxiety, or depression" in Wave 1, Wave 2, Wave 3, and Wave 4, respectively, which indicated the possible psychological problems over time.

Individual growth curve analyses were conducted to explore the developmental patterns of Internet addiction of adolescents and the predictions of economic disadvantage and family intactness on the initial level and changing rate of Internet addiction after controlling the predictions of initial age and gender. Table 4 presents the results of models.

First, Model 1 of Internet addiction indicated that around 48.5 % (ICC = .485) of the total variation were because of interindividual differences, indicating further multilevel analyses were needed (Shek and Ma 2011; Shek and Yu 2012b). Second, Model 2 of Internet addiction demonstrated a better model fit than Model 1 ($\Delta\chi^2_{(3)}$ = 248.056; ΔAIC = 242.056; ΔBIC = 219.938; $ps < .001$). Specifically, the initial level of Internet addiction was close to the medium level and it decreased linearly by an average of .117 units per year. The significance of two random-effect variances (intercepts and linear slopes) indicated that some potential interindividual factors may be able to explain the variances of the intercepts and linear slopes of Internet addiction. On average, the adolescents showed less Internet addictive behavior over time.

Finally, economic disadvantage and family intactness were included as Level 2 predictors of the intercepts and the slopes after controlling the effects of initial age and gender, since significant interindividual differences were revealed in the intercepts and slopes for Internet addiction. Model 3 of Internet addiction ($\Delta\chi^2_{(8)}$ = 8589.771; ΔAIC = 8573.771; ΔBIC = 8517.268; $ps < .001$) showed better model fit than Model 2. In terms of the predictors of the intercept of Internet addiction, it was showed that the prediction of family intactness was significant with the prediction of initial age controlled. Specifically, older adolescents reported higher levels

Table 3 Frequencies of Internet addictive behaviors in the past 1 year across four waves

Internet addictive behavior	Wave 1 (Yes)		Wave 2 (Yes)		Wave 3 (Yes)		Wave 4 (Yes)	
	N	%	N	%	N	%	N	%
1. Feeling preoccupied with the Internet or online services and thinking about it while off-line	1324	39.9	1179	40.6	933	32.7	715	26.7
2. Feeling a need to spend more and more time online to achieve satisfaction	1072	32.3	882	30.4	677	23.7	546	20.4
3. Unable to control your online use	752	22.7	669	23.1	533	18.7	513	19.1
4. Feeling restless or irritable when attempting to cut down or stop online use	484	14.6	398	13.7	304	10.7	264	9.9
5. Staying online longer than originally intended	1404	42.4	1360	46.9	1365	47.8	1310	48.9
6. Risking the loss of a significant relationship, job, or educational or career opportunity because of online use	644	19.5	609	21.0	590	20.7	561	20.9
7. Lying to family members or friends to conceal excessive Internet use	651	19.7	541	18.7	469	16.4	346	12.9
8. Going online to escape problems or relieve feelings, such as helplessness, guilt, anxiety, or depression	633	19.2	572	19.7	594	20.8	538	20.1
9. Showing withdrawal when off-line, such as increased depression, moodiness, or irritability	395	12.0	364	12.6	267	9.4	233	8.7
10. Keep on using Internet even after spending too much money on online fees	331	10.1	282	9.8	222	7.8	189	7.0
Participants can be classified as having Internet addiction (Young's criteria)	871	26.2	830	25.5	638	22.3	621	19.4

of Internet addictive behaviors than younger adolescents, and adolescents living in non-intact families displayed more Internet addictive behaviors than those adolescents living in intact families at the initial assessment. However, gender and economic disadvantage did not link to the initial level of Internet addictive behaviors. Predictors at Level 2 explained 4.3 % of the intercept variance of Internet addictive behaviors.

As to the predictors of slopes, it was showed that economic disadvantage and family intactness were both related to the decreasing rate of Internet addiction after controlling the effects of initial age and gender. Students from non-intact families

Table 4 Results of individual growth curve of Internet addictive behavior for all models

		Model 1		Model 2		Model 3	
		Estimate	SE	Estimate	SE	Estimate	SE
Fixed effects							
Intercept	β_{0j}						
Initial status	γ_{00}	2.223***	.033	2.381***	.401	2.483***	.084
Age	γ_{01}					.149*	.061
Gender[a]	γ_{02}					.056	.043
Economic disadvantage[b]	γ_{03}					.010	.087
Family intactness[c]	γ_{04}					−.203**	.065
Linear slope	β_{1j}						
Initial status	γ_{10}			−.117***	.016	−.104**	
Age	γ_{11}					−.069**	.024
Gender[a]	γ_{12}					.051**	.017
Economic disadvantage[b]	γ_{13}					.100**	.035
Family intactness[c]	γ_{14}					.107***	.026
Random effects							
Level 1 (within)							
Residual	r_{ij}	2.871***	.044	2.410***	.046	2.339***	.049
Level 2 (between)							
Intercept	u_{0j}	2.707***	.090	3.571***	.136	3.417***	.144
Time	u_{1j}			.270***	.023	.237***	.024
Fit statistics							
Deviance		50,602.185		50,354.129		41,764.358	
AIC		50,608.185		50,366.129		41,792.358	
BIC		50,630.305		50,410.367		41,893.099	
df		3		6		14	

Model 1 unconditional mean model, *model 2* unconditional growth model, *model 3* conditional model

*p<.05; **p<.01; ***p<.001

[a]Male=1, female=−1

[b]Receiving CSSA=1, not receiving CSSA=−1

[c]Intact=1, non-intact=−1

and experiencing economic advantage decreased faster in Internet addictive behaviors. Initial age and gender were also associated with the slope, with older and female adolescents decreasing faster. Level 2 predictors explained 12.2 % of the slope variance in Internet addictive behaviors.

For Wave 4 cross-sectional effects (see Table 5), it was revealed after controlling the effects of individual characteristics, family functioning and positive youth development were both negatively correlated with Internet addiction as predicted. Specifically, adolescents with better family functioning ($\beta=-.100$, $p<.000$) and more positive youth development attributes ($\beta=-.191$, $p<.000$) reported lower levels of Internet addictive behaviors.

Table 5 Multiple regression analyses on Internet addictive behavior at Wave 4

	Model A		Model B	
Predictors	Beta	ΔR^2	Beta	ΔR^2
Step 1		*.011****		*.010****
Gender[a]	.108***		.096***	
Economic disadvantage[b]	.019		.023	
Family intactness[c]	−.003		.002	
Step 2				*.064****
Family functioning			−.098***	
Positive youth development			−.195***	

***$p < .001$
[a]Male = 1, female = 0
[b]Receiving CSSA = 1, not receiving CSSA = 0
[c]Intact = 1, non-intact = 0

Table 6 Wave 1 variables predict Wave 4 Internet addictive behavior

	Model A		Model B		Model C	
Predictors	Beta	ΔR^2	Beta	ΔR^2	Beta	ΔR^2
Step 1		*.113****		*.125****		*.127****
Initial behavior	.337***		.354***		.357***	
Step 2				*.013****		*.015****
Gender[a]			.101***		.106***	
Economic disadvantage[b]			.061**		.067**	
Family intactness[c]			.041		.042	
Step 3						*.002*
Family functioning					.019	
Positive youth development					−.053*	

*$p < .05$; **$p < .01$; ***$p < .001$
[a]Male = 1, female = 0
[b]Receiving CSSA = 1, not receiving CSSA = 0
[c]Intact = 1, non-intact = 0

In terms of the over-time effects (see Table 6), it was found that students with Wave 1 Internet addictive behaviors more tended to show Internet addictive behaviors at Wave 4 ($\beta = .349$, $p < .001$). Those students who were male ($\beta = .106$, $p < .001$) and were from economic disadvantage ($\beta = .067$, $p < .01$) at Wave 1 were more likely to have Internet addictive behaviors. Positive youth development ($\beta = -.053$, $p < .05$) at Wave 1 negatively predicted Internet addiction at Wave 4, although the prediction was not strong when controlling initial behavior status and the effects of demographic factors. Concerning the effect of family functioning, family functioning at Wave 1 did not significantly predict Internet addiction at Wave 4.

Discussion

The present study attempted to examine the profiles of Internet addictive behaviors and the changes in a period of 4 years among Hong Kong adolescents. The study also examined several psychosocial correlates of Internet addictive behaviors concurrently and longitudinally. The results showed that Internet addiction among Hong Kong adolescents generally declined over time, which is in line with previous studies (Grohol 2005; Kraut et al. 1998; Young 1998; Yu and Shek 2013). According to Young (1998) and Kraut et al. (1998)'s views, excessive Internet use was something that could wear off over the long term in the majority of individuals. However, Grohol (2005) argued that although some people could change to be normal Internet users who used Internet with proper time over time, a small number of people would be stuck in Internet addiction and needed assistance. Our findings also echo the argument while the rate of adolescent Internet addiction generally reduced, around one-fourth to one-fifth of the participants were still classified as Internet addicts over a 4-year period. This suggests that such adolescents have become stable in Internet addiction and should be given special attention. The findings also imply the importance of early prevention of Internet addiction.

Regarding risk factors associated with Internet addiction, we found adolescents in poor families reported slower rate of decrease in Internet addiction than those adolescents in nonpoor families. We also found that adolescents experiencing economic disadvantage at Wave 1 were more likely to involve in Internet addictive behaviors at Wave 4, which is in line with the results of Yu and Shek (2013) who found that Wave 1 economic disadvantage positively predicted Wave 3 Internet addictive behaviors. The finding suggests that economic disadvantage as a risk factor hinders the decline of Internet addiction over time. This can be explained by the possibility that poor adolescents without sufficient resource, support, and experience from family in real life would keep seeking excitement, social support (e.g., chatting), and successful experience (e.g., games) from Internet in a virtual world. This finding demonstrates that family economic status plays a risk role in developmental trajectory of Internet addiction in adolescents. It is suggested that educators, social workers, and policy makers should pay more attention to Internet addiction issues in adolescents experiencing economic disadvantage. However, it is worth noting that economic disadvantage did not predict the initial status of Internet addiction and did also not predict Internet addiction at Wave 4 concurrently. The finding echoes previous research showing that family economic status was not related to Internet addiction at a single time point (Mashhor and Saad 2014; Shek and Yu 2012a; Yen et al. 2007b). In conjunction with the previous and present findings, it is conjectured that economic disadvantage may play a dynamic role in contributing to Internet addiction in adolescents. Hence, future studies in this area are warranted.

Consistent with our expectation, adolescents living in non-intact families reported higher initial level of Internet addictive behaviors, which is similar to previous findings (Shek and Yu 2012a; Xu et al. 2014). Researchers have pointed out that children living with divorced or separated parents tend to have high parent–child conflicts and low levels of parent–child involvement (Nelson et al. 1999), which may make them easier to suffer from emotional or behavioral problems. Lacking support (e.g., warmth and connectedness) from parents, adolescents living with divorced or separated parents may seek social support and connectedness on the Internet. However, adolescent excessive use of the Internet may further exacerbate their conflict or separation with parents, which forms a vicious circle between poor parent–child relationship and Internet addiction and makes the problem of Internet addiction more difficult to solve (Yen et al. 2007b; Yu and Shek 2013).

Out of our expectation, adolescents living in non-intact families reported faster rate of decrease in Internet addictive behaviors than those living in intact families did. It might be explained in terms of two possibilities. First, as parental separation or divorce is adversity which triggers resilience, some adolescents might have withdrawn from Internet addictive behaviors because of the growth experience involved (Kelly and Emery 2003). This may be the case when they receive extra support from the significant others around them. Second, some adolescents might turn to engage in more serious addictive behaviors, such as substance use due to adverse family environment and the absence of one or two of biological parents (Blankenhorn 1995). Obviously, future research is necessary to further understand the mechanisms involved. However, while adolescents in non-intact families reported faster decreasing rate of Internet addiction, the overall mean scores of Internet addictive behaviors adolescents in intact families reported were lower than adolescents in non-intact families did across 4 years. Such findings indicate that family non-intactness may serve as a risk factor in the development of adolescent Internet addiction.

As predicted, the study showed that adolescents with better family functioning reported lower level of Internet addictive behaviors concurrently. The findings are consistent with previous reports (Ary et al. 1999; Wartberg et al. 2014; Yen et al. 2007b). However, their longitudinal effects on Internet addictive behaviors were not significant in the study. In conjunction with the findings in the previous study (Yu and Shek 2013) that Wave 1 family functioning negatively predicted Wave 2 and Wave 3 adolescent Internet addictive behaviors, it might be that the longitudinal effect of family functioning was minimized in a long term. Many other factors which have played important role in life of adolescents (i.e., school environment and relationship with peers) may mediate the long-term effect of family functioning in the process (Dishion et al. 1991). Furthermore, positive youth development predicted lower level of adolescents' Internet addiction both concurrently and longitudinally, which is in agreement with the findings of Yu and Shek (2013). In other words, a high level of positive youth development contributes to the prevention of Internet addiction. As such, the present and previous findings provide strong support for the use of positive youth development approach for adolescent problem behavior prevention, including Internet addiction (Catalano et al. 2004).

In terms of the relatively weak longitudinal prediction of family functioning and positive youth development on Internet addictive behaviors, two other possible explanations in terms of the methodology should be considered. One possibility is that many adolescents dropped out in Wave 4 which may reduce the longitudinal effects. Since youths in Hong Kong are allowed to work when they reach the age of 15, students who cannot perform well in schools may leave school to work. For those who remain staying in the present study, they are likely to be students with relatively better school performance and less problem behaviors as compared to those who drop out. Another possible explanation is that we adopted a stringent longitudinal approach in the present study in which the initial level of Internet addictive behaviors of participants was controlled.

There are several strengths of this study. First, a large sample size was adopted and the developmental patterns obtained in the present study may be considered as a normative description of Internet addiction through adolescence for Hong Kong adolescents. Second, the study generates a longitudinal profile on adolescent Internet addiction in Hong Kong. While the majority of the adolescents showed declined Internet addiction over time, nearly one-fifth to one-fourth of the participants displayed a stable pattern of Internet addiction (26.2–19.4 %). Third, results showed that risk factors (family economic disadvantage and family non-intactness) did not only influence adolescent development at a single time point but also over time. Meanwhile, family functioning and positive youth development are well suggested as important protective factors to prevent and treat problem behaviors including Internet addiction among adolescents.

There are several limitations of this study. First, the researchers only collected quantitative data. As the developmental features of Internet addicts are unknown, it would be illuminating if qualitative methods such as case study and in-depth interview can be conducted. Second, Internet addiction was investigated at four time points over four school years. To understand the over-time developmental features of Internet addictive behaviors in individuals, multiple waves of data in a longer term may be included. Third, only four predictive factors relating to Internet addiction were examined. Other important indicators such as peer influence should be included in the future. Fourth, a self-reported questionnaire was used to assess Internet addiction. As adolescent respondents may underreport their Internet addictive behaviors because of social desirability, it would be useful to include parent, teacher, and/or peer report in future studies.

In short, although Internet addiction among Hong Kong adolescents tended to decline in a period of 4 years, the overall prevalence rate remained high. While economic disadvantage and family non-intactness were risk factors, family functioning and positive youth development were protective factors in the development of adolescent Internet addiction. Based on the present findings, it is suggested that more attention from the public and academia should be given to the phenomenon of Internet addiction in Hong Kong and that promotion of family functioning and positive youth development attributes in adolescents could be promising directions in preventing adolescent Internet addiction.

References

Ary, D. V., Duncan, T. E., Biglan, A., Metzler, C. W., Noell, J. W., & Smolkowski, K. (1999). Development of adolescent problem behavior. *Journal of Abnormal Child Psychology, 27*(2), 141–150.

Beard, K. W. (2005). Internet addiction: A review of current assessment techniques and potential assessment questions. *Cyberpsychology & Behavior, 8*, 7–14.

Blankenhorn, D. (1995). *Fatherless America: Confronting our most urgent social problem.* New York: Basic Books.

Catalano, R. F., Berglund, M. L., Ryan, J. A. M., Lonczak, H. S., & Hawkins, J. D. (2004). Positive youth development in the United States: Research findings on evaluations of positive youth development programs. *The Annals of the American Academy of Political Social Science, 591*, 98–124.

Catalano, R. F., Fagan, A. A., Gavin, L. E., Greenberg, M. T., Irwin, C. E., Ross, D. A., & Shek, D. T. L. (2012). Worldwide application of prevention science in adolescent health. *The Lancet, 379*(9826), 1653–1664.

Conger, R. D., & Conger, K. J. (2008). Understanding the processes through which economic hardship influences families and children. In D. R. Crane & T. B. Heaton (Eds.), *Handbook of families and poverty* (pp. 64–81). Los Angeles: Sage.

Dishion, T. J., Patterson, G. R., Stoolmiller, M., & Skinner, M. L. (1991). Family, school, and behavioral antecedents to early adolescent involvement with antisocial peers. *Developmental Psychology, 27*(1), 172–180.

Durkee, T., Kaess, M., Carli, V., Parzer, P., Wasserman, C., Floderus, B., … & Wasserman, D. (2012). Prevalence of pathological Internet use among adolescents in Europe: Demographic and social factors. *Addiction, 107*, 2210–2222.

Flay, B. R. (2002). Positive youth development requires comprehensive health promotion programs. *American Journal of Health Behavior, 26*, 407–424.

Grohol, J. M. (2005). *Internet addiction guide.* PsychCentral Website. Retrieved from http://psychcentral.com/netaddiction/

Hur, M. H. (2006). Demographic, habitual, and socioeconomic determinants of internet addiction disorder: An empirical study of Korean teenagers. *Cyberpsychology & Behavior, 9*, 514–525.

Kaltiala-Heino, R., Lintonen, T., & Rimpelä, A. (2004). Internet addiction? Potentially problematic use of the Internet in a population of 12–18 year old adolescents. *Addiction Research and Theory, 12*, 89–96.

Kelly, J. B., & Emery, R. E. (2003). Children adjustment following divorce: Risk and resilience perspective. *Family Relations, 52*, 352–362.

Kim, K., Ryu, E., Chon, M., Yeun, E., Choi, S., Seo, J., & Nam, B. (2006). Internet addiction in Korean adolescents and its relation to depression suicidal ideation: A questionnaire survey. *International Journal of Nursing Studies, 43*, 185–192.

Kraut, R., Patterson, M., Lundmark, V., Kiesler, S., Mukopadhyay, T., & Scherlis, W. (1998). Internet paradox: A social technology that reduces social involvement and psychological well-being? *American Psychologist, 53*, 1017–1031.

Kuss, D., Rooij, A. J., Shorter, G. W., Griffiths, M. D., & Mheen, D. (2013). Internet addiction in adolescents: Prevalence and risk factors. *Computers in Human Behavior, 29*, 1987–1996.

Kuss, D. J., Griffiths, M. D., Karila, L., & Billieux, J. (2014). Internet addiction: A systematic review of epidemiological research for the last decade. *Current Pharmaceutical Design, 20*, 4026–4052.

Lansford, J. E. (2009). Parental divorce and children's adjustment. *Perspectives on Psychological Science, 4*(2), 140–152.

Lempers, J. D., Clark-Lempers, D., & Simons, R. L. (1989). Economic hardship, parenting, and distress in adolescence. *Child Development, 60*, 25–39.

Li, Y., Zhang, X., Lu, F., Zhang, Q., & Wang, Y. (2014). Internet addiction among elementary and middle school students in China: A nationally representative sample study. *Cyberpsychology, Behavior and Social Networking, 17*, 111–116.

Lin, M. P., Ko, H. C., & Wu, J. Y. (2011). Prevalence and psychosocial risk factors associated with Internet addiction in a nationally representative sample of college students in Taiwan. *Cyberpsychology, Behavior and Social Networking, 14*, 741–746.

Liu, Q., Fang, X., Zhou, Z., Zhang, J., & Deng, L. (2013). Perceived parent-adolescent relationship, perceived parental online behaviors and pathological Internet use among adolescents: Gender-specific differences. *PLoS One, 8*, e75642–e75650.

Mashhor, A., & Saad, A. (2014). Internet addiction among secondary school students in Riyadh city, its prevalence, correlates and relation to depression: A questionnaire survey. *International Journal of Medical Science and Public Health, 3*(1), 10–15.

Moreno, M. A., Jelenchick, L., Cox, E., Young, H., & Christakis, D. A. (2011). Problematic Internet use among US youth: A systematic review. *Archives of Pediatrics and Adolescent Medicine, 165*, 797–805.

Muusses, L., Finkenauer, C., Kerkhof, P., & Billedo, C. J. (2014). A longitudinal study of the association between compulsive internet use and wellbeing. *Computers in Human Behavior, 36*, 21–28.

Nelson, B. V., Patience, T. H., & MacDonald, D. C. (1999). Adolescent risk behavior and the influence of parents and education. *Journal of the American Board of Family Practice, 12*, 436–443.

Park, S. K., Kim, J. Y., & Cho, C. B. (2008). Prevalence of Internet addiction and correlations with family factors among South Korean adolescents. *Adolescence, 43*, 895–909.

Quatman, T. (1997). High functioning families: Developing a prototype. *Family Therapy, 24*(3), 143–165.

Rutter, M. (1987). Psychosocial resilience and protective mechanisms. *American Journal of Orthopsychiatry, 57*(3), 316–331.

Salehi, M., Khalili, M. N., Hojjat, S. K., Salehi, M., & Danesh, A. (2014). Prevalence of internet addiction and associated factors among medical students from Mashhad, Iran in 2013. *Iranian Red Crescent Medical Journal, 16*(5), e17256–e17263.

Shek, D. T. L. (2002). Assessment of family functioning in Chinese adolescents: The Chinese Family Assessment Instrument. In N. N. Singh, T. H. Ollendick, & A. N. Singh (Eds.), *International perspectives on child and adolescent mental health* (Vol. 2, pp. 297–316). Kuala Lumpur: Elsevier.

Shek, D. T. L., & Lin, L. (2014). Personal well-being and family quality of life of early adolescents in Hong Kong: Do economic disadvantage and time matter? *Social Indicators Research, 117*(3), 795–809.

Shek, D. T. L., & Ma, C. M. S. (2010). The Chinese Family Assessment Instrument (C-FAI): Hierarchical confirmatory factor analyses and factorial invariance. *Social Indicators Research, 20*(1), 112–123.

Shek, D. T. L., & Ma, C. M. S. (2011). Longitudinal data analyses using linear mixed models in SPSS: Concepts, procedures and illustrations. *The Scientific World Journal, 11*, 42–76.

Shek, D. T. L., & Tsui, P. E. (2012). Family and personal adjustment of economically disadvantaged Chinese adolescents in Hong Kong. *The Scientific World Journal, 2012*, 142689–142697.

Shek, D. T. L., & Yu, L. (2012a). Internet addiction in Hong Kong adolescents: Profiles and psychosocial correlates. *International Journal of Disability and Human Development, 11*, 133–142.

Shek, D. T. L., & Yu, L. (2012b). Longitudinal impact of the project PATHS on adolescent risk behavior: What happened after five years? *The Scientific World Journal, 2012,* 14 pages. doi:10.1100/2012/316029.

Shek, D. T. L., Siu, A. M. H., & Lee, T. Y. (2007). The Chinese positive youth development scale: A validation study. *Research on Social Work Practice, 17*(3), 380–391.

Shek, D. T. L., Tang, V. M., & Lo, C. Y. (2008). Internet addiction in Chinese adolescents in Hong Kong: Assessment, profiles, and psychosocial correlates. *The Scientific World Journal, 8*, 776–787.

Shek, D. T. L., Sun, R. C. F., & Yu, L. (2012). Internet addiction. In D. W. Pfaff, E. Martin, & E. Pariser (Eds.), *Neuroscience in the 21st century*. New York: Springer.

Singer, J. D., & Willett, J. B. (2003). *Applied longitudinal data analysis: Modeling change and event occurrence*. London: Oxford University Press.

Sun, R. C. F., & Shek, D. T. L. (2010). Life satisfaction, positive youth development, and problem behavior among Chinese adolescents in Hong Kong. *Social Indicators Research, 95*(3), 455–474.

Tang, J., Yu, Y., Du, Y., Ma, Y., Zhang, D., & Wang, J. (2014). Prevalence of Internet addiction and its association with stressful life events and psychological symptoms among adolescent Internet uses. *Addictive Behavior, 39*, 744–747.

Van den Eijnden, R. J. J. M., Meerkerk, G. J., Vermulst, A. A., Spijkerman, R., & Engels, R. C. M. E. (2008). Online communication, compulsive internet use, and psychosocial well-being among adolescents: A longitudinal study. *Developmental Psychology, 44*, 655–665.

Wartberg, L., Kammerl, R., Rosenkranz, M., Hirschhäuser, L., Hein, S., Schwinge, C., … & Rainer, T. (2014). The interdependence of family functioning and problematic internet use in a representative quota sample of adolescents. *Cyberpsychology, Behavior, and Social Networking, 17*, 14–18.

Xu, J., Shen, L., Yan, C., Hu, H., Yang, F., Wang, L., … & Shen, X. (2014). Parent-adolescent interaction and risk of adolescent internet addiction: A population-based study in Shanghai. *BMC Psychiatry, 14*, 112–123.

Yellowlees, P. M., & Marks, S. (2007). Problematic internet use or internet addiction? *Computers in Human Behavior, 23*, 1447–1453.

Yen, J. Y., Ko, C. H., Yen, C. F., Wu, H. Y., & Yang, M. J. (2007a). The comorbid psychiatric symptoms of Internet addiction: Attention deficit and hyperactivity disorder (ADHD), depression, social phobia, and hostility. *Journal of Adolescent Health, 41*, 93–98.

Yen, J. Y., Yen, C. F., Chen, C. C., Chen, S. H., & Ko, C. H. (2007b). Family factors of internet addiction and substance use experience in Taiwanese adolescents. *Cyberpsychology & Behavior, 10*, 323–329.

Young, K. S. (1998). Internet addiction: The emergence of a new clinical disorder. *Cyberpsychology & Behavior, 1*(3), 237–244.

Yu, L., & Shek, D. T. L. (2013). Internet addiction in Hong Kong adolescents: A three-year longitudinal study. *Journal of Pediatric and Adolescent Gynecology, 26*(3S), S10–S17.

Adolescent Consumption of Pornographic Materials: Prevalence and Psychosocial Correlates Based on a Longitudinal Study

Daniel T.L. Shek, Qiuzhi Xie, and Cecilia M.S. Ma

Abstract In this study, prevalence and psychosocial correlates of consumption of pornographic materials in Chinese adolescents were examined over 4 years. Results showed that adolescent consumption of pornographic materials generally increased throughout the junior secondary school years. Compared with that of traditional pornographic materials, adolescent consumption of pornographic materials on the Internet was higher. Growth curve analyses showed that age was related to initial level of pornography consumption and gender was related to growth trajectory of the consumption; family intactness also influenced growth rate in consumption of pornography on the Internet. Initial level of pornography consumption in early adolescence, gender, positive youth development qualities, and family functioning also predicted consumption of pornographic materials in middle adolescence. The present findings suggested that positive youth development and family functioning are protective factors for adolescent consumption of pornographic materials.

Introduction

Adolescents' sexual curiosity is increasingly aroused during puberty. As commented by Ponton (2000), all adolescents have sex lives, although some of the related behavior is not conspicuous, such as consumption of pornographic materials via the Internet. The Internet makes pornography exposed more often because of its accessibility, affordability, and anonymity (Peter and Valkenburg 2006). Additionally, the Internet gives rise to unwanted pornography exposure through websites that come up in response to searching, misspelling of Web addresses or links within websites, pop-up windows, and spam emails (Wolak et al. 2007).

The preparation for this paper and the Project P.A.T.H.S. were financially supported by The Hong Kong Jockey Club Charities Trust.

D.T.L. Shek (✉) • Q. Xie • C.M.S. Ma
Department of Applied Social Sciences, The Hong Kong Polytechnic University,
11 Yuk Choi Road, Hung Hom, Kowloon, Hong Kong, China
e-mail: daniel.shek@polyu.edu.hk

© Springer Science+Business Media Singapore 2015
T.Y. Lee et al. (eds.), *Student Well-Being in Chinese Adolescents in Hong Kong*,
Quality of Life in Asia 7, DOI 10.1007/978-981-287-582-2_23

Researchers have explored the prevalence of pornography consumption among adolescents. In a survey in around 1500 adolescents in the USA between the fall of 1999 and spring of 2000, the proportion of 12–18-year-old adolescents who reported wanted or unwanted exposure to sexual materials in the past 1 year was 15 %, with 8 % of them exposing to the materials from the Internet (Ybarra and Mitchell 2005). In a similar survey conducted in the USA in 2005, the proportion of those exposed to online pornography rose to 42 %, but the majority of these teenagers (66 %) reported accidental exposure (Wolak et al. 2007). Jones et al. (2012) study showed that 25 % of 10–17-year-olds reported unwanted online pornography exposure in 2000; this proportion rose to 34 % in 2005 and fell back to 23 % in 2010. Similar surveys were also conducted in some European countries. For example, an earlier large-scale survey conducted in Netherlands among 13–18-year-olds showed that around 55 % adolescents had viewed any type of pornography in the past 6 months (Peter and Valkenburg 2006), whereas a recent survey indicated that this figure declined to 25 % among 12–17-year-olds (Peter and Valkenburg 2011). The proportion of young people who have ever viewed pornography during adolescence remain high in some Western countries, with above 90 % among males and above 60 % among females in the USA and Sweden (Sabina et al. 2008; Svedin et al. 2011). Some research additionally highlighted unwanted exposure to pornography. In Australia and Britain, over half of the adolescents had visited pornographic websites, yet a substantial proportion of them did this involuntarily (Flood 2007; Livingstone and Bober 2004).

Researchers also found ethnic differences in the consumption of sexual materials (Hennessy et al. 2009; Ybarra and Mitchell 2005). For example, Ybarra and Mitchell (2005) noticed that Hispanic adolescents were more likely to seek pornography online rather than offline, compared with non-Hispanic adolescents. Hence, the findings on adolescent pornography consumption obtained from one ethnic group may not be generalizable to other ethnic groups. Several surveys have been conducted in Asia. In an earlier survey conducted in South Korea, 43 % of adolescents had ever watched pornographic movies (Kim 2001). A study conducted in Taiwan showed that around 42 % of the teenagers aged above 14 years had consumed online pornography (Lo et al. 2010). In Dong et al.'s (2013) study conducted in Shandong Province of mainland China, 6.4 % of the 12–18-year-old respondents consumed pornography. In Hong Kong, proportion of early adolescents (Secondary One) who accessed to online pornography in the past 12 months was lower than 10 % in Shek and Ma's (2012a) study and rose to around 12 % one year later (Shek and Ma 2012b) and a little more than 15 % in the third year (Ma and Shek 2013). These findings showed that the rate of pornography consumption among Hong Kong adolescents was lower than those in Western countries (Ma and Shek 2013). In addition, Shek and Ma (2012a, b) also found that mainland Chinese migrant adolescents in Hong Kong were more likely to expose to pornographic materials than did Hong Kong local adolescents.

Although some scholars argued that exposure to sexual materials is a normative experience for adolescents following the development about sexual curiosity (Sabina et al. 2008; Svedin et al. 2011), high frequency of consumption of pornography could be regarded as problem behavior that needs parents' and teachers' attention (Svedin et al. 2011). A number of studies showed that the access to pornography materials through the Internet may adversely affect adolescents in numerous aspects, such as sexual attitudes and behavior, self-concept and body image, problem behavior, and psychological and social development (Owens et al. 2012; Svedin et al. 2011). For example, several researchers found that more exposure to sexual materials was related to more casual and permissive sexual attitudes and behaviors (Brown and L'Engle 2009; Lo and Wei 2005; Peter and Valkenburg 2006). Adolescent exposure to pornography was also found to be associated with conduct problems (Svedin et al. 2011; Tsitsika et al. 2009; Ybarra and Mitchell 2005). Löfgren-Mårtenson and Månsson's (2010) study showed that consumption of sexual materials was likely to lead to boys' concern about their sexual ability and girls' concern about their body image. Kim (2001) found that the consumption of pornographic materials was related to low self-esteem. Mesch (2009) reported that adolescents who accessed to pornography more frequently tended to have lower level of social interaction and bonding. Furthermore, some research also suggested that viewing pornography online was more likely to associate with negative consequences than viewing pornography through other means (Lo and Wei 2005; Lo et al. 2010; Ybarra and Mitchell 2005). For example, Lo and Wei (2005) reported that access to pornographic materials online exerted more influence on permissive sexual attitude. Ybarra and Mitchell (2005) found that compared with adolescents who viewed traditional pornographic material, those who viewed pornography through the Internet were more likely to display clinical features of depression.

Adolescent consumption of pornographic materials was associated with some demographic factors, especially gender and age. Adolescent boys are much more likely than girls to consume pornographic materials (Shek and Ma 2012a, b; Mattebo et al. 2014; Tsitsika et al. 2009). In addition, boys are more likely to seek pornographic materials intentionally, whereas a substantial proportion of girl pornography consumers are Internet victims who view pornographic materials accidentally (Sabina et al. 2008; Ybarra and Mitchell 2005). Mattebo et al.'s (2014) study also showed that a higher proportion of boys than girls viewed pornography more than they really wanted and a higher proportion of girls than boys viewed pornography less than they really wanted. Older adolescents were more inclined than those in early adolescence to consume pornography, and the access prior to age 14 was relatively rare (Sabina et al. 2008; Ybarra and Mitchell 2005). Longitudinal investigations further showed age effect on the access to sexual materials. Shek and Ma's (2012b) study showed an increasing trend over 1 year of early adolescent consumption of pornography. Hennessy et al. (2009) conducted a 3-year longitudinal study regarding adolescent exposure to sexual content through television, music, magazines, and video games. They found that 14-year-olds exposed to media sexual content less than their older counterparts (16 years old) and higher exposure at the initial level were associated with slower increase of exposure.

Research also showed that adolescent consumption of pornography was related to family functioning, family commitment, emotional bond with caregivers, and caregiver monitoring and discipline (Ma and Shek 2013; Mesch 2009; Shek and Ma

2012a, b, 2014; Ybarra and Mitchell 2005). In addition, Ybarra and Mitchell (2005) reported that online pornography seekers reported lower lever of coercive discipline and poorer emotional bonding with caregivers than did offline seekers. Ma and Shek (2013) reported that family functioning predicted pornography consumption among early adolescents 2 years later. Weber et al. (2012) found that adolescents who were less independent of their surroundings, in particular their parents, consumed pornography more often. Furthermore, adolescent consumption of pornographic materials was negatively related to positive youth development (Ma and Shek 2013; Shek and Ma 2012b).

Literature review shows that there are few longitudinal studies in pornography consumption among adolescents. In this study, longitudinal data collected in four waves were used to understand pornography consumption in Chinese adolescents in Hong Kong. The following research questions were raised. (1) What is the prevalence of pornography consumption in Secondary 1 to Secondary 4 secondary school students in Hong Kong? (2) What demographic factors affect the initial level and growth trajectory of pornography consumption in adolescents from Secondary 1 to Secondary 4 years? (3) Do family functioning and positive youth development qualities affect pornography consumption in Secondary 4 students?

Based on the scientific literature, several hypotheses were proposed. First, consistent with the maturation hypothesis, the proportion of secondary students who consumed pornographic materials would increase from early adolescence to middle adolescence (Hypothesis 1; Ma and Shek 2013; Shek and Ma 2012a, b). Being male, higher age, and non-intact family status would be associated with higher initial level and higher growth rate in pornography consumption (Hypotheses 2a to 2c; Ma and Shek 2013; Shek and Ma 2012a, b). Finally, family functioning and positive youth development qualities would negatively predict pornography consumption in middle adolescents (Hypothesis 3a and 3b; Shek and Ma 2012a, b).

Methods

Participants

This study was part of the extension phase of the Positive Adolescent Training through Holistic Social Program (Project PATHS) in Hong Kong that tracked adolescent development from their Secondary 1 to Secondary 6. Four waves of data were used in this study. In Wave 1, 3328 Secondary 1 students with the mean age of 12.59 years (SD = .74) participated in this study, and among these students, 2617 of them also participated in Wave 4 when these students were in their Secondary 4 with the mean age of 15.50 years (SD = .66). These students were from 28 government and aided schools that covered all districts of Hong Kong. The details of demographic background of these students are presented in Table 1. Prior to data collection, ethnical approval was obtained from The Hong Kong Polytechnic University

Table 1 Data profile across four waves

	Wave 1	%	Wave 2	%	Wave 2[a]	%	Wave 3	%	Wave 3[a]	%	Wave 4	%	Wave 4[a]	%
N (participants)	3328		3638		2905		4106		2858		3973		2682	
Gender														
Male	1719	51.7	1716	47.2	1445	49.7	1885	45.9	1433	50.1	1875	47.2	1335	49.8
Female	1572	47.2	1864	51.2	1419	48.8	2185	53.2	1405	49.2	2086	52.5	1337	49.9
Economic disadvantage														
NOT receiving CSSA	2606	78.3	2932	80.6	2377	81.8	3308	80.6	2339	81.8	3302	83.1	2267	84.5
Receiving CSSA	225	6.8	208	5.7	160	5.5	212	5.2	147	5.1	200	5.0	132	4.9
Family intactness														
Intact families	2781	83.6	2985	82.1	2415	83.1	3372	82.1	2396	83.8	3210	80.8	2211	82.4
Non-intact families	515	15.5	624	17.2	469	16.1	715	17.4	454	15.9	749	18.9	466	17.4

[a]The numbers were based on the participants who ever participated in Wave 1 assessment as only those joining Wave 1 assessment were included in data analysis. The numbers of the students who did not report the corresponding information were not presented

and written consent was obtained from schools and parents. Before data collection, students' written consent was obtained and anonymity and confidentiality was emphasized.

Instruments

Consumption of Pornographic Materials Six items were used to assess consumption of six different types of online pornographic materials, and another six items were used to assess the access to pornographic materials via six different traditional mass media. Adolescents' responses were scored from 1 to 6 indicating their frequency of accessing these materials (1 = never, 2 = less than once a month, 3 = once to three times a month, 4 = once a week, 5 = several times a week, and 6 = daily). Previous studies reported good internal consistency reliability of this questionnaire (Ma and Shek 2013; Shek and Ma 2012a, b).

Family Functioning The Chinese Family Assessment Instrument was used to assess family functioning (Shek 2002). Nine items of the original instrument were used in this study with three each examining family functioning on each of the three dimensions: mutuality, conflicts, and communication. The quality of family functioning was indicated by averaging the scores on the mutuality and communicating and the reversed mean score on conflict. The shortened nine-item CFAI has good psychometric properties (Shek and Ma 2010a).

Positive Youth Development The Chinese Positive Youth Development Scale (CPYDS: Shek et al. 2007) was used to assess positive youth development among Chinese adolescents. It has 15 subscales corresponding to 15 positive youth development attributes: bonding, resilience, social competence, recognition for positive behavior, emotional competence, cognitive competence, behavioral competence, moral competence, self-determination, self-efficacy, clear and positive identity, beliefs in the future, prosocial involvement, prosocial norms, and spirituality. General positive youth development qualities were scored by averaging the scores on each subscale. This measure has good reliability and validity (Shek et al. 2007; Shek and Ma 2010b).

Results

Tables 1, 2, and 3 present the descriptive statistics about participants' demographic background and patterns of consumption of pornographic materials. As can be seen from Table 2, the proportion of adolescents who consumed any type of pornographic materials from the Internet was generally below 7.0 % in Wave 1 and rose across the 4 years sharply to almost 14.0 % in Wave 4.

Table 2 Frequencies of exposure to pornographic materials across four waves

	Wave 1		Wave 2		Wave 3		Wave 4	
	n	%	n	%	n	%	n	%
From the Internet								
1. Pornographic stories	197	5.9	271	9.3	323	11.7	380	14.7
2. Pornographic pictures	233	7.0	308	10.6	365	13.2	418	16.2
3. Pornographic videos	208	6.3	298	10.3	380	13.8	478	18.5
4. Pictures of sexual intercourse	213	6.4	255	8.8	329	11.9	363	14.0
5. Videos of sexual intercourse	221	6.7	265	9.2	325	11.8	392	15.2
6. Websites of real people performing in porn	160	4.8	213	7.4	290	10.5	359	13.9
From traditional materials								
1. Pornographic movies	25	0.8	36	1.2	38	1.4	45	1.7
2. Pornographic videos (through renting)	15	0.5	32	1.1	34	1.2	30	1.2
3. Pornographic videos on TV	56	1.7	49	1.7	59	2.1	60	2.3
4. Pornographic magazines	42	1.3	51	1.8	53	1.9	51	2.0
5. Pornographic books	45	1.4	79	2.7	77	2.8	84	3.3
6. Pornographic comics	96	2.9	128	4.4	125	4.5	119	4.6
Total (N)	3328	100	2905	100	2764	100	2588	100

Note: % indicates valid percentage

The respondents consumed more pornographic pictures and videos as well as videos of sexual intercourse than the other three types of materials, whereas websites of real people performing in porn were least consumed across 4 years. In contrast, the percentage of adolescents who consumed traditional pornographic materials was far smaller. Except for pornographic comics, consumption rates of traditional materials were 1.7 % or below in Wave 1 and grew to 3.3 % or below in Wave 4. More students consumed pornographic comics than other traditional materials: the proportion was 2.9 % in Wave 1 which increased to 4.6 % in Wave 4.

Linear mixed models were tested to investigate individual growth curves of adolescent consumption of pornographic materials from the Internet (Table 4).

The unconditional mean models (Model 1) were firstly conducted, which estimated the initial status and the extent to which interindividual differences accounted for the total variance. Results showed that 24.8 % of the variance could be explained by within-subject factors, whereas 14.6 % of the variance could be explained by between-subject factors (i.e., interindividual predictors). Thus, results indicated that approximately 37.1 % (ICC = .371) of the total variance could be accounted for by interindividual differences. The unconditional growth model (Model 2) additionally showed that there was an annual increase by .086 units ($p < .001$) in the four consecutive years. This model fitted the data better than Model 1 ($\Delta\chi^2_{(3)} = 1925.00$; $\Delta AIC = 1919.00$; $\Delta BIC = 1896.96$; $ps < .001$). The model also showed that second-level analysis was needed to further explain the interindividual factors. The conditional model (Model 3) was built to analyze the effects of age, gender, family economic status, and family intactness on the initial level and growth of consumption

Table 3 Descriptive statistics of key variables and internal consistency coefficients of scales (Waves 1–4)

	Mean (SD)				Reliability			
	W1	W2	W3	W4	W1	W2	W3	W4
Family functioning	3.73 (.81)	3.65 (.81)	3.65 (.79)	3.66 (.77)	.90	.90	.90	.91
Positive youth development	4.51 (.70)	4.43 (.69)	4.44 (.65)	4.45 (.62)	.93	.96	.96	.96
Exposure to sexual materials (Internet)	1.09 (.36)	1.19 (.64)	1.28 (.79)	1.35 (.84)	.92	.95	.95	.94
Gender								
Male	1.13 (.44)	1.25 (.74)	1.42 (.95)	1.55 (1.01)	–	–	–	–
Female	1.05 (.24)	1.08 (.29)	1.08 (.31)	1.09 (.83)	–	–	–	–
Socioeconomic status								
NOT receiving CSSA	1.09 (.35)	1.16 (.56)	1.26 (.75)	1.32 (.79)	–	–	–	–
Receiving CSSA	1.13 (.46)	1.25 (.73)	1.25 (.73)	1.31 (.69)	–	–	–	–
Family structure								
Intact families	1.08 (.32)	1.15 (.54)	1.23 (.71)	1.30 (.77)	–	–	–	–
Non-intact families	1.14 (.53)	1.23 (.69)	1.32 (.81)	1.42 (.87)	–	–	–	–
Exposure to sexual materials (traditional mass media)	1.02 (.17)	1.06 (.38)	1.06 (.40)	1.06 (.37)	.86	.92	.93	.93
Gender								
Male	1.03 (.21)	1.06 (.39)	1.08 (.47)	1.07 (.39)	–	–	–	–
Female	1.01 (.11)	1.03 (.16)	1.02 (.13)	1.03 (.23)	–	–	–	–
Socioeconomic status								
NOT receiving CSSA	1.02 (.15)	1.04 (.27)	1.05 (.38)	1.05 (.31)	–	–	–	–
Receiving CSSA	1.04 (.26)	1.07 (.47)	1.03 (.11)	1.03 (.13)	–	–	–	–
Family structure								
Intact families	1.02 (.11)	1.04 (.29)	1.05 (.34)	1.05 (.33)	–	–	–	–
Non-intact families	1.05 (.35)	1.05 (.34)	1.07 (.39)	1.05 (.31)	–	–	–	–

W1 Wave 1, *W2* Wave 2, *W3* Wave 3, *W4* Wave 4

Table 4 Results of individual growth curve analysis of adolescent consumption of pornographic materials for all models

		Exposure to sexual materials (Internet)						Exposure to sexual materials (traditional mass media)					
		Model 1		Model 2		Model 3		Model 1		Model 2		Model 3	
		Estimate	SE	Estimate	SE	Estimate	SE	Estimate	SE	Estimate	SE	Estimate	SE
Fixed effects													
Intercept	β_{0j}												
Initial status	γ_{00}	1.200***	.008	1.089***	.007	1.105***	.014	1.039***	.003	1.025***	.004	1.031***	.008
Age	γ_{01}					.064***	.010					.016**	.006
Gender[a]	γ_{02}					.031***	.007					.006	.004
Economic disadvantage[b]	γ_{03}					.002	.015					.001	.008
Family intactness[c]	γ_{04}					−.021	.011					−.009	.006
Linear slope	β_{1j}												
Initial status	γ_{10}			.086***	.005	.099***	.010			.011***	.003	.009	.005
Age	γ_{11}					−.002	.008					−.002	.004
Gender[a]	γ_{12}					.075***	.005					.009***	.003
Economic disadvantage[b]	γ_{13}					.004	.011					.004	.006
Family intactness[c]	γ_{14}					−.018*	.008					−.001	.004
Random effects													
Level 1 (within)													
Residual	r_{ij}	.248***	.004	.166***	.003	.160***	.003	.070***	.001	.062***	.001	.062***	.001
Level 2 (between)													
Intercept	u_{0j}	.146***	.006	.030***	.004	.030***	.005	.012***	.001	.001	.001	.001	.001
Time	u_{1j}			.038***	.002	.033***	.002			.006***	.000	.006	.000

(continued)

Table 4 (continued)

	Exposure to sexual materials (Internet)						Exposure to sexual materials (traditional mass media)					
	Model 1		Model 2		Model 3		Model 1		Model 2		Model 3	
	Estimate	SE	Estimate	SE	Estimate	SE	Estimate	SE	Estimate	SE	Estimate	SE
Fit statistics												
Deviance	20,176.019		18,251.022		15,086.101		3549.632		3185.398		2603.056	
AIC	20,182.019		18,263.022		15,114.101		3555.632		3195.398		2629.056	
BIC	20,204.061		18,307.106		15,214.497		3577.671		3232.131		2722.277	
df	3		6		14		3		5		13	

Unstructured covariance structure was used for Models 2 and 3 on exposure to sexual materials (Internet). Variance components structure was used for covariance structure of Models 2 and 3 on exposure to sexual materials (traditional mass media), because unstructured covariance structure resulted in redundant covariance parameters for these two models

Model 1 unconditional mean model, *Model 2* unconditional growth model, *Model 3* conditional model

[*]$p < .05$; [**]$p < .01$; [***]$p < .001$

[a]Female = −1, male = 1

[b]Receiving CSSA = −1, not receiving CSSA = 1

[c]Non-intact = −1, intact = 1

of online sexual materials. Results showed that the effects of age and gender were significant at the initial level, with male and older adolescents consuming more online pornographic materials than did their female and younger counterparts at Wave 1. Gender and family intactness affected the growth trajectory. Specifically, boys increased the access to online pornographic materials much more than girls, and adolescents from non-intact families (not living with both married biological parents) increased more than those from intact families. Model 3 fitted the data much better than Model 2 ($\Delta\chi^2_{(8)} = 3164.92$; ΔAIC = 3148.92; ΔBIC = 3092.61; $p < .001$).

Regarding the models on adolescent consumption of traditional pornographic materials, the unconditional mean model (Model 1) indicated that some 14.6 % (ICC = .146) of the total variance could be interpreted by interindividual differences (Table 4). The unconditional growth model (Model 2) showed significant annual growth of adolescent consumption of traditional pornography materials by .011 unit ($p < .001$) across the four waves and provided better fit of the data than did Model 1 ($\Delta\chi^2_{(2)} = 364.23$; ΔAIC = 360.23; ΔBIC = 345.54; $p < .001$). The conditional model (Model 3) revealed that only age was related to the initial level of consuming traditional sexual materials and that gender was the only factor affecting the growth. Specifically, older adolescents accessed to traditional pornographic materials more than younger adolescents in Wave 1, and boys increased the access more than girls. Model 3 fitted our data better than Model 2 ($\Delta\chi^2_{(8)} = 582.34$; ΔAIC = 566.342; ΔBIC = 509.854; $p < .001$).

Hierarchical multiple regressions were used to assess the prediction of exposure to online and traditional pornographic materials in Wave 4 by demographic factors, family functioning, and positive youth development (Table 5).

Demographic factors (i.e., gender, family economic status, and family intactness) were introduced to the regression models first as independent variables.

Table 5 Hierarchical multiple regression analyses on consumption of pornographic materials at Wave 4

Predictors	Exposure to sexual materials (Internet)		Exposure to sexual materials (traditional mass media)	
	Beta	R^2	Beta	R^2
Step 1		*.090*		*.006*
Gender[a]	.296***		.074***	
Economic disadvantage[b]	.002		.007	
Family intactness[c]	.051*		.010	
Step 2		*.020*		*.008*
Family functioning	**−.061***		**−.040**	
Positive youth development	**−.104***		**−.068****	

*$p < .05$; **$p < .01$; ***$p < .001$
[a]Female = 0, male = 1
[b]Receiving CSSA = 0, not receiving CSSA = 1
[c]Non-intact = 0, intact = 1

Results showed that gender was a strong predictor of both online and traditional pornographic material consumption. Boys consumed these materials more than girls. Family intactness was also a predictor of online pornographic material consumption. Adolescents in intact families consumed the materials more than those in non-intact families. These demographic variables accounted for around 9 % variance in online sexual material consumption and 0.6 % variance in traditional sexual material consumption. Family functioning and positive youth development were introduced as the second block of independent factors. Positive youth development negatively predicted exposure to both online and traditional pornographic materials, while better family functioning also negatively predicted exposure to online pornographic materials. These two factors additionally accounted for about 2 % of the variance in consuming online sexual materials and about 0.8 % variance in consuming traditional sexual materials.

Two more hierarchical multiple regression analyses were conducted by additionally considering adolescent initial levels of sexual material consumption (Table 6).

Adolescent scores on sexual material consumption in Wave 1 entered the model first. These initial scores were significant predictors of their respective scores in the fourth year and respectively accounted for around 12.0 % and 1.3 % variance in online and traditional pornographic material exposure. Gender, family economic status, and family intactness were introduced as the second block of the predictors, while family functioning and positive youth development were introduced as the third block. The contribution of these factors were comparable to those in the above two regressions (without controlling for the initial scores). Gender, family economic status, and family intactness explained about 7.6 % variance in online sexual material consumption and 0.5% variance in traditional sexual materials access, after initial scores were controlled for. Family functioning and positive youth development

Table 6 Hierarchical multiple regression analyses on consumption of pornographic materials at Wave 4 after controlling the initial levels at Wave 1

Predictors	Exposure to sexual materials (Internet)		Exposure to sexual materials (traditional mass media)	
	Beta	R^2	Beta	R^2
Step 1		*.120*		*.013*
Initial score	.347***		.112***	
Step 2		*.076*		*.005*
Gender[a]	.274***		.072**	
Economic disadvantage[b]	−.015		.002	
Family intactness[c]	.037		.002	
Step 3		*.011*		*.007*
Family functioning	**−.045***		**−.036**	
Positive youth development	**−.077***		**−.061***	

*p<.05; **p<.01; ***p<.001
[a]Female=0, male=1
[b]Receiving CSSA=0, not receiving CSSA=1
[c]Non-intact=0, intact=1

additionally accounted for some 1.1 % and 0.7 % variance respectively in online and traditional sexual material consumption. These analyses strongly suggested that positive youth development and family functioning negatively predicted adolescent consumption of online pornographic materials.

Discussion

The current study was the first to explore pornography consumption prevalence and growth trajectories as well as the predictors of pornography consumption among secondary students from early adolescence to middle adolescence in a Chinese context. This longitudinal study was based on the data collected from a large sample which was representative of Hong Kong adolescents. Besides, validated measures were used to assess pornography consumption and the related psychosocial correlates.

Results showed that the proportion of the students who consumed online pornography was less than 10 % in Secondary 1 (i.e., early adolescence) which rose steadily to less than 20 % in Secondary 4 (i.e., middle adolescence). This observation gives support for Hypothesis 1. As the corresponding figures in Western studies were usually above 20 % (e.g., Peter and Valkenburg 2006, 2011), these findings additionally support Ma and Shek's (2013) observation that pornography consumption rate among Hong Kong adolescents was lower than those among Western adolescents. This is potentially due to the conservative attitudes toward sex in traditional Chinese culture (Ma and Shek 2013) as well as the heavy study load and intensive competition for university admission in Hong Kong that may transfer adolescent sexual curiosity to study. The results are also in line with previous findings suggesting that older adolescents are more likely than early adolescents to consume pornography (Mattebo et al. 2014; Sabina et al. 2008; Tsitsika et al. 2009; Ybarra and Mitchell 2005). In addition, online pornography was far more consumed by adolescents relative to traditional pornography. In view of the easy accessibility and anonymity of consuming pornography on the Internet, it is reasonable to expect that the odds of online pornography consumption is higher than traditional pornography consumption.

Consistent with the predictions, results of linear mixed models showed gender and age effects on the initial level and growth trajectories of pornography consumption among adolescents. At Wave 1, boys consumed more online pornography than did girls and older adolescents consumed more online and traditional pornography than did younger adolescents; boys also increasingly consumed more pornography materials than did girls. These results are consistent with the existing findings (Sabina et al. 2008; Ybarra and Mitchell 2005) and support Hypotheses 2a and 2b. In addition, adolescents in non-intact families increasingly consumed more online pornography than did those in intact families, thus supporting Hypothesis 2c.

Multiple regression analyses results showed that initial level of pornography consumption affected the consumption 3 years later: the more adolescents consumed online pornography in Wave 1, the more that they consumed pornography in Wave 4. It is possible that those who initially consumed more online pornographic materials were more likely to be addicted to pornography and thereby more increasingly consumed these materials. Hence, early consumption of pornographic material can be regarded as a risk factor for future consumption. Besides, multiple regression analyses indicated that gender strongly influenced pornography consumption among middle adolescents at Wave 4.

Finally, family functioning and positive youth development also predicted pornography consumption. Better family functioning and higher level of positive youth development predicted less consumption of pornographic materials on the Internet. These findings support Hypotheses 3a and 3b, and they are consistent with the previous findings obtained among early adolescents in Hong Kong (Shek and Ma 2012a, b; Ma and Shek 2013) and suggest the importance of family functioning and positive youth development quality in reducing adolescent pornography consumption.

The present study has practical implications. As excessive exposure to pornography has been regarded as problem behavior and is related to negative behavioral outcomes (Owens et al. 2012; Svedin et al. 2011), intervention should be considered for adolescents who view pornography frequently. This study indicated that those who consumed more pornography in early adolescence also consumed more pornography at later years. This suggests that frequent adolescent pornography viewers should be identified and corresponding intervention should be taken as early as possible. Furthermore, this study suggests that the Internet is the major channel for adolescents to consume pornography. Hence, parents should be advised to limit online time for their children and block the known pornography websites at home. In addition, as boys are more likely than girls to be frequent pornography consumers, we should pay more attention to boys' online behavior and consumption of pornography. As better family functioning and high positive youth development qualities predict less pornography consumption among adolescents, developing parenting programs to improve family functioning and launching youth development program to improve positive youth development qualities can help to reduce adolescent pornography consumption.

This study also has several limitations. First, the measures of family functioning and positive youth development qualities were based on students' self-reports. Hence, the results may only reflect their "perceived" rather than "real" family functioning and positive youth development qualities. Second, students were not asked to indicate whether their exposure to pornographic materials was wanted or unwanted. Knowing the proportion of intentional pornography exposure as opposed to that of accidental exposure can provide more accurate understanding of adolescent pornography consumption. Third, only family functioning and positive youth development qualities as the predictors of adolescent pornography consumption were examined in this study. Hence, other factors that are likely to affect adolescent pornography consumption are not suggested in the current study and should be examined in the future. This can be done by a series of quantitative studies to correlate adolescent pornography consumption with other seemingly related factors such as peer relationship and school support. Besides, qualitative studies should be conducted to understand the subjective experiences of adolescents in consuming pornographic materials.

References

Brown, J. D., & L'Engle, K. L. (2009). X-rated: Sexual attitudes and behaviors associated with U.S. early adolescents' exposure to sexually explicit media. *Communication Research, 36,* 129–151.

Dong, F., Cao, F., Cheng, P., Cui, N., & Li, Y. (2013). Prevalence and associated factors of poly-victimization in Chinese adolescents. *Scandinavian Journal of Psychology, 54*(5), 415–422.

Flood, M. (2007). Exposure to pornography among youth in Australia. *Journal of Sociology, 43*(1), 45–60.

Hennessy, M., Bleakley, A., Fishbein, M., & Jordan, A. (2009). Estimating the longitudinal association between adolescent sexual behavior and exposure to sexual media content. *Journal of Sex Research, 46*(6), 586–596.

Jones, L. M., Mitchell, K. J., & Finkelhor, D. (2012). Trends in youth internet victimization: Findings from three youth internet safety surveys 2000–2010. *Journal of Adolescent Health, 50,* 179–186.

Kim, Y.-H. (2001). Korean adolescents' health risk behaviors and their relationships with the selected psychological constructs. *Journal of Adolescent Health, 29*(4), 298–306.

Livingstone, S., & Bober, M. (2004). *UK children go online: Surveying the experiences of young people and their parents.* Swindon: Economic and Social Research Council.

Lo, V.-H., & Wei, R. (2005). Exposure to internet pornography and Taiwanese adolescents' sexual attitudes and behavior. *Journal of Broadcasting & Electronic Media, 49*(2), 221–237.

Lo, V.-H., Wei, R., & Wu, H. (2010). Examining the first, second and third-person effects of Internet pornography on Taiwanese adolescents: Implications for the restriction of pornography. *Asian Journal of Communication, 20*(1), 90–103.

Löfgren-Mårtenson, L., & Månsson, S. (2010). Lust, love, and life: A qualitative study of Swedish adolescents' perceptions and experiences with pornography. *Journal of Sex Research, 47,* 568–579.

Ma, C. M. S., & Shek, D. T. L. (2013). Consumption of pornographic materials in early adolescents in Hong Kong. *Journal of Pediatric and Adolescent Gynecology, 26*(3), S18–S25.

Mattebo, M., Tydén, T., Häggström-Nordin, E., Nilsson, K. W., & Larsson, M. (2014). Pornography and sexual experiences among high school students in Sweden. *Journal of Developmental and Behavioral Pediatrics, 35*(3), 179–188.

Mesch, G. S. (2009). Social bonds and Internet pornographic exposure among adolescents. *Journal of Adolescence, 32,* 601–618.

Owens, E. W., Behun, R. J., Manning, J. C., & Reid, R. C. (2012). The impact of internet pornography on adolescents: A review of the research. *Sexual Addition & Compulsivity, 19,* 99–122.

Peter, J., & Valkenburg, P. M. (2006). Adolescents' exposure to sexually explicit material on the internet. *Communication Research, 33*(2), 178–204.

Peter, J., & Valkenburg, P. M. (2011). The use of sexually explicit Internet material and its antecedents: A longitudinal comparison of adolescents and adults. *Archives of Sexual Behavior, 40*(5), 1015–1025.

Ponton, L. (2000). *The sex lives of teenagers: Revealing the secret world of adolescent boys and girls.* New York: Penguin Putman.

Sabina, C., Wolak, J., & Finkelhor, D. (2008). The nature and dynamics of Internet pornography exposure for youth. *Cyberpsychology & Behavior, 11,* 691–693.

Shek, D. T. L. (2002). Assessment of family functioning in Chinese adolescents: The Chinese version of the family assessment device. *Research on Social Work Practice, 12*(4), 502–524.

Shek, D. T. L., & Ma, C. M. S. (2010a). The Chinese Family Assessment Instrument (C-FAI): Hierarchical confirmatory factor analyses and factorial invariance. *Research on Social Work Practice, 20*(1), 112–123.

Shek, D. T. L., & Ma, C. M. S. (2010b). Dimensionality of the Chinese positive youth development scale: Confirmatory factor analyses. *Social Indicators Research, 98*(1), 41–59.

Shek, D. T. L., & Ma, C. M. S. (2012a). Consumption of pornographic materials among early adolescents in Hong Kong: Profiles and psychosocial correlates. *International Journal on Disability and Human Development, 11*(2), 143–150.

Shek, D. T. L., & Ma, C. M. S. (2012b). Consumption of pornographic materials among Hong Kong early adolescents: A replication. *The Scientific World Journal, 2012*, Article ID 406063. doi:10.1100/2012/406063.

Shek, D. T. L., & Ma, C. M. S. (2014). Using structural equation modeling to examine consumption of pornographic materials in Chinese adolescents in Hong Kong. *International Journal on Disability and Human Development, 13*(2), 239–245.

Shek, D. T. L., Siu, A. M. H., & Lee, T. Y. (2007). The Chinese positive youth development scale: A validation study. *Research on Social Work Practice, 17*(3), 380–391.

Svedin, C. G., Åkerman, I., & Priebe, G. (2011). Frequent users of pornography. A population based epidemiological study of Swedish male adolescents. *Journal of Adolescence, 34*(4), 779–788.

Tsitsika, A., Critselis, E., Kormas, G., Konstantoulaki, E., Constantopoulos, A., & Kafetzis, D. (2009). Adolescent pornographic internet site use: A multivariate regression analysis of the predictive factors of use and psychosocial implications. *Cyberpsychology & Behavior, 12*(5), 545–550.

Weber, M., Quiring, O., & Daschmann, G. (2012). Peers, parents and pornography: Exploring adolescents' exposure to sexually explicit material and its developmental correlates. *Sexuality & Culture, 16*(4), 408–427.

Wolak, J., Mitchell, K. J., & Finkelhor, D. (2007). Unwanted and wanted exposure to online pornography in a national sample of youth internet users. *Pediatrics, 119*(2), 247–257.

Ybarra, M., & Mitchell, K. J. (2005). Exposure to internet pornography among children and adolescents: A national survey. *Cyberpsychology & Behavior, 8*(5), 473–486.

Positive Youth Development (PYD) and Adolescent Development: Reflection on Related Research Findings and Programs

Daniel T.L. Shek and Rachel C.F. Sun

Abstract There are growing research findings showing that positive youth development (PYD) attributes (such as resilience) is negatively linked to adolescent risk behavior (such as substance abuse). In this chapter, studies on the relationships between PYD attributes and adolescent risk behavior are reviewed. First, research studies on the relationship between PYD and problem adolescent sexual behavior such as having early sex are reviewed. Second, the link between PYD and adolescent self-harm as well as suicidal behavior is examined. Third, Chinese research on the link between PYD and adolescent problem behavior with life satisfaction as a mediator is reviewed. Gaps in the existing research and possible future research directions are discussed. Besides, PYD programs designed to reduce adolescent risk behavior (particularly risky sexual behavior, self-harm, and suicidal behavior) and promote positive development are examined. Problems on the existing PYD programs and future directions for the development of PYD programs are discussed.

Introduction

In contrast to the "deficient" models focusing on adolescent problems, positive youth development approach (PYD) emphasizes the strengths and positive attributes of young people (Damon 2004). The basic argument of the PYD approach is that by strengthening the psychosocial competencies of young people, their holistic development will be fostered and risk behavior will be reduced. Obviously, research findings supporting this basic assertion are indispensable. Besides, how PYD

Author contributed equally with all other contributors

The Project P.A.T.H.S. and this work were financially supported by The Hong Kong Jockey Club Charities Trust.

D.T.L. Shek (✉)
Department of Applied Social Sciences, The Hong Kong Polytechnic University,
11 Yuk Choi Road, Hung Hom, Kowloon, Hong Kong, China
e-mail: daniel.shek@polyu.edu.hk

R.C.F. Sun
Faculty of Education, The University of Hong Kong, Pok Fu Lam, Hong Kong, China

© Springer Science+Business Media Singapore 2015
T.Y. Lee et al. (eds.), *Student Well-Being in Chinese Adolescents in Hong Kong*,
Quality of Life in Asia 7, DOI 10.1007/978-981-287-582-2_24

325

concepts can be applied in the real world is another question to be considered. Against this background, there are two main purposes of this chapter. First, it examines the relationship between PYD and adolescent development with reference to three examples – problem adolescent sexual behavior, adolescent self-harm and suicidal behavior, and mediational models on the link between PYD and adolescent problem behavior. Based on the review, research gaps and future directions of research are outlined. Second, examples of PYD programs are described and gaps as well as future directions regarding designs of PYD programs are discussed.

Positive Youth Development and Adolescent Risk Behavior

The first example on the relationship between PYD and adolescent risk behavior is risky sexual behavior. Reviews of the literature showed that positive youth development attributes were negatively related to risky sexual behavior. Primarily, cognitive competence determines the engagement of adolescents in sexual behavior. Holmbeck et al. (1994) reasoned that different cognitive factors, including reasoning ability, probabilistic thinking, and cognitive functions such as the ability to evaluate alternatives and perceptions of risk, influence sexual postponement. There is evidence showing that higher intelligence was negatively related to the onset of sexual activities (Halpern et al. 2000; Hardy et al. 1998). Sexually abstinent adolescents also reported higher GPAs than did their high-risk counterparts (Luster and Small 1994).

Positive self-representation is also conducive to healthy adolescent sexual behavior. Studies showed that low global self-worth and poor self-image were risk factors for adolescent girls to engage in risky sexual behaviors, such as having more sexual partners (Ethier et al. 2006; Wild et al. 2004a). Similarly, low self-esteem might predispose adolescents to use risky sexual behavior as a way to cope with negative emotions (Baumeister 1990), and they were more susceptible to peer pressure (McGee and Williams 2000). However, the literature on the relationship between adolescent self-esteem and adolescent sexuality is not entirely consistent in the literature. For example, Goodson et al. (2006) showed that while around 26 % of the reviewed studies reported inverse relationships between self-esteem and adolescent sexual behaviors, attitudes, and intentions, around 60 % of studies showed no relationship involved. Some researchers even found that excessive high self-esteem would create egocentric and self-centered attitudes which would in turn promote experimentation of sexual activity (Baumeister et al. 2003).

Intrapersonal and interpersonal attributes are also associated with adolescent sexual behavior and intention. At the intrapersonal level, spirituality was negatively related to initiation of sexual activity (Holder et al. 2000). Moral values are also related to adolescent sexual behavior. While identification with positive moral values and attitudes was negatively related to sexual risk behaviors (Hubbs-Tait and Garmon 1995; Kotchick et al. 2001), liberal sexual attitudes were positively related to adolescent sexual risk taking (Jemmott and Jemmott 1990). Poor emotional competence also predisposes adolescents to underestimate the effect of emotion on sexual behavior (Loewenstein 1996).

Regarding interpersonal competence, social competence such as communication with peers and social assertiveness has impact on adolescent sexual behavior. For instance, the ability to show different opinions was associated with lower sexual risk behavior (Magnani et al. 2001). Besides, students who had a strong bondage with their school or family reported lower levels of sexual behavior (Catalano et al. 2004b; Magnani et al. 2001).

Social norms are also important for reducing sexual risk taking among adolescents. Kirby (2001a) reviewed several education programs on sexuality and HIV and found that focus on clear norms about avoiding unprotected sex is an important element. Adolescents who are involved in prosocial activities are more likely to interact with positive role models who embrace conventional values such as delayed pregnancy and higher career aspirations.

The second example is about the relationship between positive youth development and adolescent self-harm and suicidal behavior. Research findings showed that good bonding with healthy peers and adults are protective factors against self-harm. There is evidence showing that bonding or connectedness in the family (e.g., Borowsky et al. 2001; Tatnell et al. 2013), peers (e.g., Rubenstein et al. 1989), school (e.g., Pisani et al. 2013; Sun and Hui 2007), and community (Pisani et al. 2013) contexts was negatively related to adolescent self-harm behavior. Kaminski and colleagues (2010) examined the role of connectedness in adolescent self-harm and suicidal behavior in secondary school students in a high-risk community characterized by high-rate poverty, unemployment, single-parent households, and serious crimes. They showed that different types of connectedness were negatively related to self-harm and suicidal behavior – family connectedness was the strongest predictor of deliberate self-harm and suicidal behavior; school connectedness predicted deliberate self-harm and suicidal signs except suicidal injury; connectedness with adults at school predicted deliberate self-harm and suicidal behavior; peer connectedness predicted suicidal attempt.

Resilience was also negatively related to self-harm. Conceiving resilience in terms of personal competence, social competence, and structured living style, von Soest et al. (2010) showed that these three factors of resilience were associated with a lower level of suicidal ideation and suicidal attempts in 9,085 Norway late adolescents. Besides, resilience helps high-risk adolescents to deal with the negative impact of adversity on suicidal attempt. For example, Nrugham et al. (2010) found the inverse link of resilience and suicidal attempt in adolescents experiencing depression and violent life events. However, there is no known scientific study on resilience and deliberate self-harm.

In addition, adolescents who display self-harm often have poor social-emotional control and maladaptive coping strategies (Lloyd-Richardson et al. 2007; Muehlenkamp et al. 2013). From the positive youth development literature, it can be conjectured that high emotional and social competences are protective factors. Baetens et al. (2012) found that adolescents with deliberate self-harm history reported a lower level of social competence than did those without such history.

Mikolajczak et al. (2009) similarly found that emotional intelligence and maladaptive coping strategies were inversely related to adolescent self-harm and suicide through maladaptive coping strategies. According to Cha and Nock (2009), emotional intelligence served as a buffer to attenuate the harmful impact of child abuse on suicidal ideation and attempt.

Furthermore, negative identity and low self-esteem were related to adolescent self-harm. Based on the responses of 455 Norway adolescents, Grøholt et al. (2005) showed that non-suicidal attempters reported higher levels of self-concept, global self-worth, and self-concept stability than did suicidal attempters. Wild et al. (2004b) similarly showed that self-esteem differentiated adolescents with suicidal ideation and suicidal attempts from those without suicidal behavior. Based on a survey of 6,020 adolescents, Hawton et al. (2002) showed that adolescents with deliberate self-harm and those without self-harm history were different in self-esteem, with higher self-esteem predicting lower deliberate self-harm.

Adolescents who possess positive beliefs in the future are also less likely to engage in self-harm behavior. There are research findings showing the positive link between adolescent hopelessness and self-harm (Lee et al. 2009; McLaughlin et al. 1996; Taliaferro et al. 2012). For example, O'Connor et al. (2009) showed that optimism defined in terms of generalized positive expectations for the future was negatively related to deliberate self-harm in girls.

Finally, spirituality has been proposed to be negatively related to adolescent developmental problems (Shek 2010) and lack of purpose in life can be regarded as a warning sign for adolescent suicide (Rudd et al. 2006). Wang and colleagues (2007) showed that purpose in life was negatively associated with suicidal ideation and attempt and it predicted lower level of suicidal ideation and attempt through decreased depression. However, there is paucity of research examining the role of purpose in life in preventing deliberate self-harm.

With specific reference to the Hong Kong context, there are several studies showing that PYD attributes are related to adolescent self-harm and suicidal behavior. Shek and Yu (2012) examined the influence of cognitive-behavioral competence, positive identity, prosocial attributes, and general positive youth development on self-harm. Results showed that general positive youth development predicted lower occurrence of suicidal behavior and deliberate self-harm. Contrary to the expectation, cognitive-behavioral competence was positively associated with suicidal behavior and deliberate self-harm. The above findings were basically replicated by Law and Shek (2013) who found that positive youth development attributes were associated with suicidal behavior and deliberate self-harm in Secondary 2 students. The unexpected reverse patterns were found again in the link between cognitive-behavioral competence and suicidal behavior and that between prosocial attributes and both forms of self-harm. Finally, Law and Shek (2014) showed that over three years, positive youth development mediated the relationship between family functioning and adolescent deliberate self-harm and suicidal behavior. Specifically, family mutuality and communications at Wave 1 predicted increased positive youth development at Wave 2, which further predicted lower levels of suicidal behavior and deliberate self-harm at Wave 3.

The third example on the linkage between PYD and adolescent problem behavior is on the mediating role of life satisfaction between PYD and problem behavior. Based on the data collected from the Project P.A.T.H.S., Sun and Shek (2010) showed that PYD influenced adolescent problem behavior via life satisfaction. The related findings were replicated in another study involving three datasets of the study. Finally, using another three waves of data, findings similarly showed that PYD influenced adolescent problem behavior via life satisfaction.

Several observations can be highlighted from the existing research studies. First, there is a need to step up research on the relationship between PYD constructs and adolescent risk behavior. Generally speaking, compared with research on risk factors, there are relatively few studies on protective factors of adolescent risk behavior with respect to the PYD framework. For example, there are few studies on the linkage between PYD and adolescent self-harm and suicidal behavior.

Second, there are inconsistent research findings on the linkage between PYD and adolescent risk behavior. In the area of adolescent sexual behavior, research showed that positive identity (such as overconfidence) and social competence (such as over-engagement in social activities) might promote risky adolescent sexual behavior. In the area of self-harm and suicidal behavior, the available findings on the links between positive youth development attributes and adolescent self-harm are also not entirely consistent. Some positive relationships between these two domains have been found by researchers (Kaminski et al. 2010; Shek and Yu 2012; Law and Shek 2013).

Third, there are few validated measures of PYD constructs in the field. While there are some isolated measures of different aspects of PYD such as positive identity, resilience, and self-efficacy, there are few scales which examine multiple dimensions of PYD in a study. Besides, few researchers have used multiple measures of PYD in their study. The inclusion of multiple measures in a study is important because this can enable researchers to understand the differential relationships between PYD constructs and adolescent risk behavior.

Fourth, most of the existing studies on the link between PYD and adolescent risk behavior were conducted in the Western contexts and few studies have been carried out in Asian contexts, particularly China. As Chinese people constitutes roughly one-fourth of the world's population, there is a need to examine the generalizability of Western findings to the Chinese contexts. In addition, with rapid transformations in the socioeconomic and cultural environment in China, there has been a change in collectivistic values toward a more individualistic direction. Hence, it would be both theoretically and practically exciting to look at the relationships between these two domains in the fast-changing Chinese context.

Fifth, PYD concepts such as self-efficacy and self-determination are largely based on Western ideas. Besides, indigenous Chinese concepts can also be enlightening. For example, Confucian virtues can be examined within the context of moral competence and Buddhist and Taoist thoughts can be examined within the context of spirituality.

Sixth, most of the existing studies adopted cross-sectional designs. Although cross-sectional research can be easily conducted, the related findings cannot give definitive conclusions on the cause-effect relationships between PYD and adolescent risk behavior. Furthermore, overreliance on cross-sectional design in the studies also limits the ability to examine the complex relationships between PYD and adolescent risk behavior over time. While positive youth development can reduce the risk of self-harm, self-harm can also lead to a reduction in positive youth development. Therefore, there is a need to call for investigation in protective positive youth development factors with longitudinal design in the future studies.

Finally, besides direct models on the linkage between PYD and adolescent risk behavior, more complex models with mediating and/or moderating mechanisms should be considered. Primarily, it is theoretically interesting to ask whether there are any mediating mechanisms involved in the linkage between PYD constructs and adolescent risk behavior. With specific reference to the Chinese context, it was found that PYD influenced adolescent problem behavior through the influence of life satisfaction in a series of studies (Sun and Shek 2010, 2013). Besides, very few studies have examined the factors that moderate the relationships between PYD constructs and adolescent risk behavior. For example, it is theoretically interesting to ask how spirituality moderates the relationship between stress and adolescent risk behavior. It is also important to ask how prosocial behavior moderates the relationship between moral competence and adolescent risk behavior.

Positive Youth Development Programs

Positive youth development programs have been designed with reference to the two adolescent risk behavior outlined in this chapter. With reference to adolescent sexual problems, positive youth development programs have been developed to delay the onset of sexual behavior in adolescents. As pointed out by House et al. (2010), "competence can be a protective factor for adolescent sexual and reproductive health outcomes. Positive youth development programs that provide a safe setting in which youth can learn and use social and cognitive skills may have a positive impact on sexual and reproductive health as well as other youth outcomes" (p. S19). Positive youth development programs have been shown to be effective in promoting healthy adolescent sexual and reproductive health (Gavin et al. 2010).

Promotion of psychosocial competence prevents the development of risky sexual behavior in adolescents. Intervention programs focusing on the promotion of cognitive-behavioral skills in adolescents, such as sexual assertion, refusal, self-management, problem solving, and risk recognition, were found to reduce adolescent risky sexual behavior and delay the onset of sexual activity (Lawrence et al. 1995). Incorporating emotional education component into intervention programs such as helping students identify, anticipate, and deal with emotions in a healthy manner facilitated sexual risk reduction among adolescents (Ferrer et al. 2011). Programs emphasizing sexual assertiveness, communication, and negotiation skills were effective in reducing sexual risk behaviors enabling youths to cope with partner pressure (Pedlow and Carey 2004).

Besides, there are programs which attempted to promote adolescent sexual health by targeting different aspects of adolescent identity. For example, promotion of self-efficacy and refusal self-efficacy was effective in delaying risky sexual behavior among adolescents (Guse et al. 2012). Besides, positive beliefs in the future served as a protective factor for adolescent risky sexual behavior (Mueller et al. 2010; Vesely et al. 2004). Furthermore, there are views suggesting that helping young people to develop a sense of purpose is important. As pointed out by Bolland (2003), "it is important that prevention and intervention programmes also attempt to build skills that allow participants to better understand their cognitive-affective responses to adversity, or that provide them with the ability to take advantage of life opportunities that they encounter; both of these approaches may allow individual adolescents to overcome the limitations of hopelessness" (p. 156).

Reinforcement of prosocial norms and providing students with the opportunities to engage in youth activities to personalize these norms are important (Kirby 2001b). Indeed, youths' participation in prosocial activities in school, church, or community was found to be negatively associated with sexual behavior (Ramirez-Valles et al. 1998). Finally, there are views suggesting that prevention programs should not reinforce individualistic and egotistic values in young people (Hughes et al. 2001).

There are also programs showing that PYD intervention components are effective to reduce adolescent self-harm and suicide. For example, according to the 2012 National Strategy for Suicide Prevention in the USA, promoting connectedness was identified as an effective means to prevent suicide (USHHS and National Action Alliance for Suicide Prevention 2012).

In addition to the above programs which are specifically related to adolescent sexuality as well as self-harm and suicidal behavior, there is research evidence showing that PYD programs promote positive youth behavior and reduce adolescent risk behavior. Catalano et al. (2004a) reviewed 77 programs in the USA. They found that among the 25 successful programs, 15 positive youth development constructs could be identified. These included bonding, resilience, psychosocial competence (cognitive, emotional, social, behavioral, and moral competencies), self-determination, self-efficacy, clear and positive identity, spirituality, beliefs in the future, promotion of prosocial norms, opportunities for prosocial involvement, and recognition for positive behavior.

There are also many programs targeting social-emotional skills in students. The basic argument of such programs is that a lack of social-emotional skills in students would make them disconnected which eventually impair their academic achievement. Research findings have shown that young people generally lack psychosocial skills. For example, based on roughly 150,000 students in Grade 6 to Grade 12, Benson (2006) showed that less than half of the students reported that they possessed psychosocial skills such as empathy, rational decision-making and ability to resolve interpersonal conflicts. In a recent meta-analysis study based on 213 social-emotional learning programs involving roughly 270,000 students, Durlak et al. (2011) showed that relative to the control students, participants joining social-emotional learning programs showed better psychosocial skills, attitudes, and behavior as well as higher academic performance.

With specific reference to Hong Kong, positive evaluation findings are also intrinsic to a large-scale positive youth development program entitled "Positive Adolescent Training through Holistic Social Programmes" (Project P.A.T.H.S.). There are two tiers of programs in the project (Tier 1 and Tier 2 Programs). For the Tier 1 Program, systematic and curricular-based programs were designed based on the positive youth development constructs identified from the successful PYD programs in the West. Utilizing multiple evaluation strategies including objective outcome evaluation, subjective outcome evaluation, process evaluation, qualitative evaluation, and personal construct psychology evaluation and results generally showed that different stakeholders had positive evaluation of the program. In particular, the longitudinal evaluation using a randomized group trial showed that compared to the control school students, students in the experimental group showed better positive development (e.g., resilience), slower development in drinking, smoking, and consumption of psychotropic substances, and slower development of delinquent behavior and intention to engage in risky behavior.

Several observations can be highlighted from the PYD programs in the scientific literature. First, the development of PYD programs with reference to different adolescent developmental problems is rather uneven. For example, while there are many programs on promoting the social skills of adolescents to prevent adolescent substance abuse, there are comparatively fewer PYD programs developed to help adolescents in dealing with adolescent deliberate self-harm behavior. Similarly, there are few PYD programs targeting compensated dating behavior in adolescents. Furthermore, there are few generic PYD programs that attempt to strengthen multiple PYD attributes.

Second, compared with the PYD programs in the West, there are comparatively fewer PYD programs in different Chinese contexts. In a review of adolescent prevention and PYD programs in the Chinese context, Shek and Yu (2011) reported that there were very few validated PYD programs in different Chinese communities. As the development of Chinese adolescents is shaped by Chinese influences such as Confucian and Buddhist values, Western programs may need adaptation when they are used in Chinese adolescents. Besides, indigenous concepts should also be incorporated in the Chinese PYD programs. As pointed out by Shek and Sun (2013a, b), different cultural issues should be considered when implementing PYD programs in Chinese cultural contexts.

Third, different mechanisms have been included in existing PYD programs. For example, based on the assumption that positive self-identity is the foundation of healthy adolescent development, some programs attempt to promote self-confidence, self-esteem, and self-image in adolescents. On the other hand, based on social learning theories, some theorists focus on promotion of self-efficacy in adolescents. Hence, there is a need to clarify the theoretical mechanisms which are conducive to enhancement of positive youth development. For some of the PYD constructs such as resilience and spirituality, there can be different theoretical accounts and explanations involved in conceptualizing the positive influence of PYD constructs. Hence, delineation and clarification of the related mechanisms are in order.

Fourth, closely related to the issue of theoretical mechanisms is how the theoretical mechanisms can be translated into practice. Primarily, there is a great "leap of faith" in the translation of validated theoretical mechanisms to practice in the real world. There are at least two issues that require consideration here. The first issue is how the theoretical mechanisms are adequately included in the program materials. Without a good program, good theory alone is not adequate. The second issue is how the developed program can be effectively implemented. Basically, translation of "good" theoretical mechanisms to "good" program and "good" implementation is not simple. In reality, there are different degrees of sophistication in translating the effective mechanism into practice.

Fifth, there are wide variations in the training of potential program implementers. Effective training is very important because it is the link between the theory behind the program, the developed program, and the program to be delivered. Without dedicated trainers who have good understanding of and identification with the program, program success would not be possible. In the training programs, the potential program implementers should be trained to understand and identify with the program philosophy, have correct understanding of the curriculum, understand the teaching and learning processes and ways to promote student involvement and teacher teaching effectiveness, be familiar with the ways to deal with classroom misbehavior, and appreciate the importance of evaluation of program implementers' own practice.

Sixth, the quality of evaluation in the existing PYD programs varies much across different programs. Subjective outcome evaluation and qualitative evaluation were carried out to evaluate most programs. While these evaluation strategies are easily conducted, they are commonly criticized as subjective and unable to give a true picture of the effectiveness of the program as far as objective outcomes are concerned. In the context of adolescent prevention and PYD programs, randomized group trials are usually regarded as the "gold standard" in evaluating program effectiveness. With specific focus on different Chinese communities, randomized groups trials are seldom conducted which has adversely affected the development of evidence-based PYD programs.

Finally, the degree of dissemination and sustainability in the PYD programs varies. For some successful programs such as the Life Skills Training Program, they are incorporated in the formal service delivery system and they receive funding from the government. For some programs, they might simply be terminated after the funding becomes exhausted. Hence, it is important to consider how the successful experiences can be disseminated and the long-term sustainability of the successful programs can be ensured. Besides, how to link the successful programs to government policies is an important issue to be considered. To get things done, soliciting support from different political parties is an important task to be done.

Summary and Conclusion

In this chapter, empirical evidence on the influence of positive youth development on adolescent risk behavior indexed by risky sexual behavior and self-harm as well as suicidal behavior is reviewed. Generally speaking, research findings showed that

PYD constructs are negatively linked to adolescent risk behavior. However, there are several gaps and problems in this field of research. In this chapter, generic PYD programs and specific PYD programs with reference to risky sexual behavior and self-harm as well as suicidal behavior are outlined. Similar to PYD research, there are several gaps and issues in the field of PYD programs which deserve future research.

References

Baetens, I., Claes, L., Muehlenkamp, J., Grietens, H., & Onghena, P. (2012). Differences in psychological symptoms and self-competencies in non-suicidal self-injurious Flemish adolescents. *Journal of Adolescence, 35*(3), 753–759.

Baumeister, R. F. (1990). Suicide as escape from self. *Psychological Review, 97*(1), 90–113.

Baumeister, R. F., Campbell, J. D., Krueger, J. I., & Vohs, K. D. (2003). Does high self-esteem cause better performance, interpersonal success, happiness, or healthier lifestyles? *Psychological Science in the Public Interest, 4*(1), 1–44.

Benson, P. L. (2006). *All kids are our kids: What communities must do to raise caring and responsible children and adolescents* (2nd ed.). San Francisco: Jossey-Bass.

Bolland, J. M. (2003). Hopelessness and risk behavior among adolescents living in high-poverty inner-city neighborhoods. *Journal of Adolescence, 26*(2), 145–158.

Borowsky, I. W., Ireland, M., & Resnick, M. D. (2001). Adolescent suicide attempts: Risks and protectors. *Pediatrics, 107*(3), 485–493.

Catalano, R. F., Berglund, M. L., Ryan, J. A. M., Lonczak, H. S., & Hawkins, J. D. (2004a). Positive youth development in the United States: Research findings on evaluations of positive youth development programs. *Annals of the American Academy of Political and Social Science, 591*, 98–124.

Catalano, R. F., Oesterle, S., Fleming, C. B., & Hawkins, J. D. (2004b). The importance of bonding to school for healthy development: Findings from the Social Development Research Group. *Journal of School Health, 74*(7), 252–261.

Cha, C. B., & Nock, M. K. (2009). Emotional intelligence is a protective factor for suicidal behavior. *Journal of the American Academy of Child and Adolescent Psychiatry, 48*(4), 422–430.

Damon, W. (2004). What is positive youth development? *Annals of the American Academy of Political and Social Science, 591*(1), 13–24.

Durlak, J. A., Weissberg, R. P., Dymnicki, A. B., Taylor, R. D., & Schellinger, K. B. (2011). The impact of enhancing students' social and emotional learning: A meta-analysis of school-based universal interventions. *Child Development, 82*(1), 405–432.

Ethier, K. A., Kershaw, T. S., Lewis, J. B., Milan, S., Niccolai, L. M., & Ickovics, J. R. (2006). Self-esteem, emotional distress and sexual behavior among adolescent females: Interrelationships and temporal effects. *Journal of Adolescent Health, 38*(3), 268–274.

Ferrer, R. A., Fisher, J. D., Buck, R., & Amico, K. R. (2011). Pilot test of an emotional education intervention component for sexual risk reduction. *Health Psychology, 30*(5), 656–660. doi:10.1037/a0023438.

Gavin, L. E., Catalano, R. F., David-Ferdon, C., Gloppen, K. M., & Markham, C. M. (2010). A review of positive youth development programs that promote adolescent sexual and reproductive health. *Journal of Adolescent Health, 46*(3), S75–S91.

Goodson, P., Buhi, E. R., & Dunsmore, S. C. (2006). Self-esteem and adolescent sexual behaviors, attitudes, and intentions: A systematic review. *Journal of Adolescent Health, 38*(3), 310–319.

Grøholt, B., Ekeberg, Ø., Wichstrøm, L., & Haldorsen, T. (2005). Suicidal and nonsuicidal adolescents: Different factors contribute to self-esteem. *Suicide and Life-Threatening Behavior, 35*(5), 525–535.

Guse, K., Levine, D., Martins, S., Lira, A., Gaarde, J., Westmorland, W., & Gilliam, M. (2012). Interventions using new digital media to improve adolescent sexual health: A systematic review. *Journal of Adolescent Health, 51*(6), 535–543. doi:10.1016/j.jadohealth.2012.03.014.

Halpern, C. T., Joyner, K., Udry, J. R., & Suchindran, C. (2000). Smart teens don't have sex (or kiss much either). *Journal of Adolescent Health, 26*(3), 213–225.

Hardy, J. B., Astone, N. M., Brooks-Gunn, J., Shapiro, S., & Miller, T. L. (1998). Like mother, like child: Intergenerational patterns of age at first birth and associations with childhood and adolescent characteristics and adult outcomes in the second generation. *Developmental Psychology, 34*(6), 1220–1232.

Hawton, K., Rodham, K., Evans, E., & Weatherall, R. (2002). Deliberate self harm in adolescents: Self report survey in schools in England. *BMJ, 325*(7374), 1207–1211.

Holder, D. W., DuRant, R. H., Harris, T. L., Daniel, J. H., Obeidallah, D., & Goodman, E. (2000). The association between adolescent spirituality and voluntary sexual activity. *Journal of Adolescent Health, 26*(4), 295–302.

Holmbeck, G. N., Crossman, R. E., Wandrei, M. L., & Gasiewski, E. (1994). Cognitive development, egocentrism, self-esteem, and adolescent contraceptive knowledge, attitudes, and behavior. *Journal of Youth and Adolescence, 23*(2), 169–193.

House, L. D., Bates, J., Markham, C. M., & Lesesne, C. (2010). Competence as a predictor of sexual and reproductive health outcomes for youth: A systematic review. *Journal of Adolescent Health, 46*(3), S7–S22. doi:10.1016/j.jadohealth.2009.12.003.

Hubbs-Tait, L., & Garmon, L. C. (1995). The relationship of moral reasoning and AIDS knowledge to risky sexual behavior. *Adolescence, 30*(119), 549–564.

Hughes, J. N., Cavell, T. A., & Prasad-Gaur, A. (2001). A positive view of peer acceptance in aggressive youth risk for future peer acceptance. *Journal of School Psychology, 39*(3), 239–252.

Jemmott, L. S., & Jemmott, J. B., III. (1990). Sexual knowledge, attitudes, and risky sexual behavior among inner-city Black male adolescents. *Journal of Adolescent Research, 5*(3), 346–369.

Kaminski, J. W., Puddy, R. W., Hall, D. M., Cashman, S. Y., Crosby, A. E., & Ortega, L. A. (2010). The relative influence of different domains of social connectedness on self-directed violence in adolescence. *Journal of Youth and Adolescence, 39*(5), 460–473.

Kirby, D. (2001a). *Emerging answers: Research findings on programs to reduce teen pregnancy.* Washington, DC: National Campaign to Prevent Teen Pregnancy.

Kirby, D. (2001b). Understanding what works and what doesn't in reducing adolescent sexual risk-taking. *Family Planning Perspectives, 33*(6), 276–281.

Kotchick, B. A., Shaffer, A., Forehand, R., & Miller, K. S. (2001). Adolescent sexual risk behavior: A multi-system perspective. *Clinical Psychology Review, 21*(4), 493–519.

Law, B. M. F., & Shek, D. T. L. (2013). Self-harm and suicide attempts among young Chinese adolescents in Hong Kong: Prevalence, correlates, and changes. *Journal of Pediatric and Adolescent Gynecology, 26*(3), S26–S32.

Law, B. M. F., & Shek, D. T. L. (2014). A longitudinal study on deliberate self-harm and suicidal behaviors among Chinese adolescents. In D. T. L. Shek, R. C. F. Sun, & C. M. S. Ma (Eds.), *Chinese adolescents in Hong Kong: Family life, psychological well-being and risk behavior* (pp. 155–172). Singapore: Springer.

Lawrence, J. S. S., Brasfield, T. L., Jefferson, K. W., Alleyne, E., O'Bannon, R. E., III, & Shirley, A. (1995). Cognitive-behavioral intervention to reduce African American adolescents' risk for HIV infection. *Journal of Consulting and Clinical Psychology, 63*(2), 221–237.

Lee, A., Wong, S. Y. S., Tsang, K. K., Ho, G. S. M., Wong, C. W., & Cheng, F. (2009). Understanding suicidality and correlates among Chinese secondary school students in Hong Kong. *Health Promotion International, 24*(2), 156–165.

Lloyd-Richardson, E. E., Perrine, N., Dierker, L., & Kelley, M. L. (2007). Characteristics and functions of non-suicidal self-injury in a community sample of adolescents. *Psychological Medicine, 37*(8), 1183–1192.

Loewenstein, G. (1996). Out of control: Visceral influences on behavior. *Organizational Behavior and Human Decision Processes, 65*(3), 272–292.

Luster, T., & Small, S. A. (1994). Factors associated with sexual risk-taking behaviors among adolescents. *Journal of Marriage and Family, 56*(3), 622–632.

Magnani, R. J., Seiber, E. E., Gutierrez, E. Z., & Vereau, D. (2001). Correlates of sexual activity and condom use among secondary school students in urban Peru. *Studies in Family Planning, 32*(1), 53–66.

McGee, R., & Williams, S. (2000). Does low self-esteem predict health compromising behaviors among adolescents? *Journal of Adolescence, 23*(5), 569–582.

McLaughlin, J. A., Miller, P., & Warwick, H. (1996). Deliberate self-harm in adolescents: Hopelessness, depression, problems and problem-solving. *Journal of Adolescence, 19*(6), 523–532.

Mikolajczak, M., Petrides, K. V., & Hurry, J. (2009). Adolescents choosing self-harm as an emotion regulation strategy: The protective role of trait emotional intelligence. *British Journal of Clinical Psychology, 48*(2), 181–193.

Muehlenkamp, J., Brausch, A., Quigley, K., & Whitlock, J. (2013). Interpersonal features and functions of nonsuicidal self-injury. *Suicide and Life-Threatening Behavior, 43*(1), 67–80.

Mueller, T., Gavin, L., Oman, R., Vesely, S., Aspy, C., Tolma, E., & Rodine, S. (2010). Youth assets and sexual risk behavior: Differences between male and female adolescents. *Health Education & Behavior, 37*(3), 343–356.

Nrugham, L., Holen, A., & Sund, A. M. (2010). Associations between attempted suicide, violent life events, depressive symptoms, and resilience in adolescents and young adults. *Journal of Nervous and Mental Disease, 198*(2), 131–136.

O'Connor, R. C., Rasmussen, S., Miles, J., & Hawton, K. (2009). Self-harm in adolescents: Self-report survey in schools in Scotland. *The British Journal of Psychiatry, 194*(1), 68–72.

Pedlow, C. T., & Carey, M. P. (2004). Developmentally appropriate sexual risk reduction interventions for adolescents: Rationale, review of interventions, and recommendations for research and practice. *Annals of Behavioral Medicine, 27*(3), 172–184.

Pisani, A. R., Wyman, P. A., Petrova, M., Schmeelk-Cone, K., Goldston, D. B., Xia, Y., & Gould, M. S. (2013). Emotion regulation difficulties, youth–adult relationships, and suicide attempts among high school students in underserved communities. *Journal of Youth and Adolescence, 42*(6), 807–820.

Ramirez-Valles, J., Zimmerman, M. A., & Newcomb, M. D. (1998). Sexual risk behavior among youth: Modeling the influence of prosocial activities and socioeconomic factors. *Journal of Health and Social Behavior, 39*(3), 237–253.

Rubenstein, J. L., Heeren, T., Housman, D., Rubin, C., & Stechler, G. (1989). Suicidal behavior in "normal" adolescents: Risk and protective factors. *American Journal of Orthopsychiatry, 1*, 59–71.

Rudd, M. D., Berman, A. L., Joiner, T. E. Jr., Nock, M. K., Silverman, M. M., Mandrusiak, M., … & Witte, T. (2006). Warning signs for suicide: Theory, research, and clinical applications. *Suicide and Life-Threatening Behavior, 36*(3), 255–262.

Shek, D. T. L. (2010). The spirituality of Chinese people. In M. H. Bond (Ed.), *Oxford handbook of Chinese psychology* (pp. 343–366). New York: Oxford University Press.

Shek, D. T. L., & Sun, R. C. F. (Eds.). (2013a). *Development and evaluation of positive adolescent training through holistic social programs (P.A.T.H.S.)*. Heidelberg: Springer.

Shek, D. T. L., & Sun, R. C. F. (2013b). The Project P.A.T.H.S. in Hong Kong: Development, training, implementation, and evaluation. *Journal of Pediatric and Adolescent Gynecology, 26*(3S), S2–S9.

Shek, D. T. L., & Yu, L. (2011). A review of validated youth prevention and positive youth development programs in Asia. *International Journal of Adolescent Medicine and Health, 23*(4), 317–324.

Shek, D. T. L., & Yu, L. (2012). Self-harm and suicidal behaviors in Hong Kong adolescents: Prevalence and psychosocial correlates. *The Scientific World Journal, 2012*, Article ID 932540, 14 pages. doi:10.1100/2012/932540.

Sun, R. C. F., & Hui, E. K. P. (2007). Psychosocial factors contributing to adolescent suicidal ideation. *Journal of Youth and Adolescence, 36*(6), 775–786.

Sun, R. C. F., & Shek, D. T. L. (2010). Life satisfaction, positive youth development, and problem behavior among Chinese adolescents in Hong Kong. *Social Indicators Research, 95*(3), 455–474.

Sun, R. C. F., & Shek, D. T. L. (2013). Longitudinal influences of positive youth development and life satisfaction on problem behaviour among adolescents in Hong Kong. *Social Indicators Research, 114*, 1171–1197.

Taliaferro, L. A., Muehlenkamp, J. J., Borowsky, I. W., McMorris, B. J., & Kugler, K. C. (2012). Factors distinguishing youth who report self-injurious behavior: A population-based sample. *Academic Pediatrics, 12*(3), 205–213.

Tatnell, R., Kelada, L., Hasking, P., & Martin, G. (2013). Longitudinal analysis of adolescent NSSI: The role of intrapersonal and interpersonal factors. *Journal of Abnormal Child Psychology, 42*, 885–896.

U.S. Department of Health and Human Services (HHS), Office of the Surgeon General and National Action Alliance for Suicide Prevention. (2012). *2012 National strategy for suicide prevention: Goals and objectives for action.* Washington, DC: HHS.

Vesely, S. K., Wyatt, V. H., Oman, R. F., Aspy, C. B., Kegler, M. C., Rodine, S., Marshall, L., & McLeroy, K. R. (2004). The potential protective effects of youth assets from adolescent sexual risk behaviors. *Journal of Adolescent Health, 34*(5), 356–365.

von Soest, T., Mossige, S., Stefansen, K., & Hjemdal, O. (2010). A validation study of the Resilience Scale for Adolescents (READ). *Journal of Psychopathology and Behavioral Assessment, 32*(2), 215–225.

Wang, M. C., Lightsey, O. R., Pietruszka, T., Uruk, A. C., & Wells, A. G. (2007). Purpose in life and reasons for living as mediators of the relationship between stress, coping, and suicidal behavior. *The Journal of Positive Psychology, 2*(3), 195–204.

Wild, L. G., Flisher, A. J., Bhana, A., & Lombard, C. (2004a). Associations among adolescent risk behaviours and self-esteem in six domains. *Journal of Child Psychology and Psychiatry, 45*(8), 1454–1467.

Wild, L. G., Flisher, A. J., & Lombard, C. (2004b). Suicidal ideation and attempts in adolescents: Associations with depression and six domains of self-esteem. *Journal of Adolescence, 27*(6), 611–624.

Index